Farm Animal Anesthesia

Farm Animal Anesthesia

Cattle, Small Ruminants, Camelids, and Pigs

Edited by

HuiChu Lin, DVM, MS

Diplomate of American College of Veterinary Anesthesia and Analgesia,
Professor,
Department of Clinical Sciences,
College of Veterinary Medicine,
Auburn University, USA

Paul Walz, DVM, MS, PhD

Diplomate of American College of Veterinary Internal Medicine
Associate Professor,
Department of Pathobiology,
College of Veterinary Medicine,
Auburn University, USA

WILEY Blackwell

Editorial Offices
1606 Golden Aspen Drive, Suites 103 and 104, Ames, Iowa 50014-8300, USA
The Atrium, Southern Gate, Chichester, West Sussex, PO19 8SQ, UK
9600 Garsington Road, Oxford, OX4 2DQ, UK

For details of our global editorial offices, for customer services and for information about how to apply for permission to reuse the copyright material in this book please see our website at www.wiley.com/wiley-blackwell.

Library of Congress Cataloging-in-Publication Data

Lin, HuiChu, 1958– author.
Farm animal anesthesia : cattle, small ruminants, camelids, and pigs / HuiChu Lin and Paul Walz.
p. ; cm.
Includes bibliographical references and index.
ISBN 978-1-118-47435-8 (pbk.)
1. Animal anesthesia. 2. Pain in animals–Treatment. I. Walz, Paul, 1967– author. II. Title.
[DNLM: 1. Anesthesia–veterinary. 2. Animals, Domestic. 3. Ruminants. SF 914]
SF910.P34L56 2014
636.089′796–dc23

2014001177

A catalogue record for this book is available from the British Library.

Wiley also publishes its books in a variety of electronic formats. Some content that appears in print may not be available in electronic books.

Cover image: #13757427 © Frank Leung, #2432613 © clintscholz, #3197681 © lesliejmorris and #16204673 © steverts, iStockphoto.com

Set in 10/12.5 pt Times by SPi Publisher Services, Pondicherry, India

Printed in the UK

For the unconditional support of my father, Pin-Kuo, who passed away in 2010; my mother, Yao-Hwa; and my son, Dow, who have given me support to pursue my dream and to do what I love to do.

–HuiChu Lin

To my wife, Heather, and children, Jacob, Madison, and Kaitlyn, for their encouragement and support and to my veterinary colleagues and students, who have continually provided me inspiration.

–Paul Walz

Contents

Contributing Authors

Dr. Misty A. Edmondson, DVM, MS
Diplomate of American College of Theriogenologists
Associate Professor
Department of Clinical Sciences
College of Veterinary Medicine
Auburn University, USA

Dr. Benjamin Newcomer, DVM, PhD
Diplomate of American College of Veterinary Internal Medicine,
Diplomate of American College of Veterinary Preventive Medicine
Assistant Professor
Department of Pathobiology
College of Veterinary Medicine
Auburn University, USA

Dr. Thomas Passler, DVM, PhD
Diplomate of American College of Veterinary Internal Medicine
Assistant Professor
Department of Clinical Sciences
College of Veterinary Medicine
Auburn University, USA

Preface

This book covers both the basic knowledge of commonly used anesthetics and analgesics and practical use of these drugs to prevent farm animal pain caused by surgery and/or disease processes. We hope farm animal veterinarians find this book useful and practical for the anesthetic techniques and pain management aspect of their daily practice. There are few anesthetics and analgesics approved by the Food and Drug Administration. As consumers demand healthy and safe food products, it is imperative that farm animal veterinarians and producers are aware of the regulatory and legal guidelines of extralabel use of these drugs to ensure edible animal products are free of harmful pharmaceutical residues.

My appreciation to my coeditor, Dr. Paul Walz; contributing authors, Drs. Misty Edmondson, Benjamin Newcomer, and Thomas Passler (their chapters make this book a complete book on farm animal anesthesia); illustrators, Kim Crosslin and Katlyn King, for their picture-perfect artworks; and my colleagues, Drs. Fred Caldwell, John Schumacher, and Jennifer Taintor, for reading and editing several chapters of this book.

Special thanks to my mentors, Drs. John Benson, John Thurmon, and William Tranquilli, for laying the foundation during my residency training at the University of Illinois that has benefited me throughout my career.

Most of all, I thank my colleagues in the Food Animal Section of Auburn University for being always kind and helpful; you make my job so much easier and **fun**.

HuiChu Lin

Chapter 1

Preanesthetic considerations

HuiChu Lin
Department of Clinical Sciences, College of Veterinary Medicine, Auburn University, USA

General anesthesia in farm animals, like cattle, sheep, goats, llamas, alpacas, and pigs, requires special attention due to the uniqueness of the anatomical and physiological characteristics as compared to dogs, cats, and horses. Camelids (llamas and alpacas) only have two forestomachs but are otherwise similar in many ways to cattle and small ruminants. Although some farm animals may cost as much as purebred companion animals, farm animal veterinarians are often faced with economic constraints and a limited number of approved drugs for use in surgical procedures requiring anesthesia. Physical restraint and local anesthetic techniques are most commonly employed to produce immobility and analgesia for these species. Ruminants generally tolerate physical restraint and recumbency well. This, along with local and/or regional anesthetic techniques, allows many minor surgical procedures to be performed in the standing position and under field conditions. General anesthesia is more frequently performed in camelids and swine for even minor surgical procedures due to their intolerance of physical restraint. It is important to remember that farm animals perceive pain no differently than other species; therefore, analgesia for prevention and easing of pain is just as important as it is for companion animals. With surgical procedures requiring general anesthesia, balanced anesthetic technique should be employed to provide narcosis, analgesia, and muscle relaxation, thereby minimizing the stress response induced by surgery and anesthesia. Most of the anesthetics and anesthetic adjuncts commonly used in farm animal practice do not have Food and Drug Administration (FDA) approval for use in ruminants, camelids, and swine [1, 2]. However, per the Animal Medicinal Drug Use Clarification Act (AMDUCA) of 1994, extralabel use of drugs is permitted when animal health is threatened or death may result if not treated [3]. While prevention of violative residues should always be considered, anesthetics are usually used for a short duration, and anesthetized animals are unlikely to be marketed immediately after surgery. Furthermore, anesthetics used today tend to have very short half-lives ($t½$), and they are potent enough that only low doses are required to produce general anesthesia.

Farm Animal Anesthesia: Cattle, Small Ruminants, Camelids, and Pigs, First Edition.
Edited by HuiChu Lin and Paul Walz.

The possibility of an animal carrying anesthetic residues within its edible tissues after the surgical incision has healed, which normally occurs within an average of 14 days, is extremely low. Thus, problems with anesthetic drug residues appear to be rare [4]. Nevertheless, veterinarians should consult the Food Animal Residue Avoidance Databank (FARAD) for meat and milk withdrawal intervals for extralabel use of analgesics, sedatives, and injectable anesthetics as well as for updates of drugs prohibited from extralabel use [1, 2].

Prior to anesthesia, an appropriate patient history including breed, age, sex, condition, and temerament of the patient, and a complete physical examination, are indicated. Due to economic reasons, blood work including complete blood count and chemistry profile is performed only in farm animals with significant systemic diseases and those considered to have a higher anesthetic risk. For example, animals with severe gastrointestinal (GI) abnormalities often suffer extreme dehydration with or without electrolyte alteration, which may require intervention to optimize the patient's condition with fluid therapy prior to the induction of anesthesia [5]. In healthy animals, total plasma protein and packed cell volume are sufficient indicators of a patient's hydration status.

Most of the sedatives and general anesthetics cause some degree of cardiovascular depression, which may not be a great concern for healthy patients. However, normal cardiovascular protective mechanisms or reflexes in response to the depressing effects of anesthetics may be obtunded in animals with compromised cardiac function or severe electrolyte imbalances as a consequence of disease conditions. Maintaining balance of concentrations of electrolytes like calcium, sodium, and potassium across the cell membranes is essential in establishing normal cell membrane potential and contractility. Disturbance of these electrolyte balances across cell membranes changes cellular resting membrane potentials and subsequent initiation and propagation of cellular depolarization and repolarization. Acidosis has been shown to cause electrolyte imbalances resulting in decreased myocardial contractility and increased response of the myocardial cells to circulating catecholamines. Therefore, anesthetic-induced cardiovascular depression combined with severe preexisting acidosis and electrolyte imbalances can lead to detrimental side effects like severe cardiac arrhythmias, bradycardia, decreased myocardial and vascular cellular contractility, reduced cardiac output, and hypotension. As a result, anesthetized animals may not be able to maintain adequate cardiac output or arterial blood pressure leading to significantly decreased peripheral tissue and muscle perfusion with subsequent development of severe adverse effects such as irreversible postanesthetic neuromyopathy [6].

Positioning

Ruminants, camelids, and swine are susceptible to complications associated with anesthesia and recumbency. Positioning of these animals, particularly adult cattle, in dorsal or lateral recumbency for surgery allows for the weight of abdominal viscera to shift ventrally and cranially, causing the diaphragm to be pushed further into the thoracic cavity, thereby reducing the functional residual capacity of the lungs (Figure 1.1). As a result, an increased ventilation/perfusion mismatch may lead to significant hypoventilation and hypoxemia during anesthesia. Furthermore, the weight of the abdominal viscera may compress great vessels such as the vena cava leading to decreased venous return, cardiac output, and

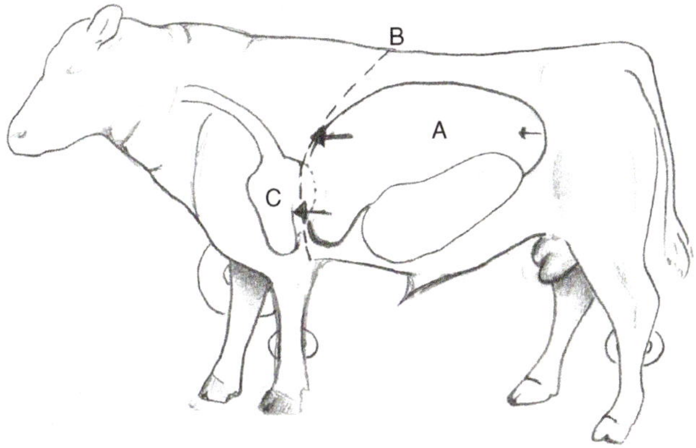

Figure 1.1 The effect of lateral recumbency on the position of the diaphragm in ruminants; A, rumen; B, diaphragm; and C, lungs. (Source: Illustration by Kim Crosslin.)

arterial blood pressures [7]. Therefore, close monitoring of cardiovascular and pulmonary functions and institution of appropriate treatments to ensure normal arterial blood pressure and adequate ventilation are important parts of perioperative anesthetic management.

Ruminal tympany

Ruminal tympany, bloat, regurgitation, and aspiration pneumonia are common problems associated with general anesthesia in farm animal species that should be anticipated and addressed with proper precautions. Ruminal fermentation continues even in anesthetized animals. Postprandial gas production at an average of 30 L per hour has been reported in cattle [8]. Normal, awake animals are able to relieve the gas produced by fermentation through the eructation. Sedatives and anesthetics tend to inhibit GI motility and prohibit eructation, thus allowing gas to accumulate in the rumen. The rumen of an adult large ruminant has a capacity of 115–150 L [9]. An average capacity of 15–18 L has been reported in small ruminants [10]. Bloating, especially in nonfasted animals, can occur during anesthesia and compromise the cardiopulmonary systems by increasing intra-abdominal pressure resulting in compression of the diaphragm and great vessels such as the vena cava in the abdominal cavity, thus further complicating the already compromised cardiopulmonary function resulting from abnormal positioning required by the surgery. Fasting of these animals prior to anesthesia reduces the amount of gas produced by fermentation and minimizes its detrimental effect on the cardiopulmonary systems.

Regurgitation

Regurgitation and aspiration of stomach content can occur in farm animal species during anesthesia, especially in nonfasted animals. The risk of regurgitation decreases significantly when water is withheld for 6–12 hours and feed is withheld for 12–24 hours prior to anesthesia in small ruminants. Pigs are monogastrics. It has been indicated that alfalfa or any type of hay delays gastric emptying time, and vomiting with possible aspiration may occur during induction of anesthesia after a recommended fasting period of 12 hours. Thus, removal of alfalfa or other types of hay from their routine diet should be instituted 2–3 days prior to anesthesia [11].

Domestic ruminants have a large rumen that is usually full of liquid materials, and it does not empty completely even after 24–48 hours of fasting. Regurgitation can occur either during light (active regurgitation) or deep (passive regurgitation) anesthesia in ruminants and camelids in spite of preoperative fasting and withholding of water. Active regurgitation usually occurs during light anesthesia and is characterized by explosive discharge of large quantities of ruminal materials. Passive regurgitation occurs during deeper planes of anesthesia when the esophageal muscles and transluminal pressure gradients relax as a result of anesthetic-induced muscle relaxation. If the airway is not protected, a large amount of ruminal materials can be aspirated into the trachea and reach the small airways. Aspiration of acidic stomach fluid causes immediate reflex airway closure and destruction of type II alveolar cells and pulmonary capillary lining cells. Consequently, pulmonary edema and hemorrhage, hypoxemia, and arterial hypotension develop due to loss of alveolar and capillary integrity leading to reflex airway closure, bronchospasm, dyspnea, hypoxemia, and cyanosis. Recovery from aspiration pneumonia depends on the pH and amount of ruminal materials aspirated [10]. Pigs tend to have very acidic stomach fluid with a pH as low as 1.5–2.5 [12], whereas the rumen pH remains within 5.5–6.5 in cattle, sheep, and goats [13] and 6.4–7.0 for C1 of camelids [14]. Thus, the greater impact of aspirating rumen contents lies in the amount of bacterial microflora and solid food materials aspirated. In pigs, the level of acidity of stomach fluid is the primary factor affecting the severity of damage to the pulmonary tissues upon aspiration. Severe consequences like reflex airway constriction, mechanical airway obstruction, and aspiration of bacteriologically active materials can still occur in the presence of a neutral pH in ruminants [10]. Animals may die before an endotracheal tube can be placed to protect the airway in extreme cases. Please refer to Chapter 7 for prevention and treatment of aspiration pneumonia. Preoperative withholding of feed and endotracheal intubation with an adequately inflated cuff immediately following induction of anesthesia are recommended in all anesthetized farm animals.

Salivation

Ruminants normally salivate profusely during anesthesia. Total amounts of saliva secretion in conscious adult cattle and sheep have been reported to be 50 L and 6–16 L per 24 hours, respectively [15, 16]. In the past, anticholinergics like atropine were used routinely as part of the anesthetic induction regimen in an effort to prevent salivation. However, atropine only reduces the water content of the saliva [17], thus causing the saliva to become more viscous and increasing the potential of airway obstruction, particularly in neonates. If the trachea is left unprotected during anesthesia, large amounts of saliva may be aspirated.

Thus, tracheal intubation with appropriate inflation of the cuff immediately following induction should be instituted to protect the airway. For large ruminants, setting up the surgery table in a way that the head is lower and the throatlatch area is elevated relative to the mouth and thoracic inlet will help drainage and prevent pooling of the saliva and ruminal contents in the oral cavity (Figure 1.2). Placing a sandbag or rolled-up towel under the neck of a small ruminant or camelid patient to elevate the throatlatch so that the mouth opening is lower than the occiput allows saliva to escape, avoiding the potential for aspiration (Figure 1.3). This technique also helps to minimize the flow of passive regurgitation during deep anesthesia [18].

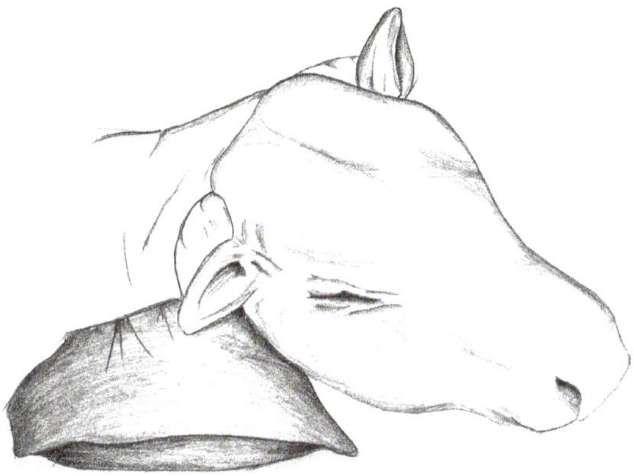

Figure 1.2 Lateral recumbency of an adult bovid; note the elevation of the throatlatch. (Source: Illustration by Kim Crosslin.)

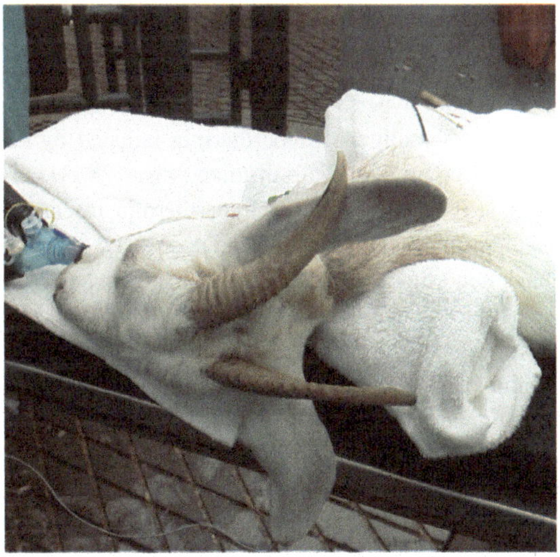

Figure 1.3 Lateral recumbency of a small ruminant; note the elevation of the throatlatch.

Malignant hyperthermia

Malignant hyperthermia, also referred to as **porcine stress syndrome**, is a genetic disorder that occurs due to mutation of the ryanodine receptors (ryr-1 locus) of the calcium channels in the skeletal muscles [19–21]. The presence of abnormal ryanodine receptors allows a massive amount of calcium to be released from the cells into the sarcoplasmic reticulum resulting in generalized extensive skeletal muscle contraction. Though malignant hyperthermia has been reported in other animal species, pigs and humans seem to be the most susceptible. Certain breeds of pigs like Pietrain, Portland China, or Landrace are very susceptible to this syndrome, while Large White, Yorkshire, and Hampshire, on the other hand, are much less so [22, 23]. The clinical signs of malignant hyperthermia syndrome are manifested in a sudden and dramatic rise in body temperature and end-tidal CO_2 followed by muscle fasciculation, muscle rigidity, tachypnea, tachycardia, arrhythmias, myoglobinuria, metabolic acidosis, renal failure, and often death. The prognosis is usually poor once the episode is initiated. The triggering agents of malignant hyperthermia include stress (e.g., excitement, transportation, or preanesthetic handling), halogenated inhalation anesthetics (e.g., halothane, isoflurane, sevoflurane, and desflurane), and depolarizing neuromuscular blocking drugs (e.g., succinylcholine). Lidocaine and ketamine have been indicated as triggering agents, but there is no evidence to support this theory [24]. Halogenated inhalation anesthetics are known triggers for malignant hyperthermia, and halothane has been indicated to be the most potent trigger [25]. A report in humans demonstrated that in a total of 75 malignant hyperthermia cases, 42 were isoflurane related, 12 were sevoflurane related, 11 were halothane related, and 8 were enflurane related [26]. Further study showed that the augmentation of caffeine-induced contractures of frog sartorius muscle by isoflurane is 3 times and by enflurane is 4 times, whereas by halothane is 11 times [27]. Similarly, halothane appears to be the most potent and most frequently reported trigger of malignant hyperthermia in pigs. Isoflurane has been reported to trigger malignant hyperthermia in susceptible pigs like Pietrain or Pietrain-mixed pigs [28]. Only one incidence of isoflurane-induced malignant hyperthermia has been reported in a potbellied pig [29]. Sevoflurane-induced malignant hyperthermia also has been reported in purebred Portland China pigs [30]. Episodes of malignant hyperthermia induced by desflurane have been reported in Large White, Pietrain, and Pietrain-mixed pigs [28, 31]. There is no report of isoflurane- or sevoflurane-induced malignant hyperthermia in cattle. In 1981, McGrath *et al.* [32] reported that intramuscular (IM) acepromazine at 1.1 and 1.65 mg/kg reduced the incidence of malignant hyperthermia by 40% and 73%, respectively. A lower dose of 0.55 mg/kg IM was only able to delay but not prevent the onset of the episode [32]. Because of limited availability of effective drugs for treatment, minimizing the stress prior to anesthesia and avoiding using anesthetics that are known triggers are imperative in susceptible animals to prevent a malignant hyperthermia episode.

Differences in sensitivity to anesthetics

Xylazine is a potent sedative, analgesic, and muscle relaxant that is frequently used as a preanesthetic or anesthetic adjunct in farm animal species. Cattle are more sensitive to xylazine than horses, and they require only one-tenth of the dose needed in horses to produce equipotent sedation [33]. Apparently, there are differences in the level of sensitivity to xylazine among breeds and species of these animals. It appears that Brahmans are the most sensitive, Herefords intermediate, and Holsteins are the least sensitive [34, 35]. Small ruminants are more sensitive to xylazine than camelids, whereas goats tend to be more sensitive than sheep and llamas are more sensitive than alpacas. Administration of xylazine to pregnant ruminants in the final trimester may cause premature parturition and retention of fetal membranes [36, 37]. In pregnant dairy cows during late gestation, intravenous (IV) administration of xylazine (0.04 mg/kg) resulted in a significant increase in uterine vascular resistance (118–156%) and a decrease in uterine blood flow (25–59%), which were accompanied by a drastic decrease in O_2 delivery to the fetus (59%) [38]. Therefore, the use of xylazine during late gestation in pregnant ruminants is not recommended to avoid detrimental effects to the fetus. Fayed *et al.* (1989) [39] had observed pronounced and prolonged response when xylazine was administered to cattle under high ambient temperature. Interestingly, camelids are less sensitive to xylazine than ruminants; thus, higher doses are required to produce a similar degree of sedation in ruminants. In addition, the dose requirement is higher for alpacas than llamas. Compared to other farm animal species, pigs are the least sensitive to xylazine and other α_2 agonists. These drugs when used alone in pigs are not effective in producing adequate sedation. Vomiting has been observed following the administration of xylazine to pigs with digestive disturbances [11]. In addition to α_2 agonists, pigs are also less sensitive to the pharmacologic effects of opioids [40, 41]. Benzodiazepines, for example, diazepam and midazolam, seem to produce reliable sedation in pigs even at doses that do not produce effective sedation in other species [42].

In regard to α_2 antagonists, ruminants and camelids are more sensitive to tolazoline than other species [43, 44]. When administered intravenously alone at 1.5 mg/kg to non-sedated Holstein calves, tolazoline caused coughing, increased frequency of defecation, and a mild increase in breathing effort. At higher IV doses from 2 to 10 mg/kg, adverse effects including bright red conjunctival mucous membrane, coughing, nasal discharge, profuse salivation, labored breathing, CNS depression, signs of abdominal pain, straining, head pressing, restlessness, and severe diarrhea were observed. However, there were no long-lasting adverse effects observed in those calves [44]. Currently, lower doses of tolazoline at 0.5–1.5 mg/kg IV are recommended for use in all ruminants including camelids. Others have suggested that IV administration of tolazoline should be avoided, except in emergency situations, to prevent adverse effects such as cardiac asystole [45].

There are concerns from potbellied pig owners and breeders regarding the statement that "injectable anesthetics should not be used in young pigs" and that "ketamine in particular should not be used in potbellied pigs of any age" [46]. These statements have never been proven or supported by controlled, scientific studies. Furthermore, the clinical experiences of this author and of most practicing veterinarians indicate otherwise.

Ruminants recover gradually but smoothly from Telazol anesthesia as a result of the slower metabolism and longer-lasting effect of zolazepam [47, 48]. Pigs, on the other hand, often experience prolonged and stormy recovery characterized by swimming and paddling with repeated attempts to right themselves when recovering from Telazol anesthesia, similar to that observed when ketamine was used alone [42, 49]. Studies have shown that tiletamine and zolazepam are both eliminated slower in pigs than in other species [49] and tiletamine apparently outlasted zolazepam in pigs [47].

Preanesthetic preparation

When possible, adult cattle should be fasted for 24–48 hours and water withheld for 24 hours before induction of anesthesia. Small ruminants, camelids, and swine should be fasted for 12–24 hours and water withheld for 8–12 hours before induction of anesthesia. Preanesthetic fasting may not completely prevent regurgitation, but it will decrease the amount of solid matter in the rumen content. Fasting also does not prevent bloating during anesthesia, but it reduces the rate of fermentation, thus reducing the amount of gas formation, the severity of bloating, and its effect on ventilation. Removal of alfalfa or other types of hay from their routine diet should be instituted 2–3 days prior to anesthesia to avoid prolonged gastric emptying time caused by this type of diet [11]. A shorter fasting period of 6–8 hours is sufficient for pigs undergoing most elective surgeries due to rapid intestinal transport times in the upper GI tract and less time required to empty the stomach [50]. Ruminants are born without a developed forestomach system and thus can be treated as monogastrics until 3 weeks of age [51]. Fasting of young ruminants less than 4 months old is not recommended because of the potential for hypoglycemia and prolonged recovery. Fasting may not be possible under emergency situations, and precautions should be taken to avoid aspiration of gastric fluid and ingesta. Prevention of regurgitation and aspiration of ruminal content can be achieved effectively by placing the animal in sternal recumbency and endotracheal intubation instituted immediately following induction. However, some practices may induce anesthesia with adult cattle already strapped to the table and in lateral recumbency. In this case, it is even more important to ensure animals are under an adequate plane of anesthesia to prevent stimulation of active regurgitation and allow immediate intubation. Regurgitation does not occur in pigs as commonly as in ruminants. However, vomiting can result from nonfasting prior to induction of anesthesia and following administration of xylazine. In general, removal of hay or alfalfa and withholding food for 12 hours and water for 6–8 hours the night before anesthesia should be sufficient for most elective surgeries [23].

In adult cattle, a 14-gauge and 2- to 3-in. needle is placed in the jugular vein for administration of IV anesthetics for induction of anesthesia and for maintenance of fluid therapy. A 14-gauge, 5¼-in. indwelling catheter can be used if postoperative IV medication or fluid therapy is needed. Cutdown of the skin at the catheterization site may be helpful to facilitate insertion of the catheter. A 16- or 18-gauge catheter is appropriate for younger animals. The technique for IV catheterization in sheep and goats is similar to that used in calves. Venipuncture can be difficult in camelids because they have thick fiber coats and neck skin and, a less-apparent jugular groove. The jugular vein lies deep to the sternomandibularis and brachiocephalicus muscles, ventral to the cervical vertebral transverse processes, and superficial to the carotid artery and vagosympathetic trunk within the carotid sheath for most of its length [52–56]. The jugular vein of camelids is not always visible even after occlusion of the vessels, particularly in adult males. The right internal jugular vein is the best choice for catheterization in these animals. A 14- or 16-gauge indwelling catheter is appropriate for adult camelids, and an 18-gauge catheter is suitable for younger animals. Catheters should be secured with suture or bandage. Skin cut down with a #15-scalpel blade or a sharp 14-gauge needle is helpful in passing the catheter into the vein [57]. An ear vein can be an alternative site for IV injection using a 25-gauge needle or butterfly catheter to deliver a small volume of chemical restraint drugs in camelids. Also, camelids have four or five jugular valves that prevent flow of venous blood into the head when they lower their head during grazing. These valves may occlude the IV catheter and prevent backflow of the blood into the catheter, giving a false impression that the catheter may not be correctly placed in the vessel.

In swine, IV injection poses a greater challenge than in other species because pigs resist restraint and they have very few superficial veins accessible for IV injection or catheterization for administration of drugs or fluid therapy. In Vietnamese potbellied pigs, IV catheterization has been even more difficult because they have small ears with small vessels and their skin is usually dark colored. In large adult pigs with proper restraint, a central dorsal ear vein can be used for IV injection and/or catheterization. An 18- or 20-gauge, 1- to 1½-in. hypodermic needle or butterfly catheter can be used for large adult pigs. A 21- or 23-gauge butterfly catheter will be suitable for smaller-sized pigs with small ears. This author prefers a butterfly catheter because it has a shorter needle and tends to stay in the vessel better than hypodermic needles, especially when the animal struggles during injection. Shorter needles are easier to hold in place and decrease the chance of perivascular injection. IM injection of anesthetics or anesthetic combinations to pigs has been shown to produce short-term anesthesia effectively. Always keep in mind that pigs have a thick subcutaneous layer of fat, and thus, to ensure the drug is deposited into the muscle, a longer needle (>1½ in. for large, mature pigs; 1 in. for piglets) should be used [23].

Tracheal intubation is somewhat difficult in ruminants, camelids, and pigs. Blind intubation as in horses is less likely to be successful. For large ruminants, this author's preference is to use digital palpation to guide the endotracheal tube into the trachea immediately following induction of anesthesia with the animal in either sternal or lateral recumbency (Figure 1.4a). Another technique involves use of a stomach tube as a stylet with the aid of digital palpation to place the stomach tube in the trachea; the stomach tube then serves as a guide tube (Figure 1.4b). The endotracheal tube is threaded into the trachea and the stomach tube removed once the endotracheal tube is in place. Intubation should be performed immediately after induction. In calves, intubation is easier when placing the animal in sternal recumbency and an assistant pulls the mouth open by placing a loop of gauze around the upper jaw and a second loop around the lower jaw and tongue. An assistant should lift the head and keep the head and neck in a straight line to allow visualization of the epiglottis and the larynx. If the larynx cannot be visualized, the neck should be extended further. A long laryngoscope blade (250–350 mm) can be used to suppress the tongue base and epiglottis to enable visualization of the larynx. A guide tube or stylet (preferably a 10-French, 22-in.-long polyethylene canine urethral catheter that is three times the length of the endotracheal tube) can be used (Figure 1.5). A cuffed endotracheal tube will prevent regurgitation and aspiration of ruminal contents, and the calf should be maintained in sternal recumbency until the cuff is inflated.

Intubation is more difficult in small ruminant and camelids as compared to large ruminants and other animal species because their mouths do not open widely, the intermandibular space is narrow, and the laryngeal opening is distant to the thick base of the tongue (Figure 1.6). In camelids, the presence of glottal folds adds to the difficulty in visualizing the epiglottis. The technique used for tracheal intubation of small ruminants and camelids

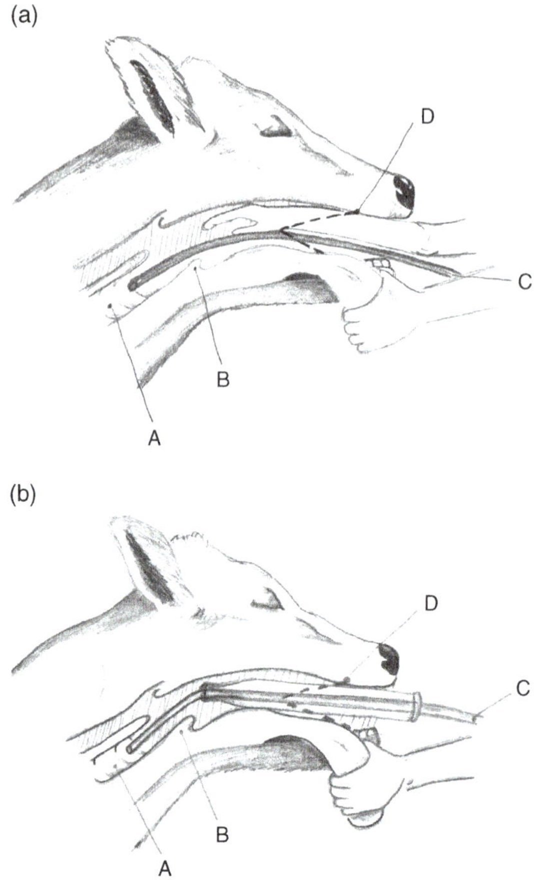

Figure 1.4 (a) Intubation in an adult bovid using digital palpation technique: A, trachea; B, epiglottis; C, endotracheal tube/guide tube; and D, wedge. (b) Intubation in an adult bovid using a guide tube technique: A, trachea; B, epiglottis; C, guide tube; and D, wedge. (Source: Illustration by Kim Crosslin.)

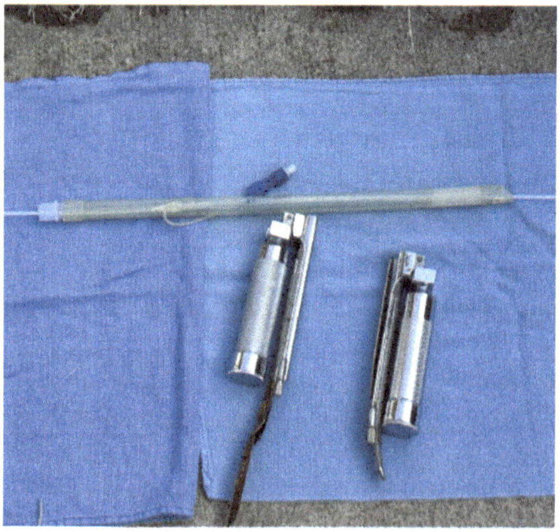

Figure 1.5 Guide tube/stylet and laryngoscope used for endotracheal intubation for small ruminants, camelids, and pigs.

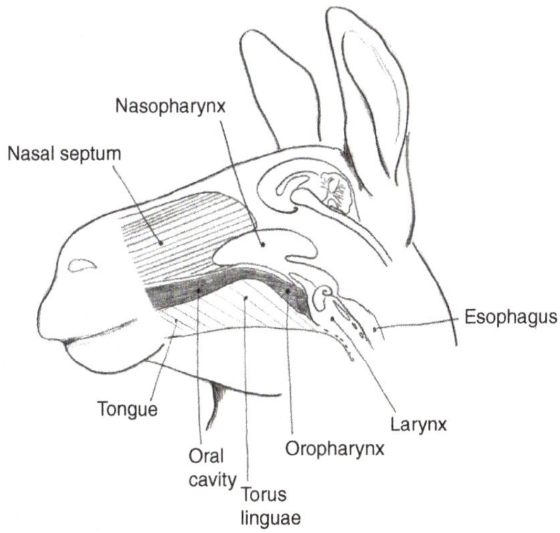

Figure 1.6 Anatomic structures for endotracheal intubation in camelids. (Source: Illustration by Kim Crosslin.)

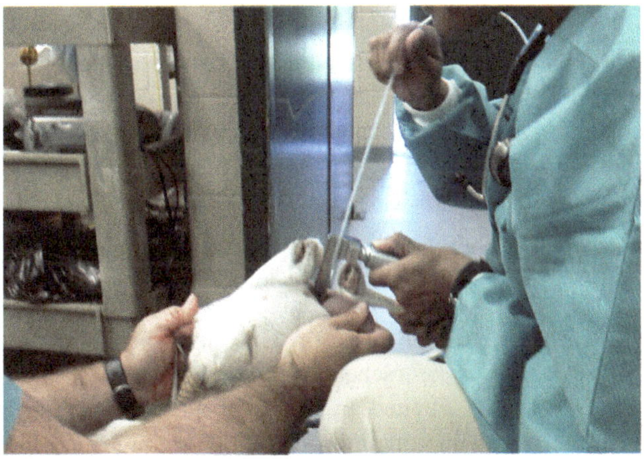

Figure 1.7 Endotracheal intubation in anesthetized goats.

is similar to the technique used in calves. It is easier when the animal is placed in sternal recumbency immediately after induction of anesthesia. Intubation is best accomplished with the help of a guide tube/stylet and long-bladed laryngoscope (250–350 mm) as described for intubation in calves. Hyperextending the animal's neck helps visualization of the larynx (Figure 1.7). The method makes endotracheal intubation in small ruminants and camelids much easier to achieve than with other methods. A cuffed endotracheal tube should be used to provide an adequate seal between the tube and the tracheal mucous membrane so to prevent aspiration of saliva and regurgitated ruminal contents. The animal should be maintained in sternal recumbency until the cuff is inflated. Blind intubation, similar to that used in horses, has been used for intubation in sheep and goats; however,

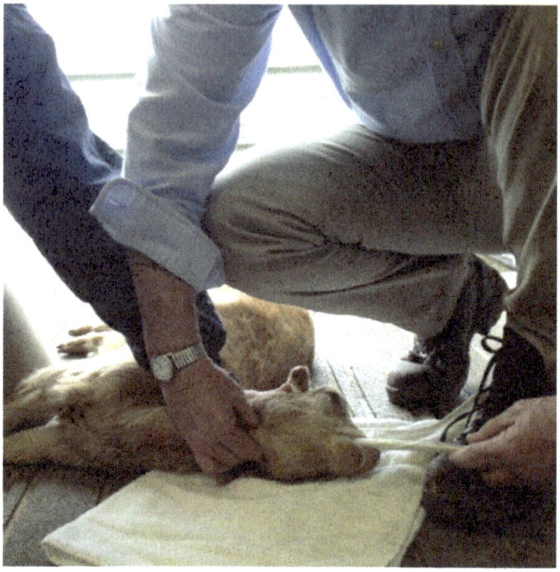

Figure 1.8 "Stick intubation" (blind intubation) in anesthetized goats.

it may require multiple attempts in order to successfully place the endotracheal tube in the trachea. Another technique described as **stick intubation** has been used effectively at Auburn University. With the animal in lateral recumbency, a small-diameter rod made of wood or stainless steel can be used as a stylet to stiffen the endotracheal tube. One hand occludes the esophagus, and the other hand manipulates the endotracheal tube into the trachea (Figure 1.8). Care and gentle maneuvering should be used to prevent initiating laryngeal spasm and to minimize trauma to the oral mucous membrane.

Similar to small ruminants and camelids, pigs' mouths cannot be opened wide, the epiglottis is often entrapped behind the soft palate, and the small larynx slopes downward creating a sharp angle to the tracheal opening (ventral floor fornix) (Figure 1.9). Laryngeal spasms are easily elicited by repeated attempts at tracheal intubation. Vomiting can also occur if attempting intubation while the pig is under a light plane of anesthesia, especially when the animal is not appropriately fasted prior to anesthesia. Spraying a small amount of local anesthetic to desensitize the larynx will reduce the potential for laryngeal spasm. In larger or adult pigs, tracheal intubation is easier to accomplish with the pigs placed in sternal recumbency. Using the same technique as in small ruminants and camelids, with the aid of laryngoscope and guide tube/stylet, the epiglottis and laryngeal aperture can be visualized. Be aware of the sharp angle between the larynx and tracheal opening; it is helpful to apply some pressure to the end of the endotracheal tube as it enters the larynx. This technique keeps the tip of the tube slightly elevated and enables passing the sharp angle to enter the trachea. Another helpful tip for successful endotracheal intubation in pigs is to spin the tube 180° or in a screwlike fashion and advancing it in a dorsal direction while the tube passes through the arytenoid cartilages into the trachea [58].

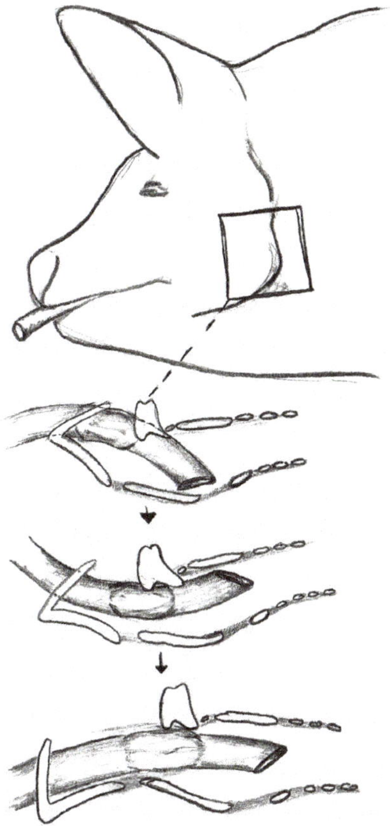

Figure 1.9 Technique for endotracheal intubation in swine. (Source: Illustration by Kim Crosslin.)

It is important to understand the anatomical and physiological differences of ruminants, camelids, and pigs as compared to other species. Veterinarians should incorporate this knowledge with proper preanesthetic preparations and appropriate perioperative management to ensure successful outcome of anesthesia in these animals.

References

1. Craigmill, A., Rangel-Lugo, M., Damian, P. and Riviere, J. (1997) Extralabel use of tranquilizers and general anesthetics. *Journal of the American Veterinary Medical Association*, **211**, 302–304.
2. Davis, J., Smith, G., Baynes, R. *et al.* (2009) Update on drug prohibited for extralabel use in food animals. *Journal of the American Veterinary Medical Association*, **235**, 528–534.
3. US Food and Drug Administration. *Animal Medicinal Drug Use Clarification Act of 1994 (AMDUCA)*, http://www.fda.gov/RegulatoryInformation/Legistration/FederalFoodDrugandCosmeticActFDCAct/SignificantAmendamentstotheFDCAct/AnimalMedicinalDrugUseClarificationActAMDUCAof1994/default.htm (accessed January 21, 2014).
4. Papich, M. (1996) Drug residue considerations for anesthetics and adjunctive drugs in food-producing animals. *Veterinary Clinics of North America: Food Animal Practice*, **12**, 693–706.

5. Perkins, G. (2004) Examination of the surgical patient, in *Farm Animal Surgery* (eds S. Fubini and N. Ducharme), Saunders-Elsevier, St. Louis, pp. 3–14.
6. Lee, D. and Swanson, C. (1996) General principles of anesthesia and sedation in food animals. *Veterinary Clinics of North America: Food Animal Practice*, **12**, 473–480.
7. Klein, L. and Fisher, N. (1988) Cardiopulmonary effects of restraint in dorsal recumbency on awake cattle. *American Journal of Veterinary Research*, **49**, 1605–1608.
8. Dyce, K., Sack, W. and Wensing, C. (1987) The abdomen of the ruminants, in *Textbook of Veterinary Anatomy* (eds K. Dyce, W. Sack and C. Wensing), WB Saunders, Philadelphia, pp. 633–656.
9. Habel, R. (1975) Ruminants digestive system, in *Sisson and Grossman's the Anatomy of the Domestic Animals*, 5th edn (ed S. Getty), WB Saunders, Philadelphia, pp. 861–915.
10. Steffey, E. (1986) Some characteristics of ruminants and swine that complicate management of general anesthesia. *Veterinary Clinics of North America: Food Animal Practice*, **2**, 507–516.
11. Wolff, P. (2009) Pet pig problems. *North American Veterinary Community Conference,* pp. 416–419.
12. DeRouchey, J. Goodband, B. Tokach, M. *et al.* (2009) Digestive system of the pig-anatomy and function. *North American Veterinary Community Conference*, pp. 375–376.
13. Hinchcliff, K., Jernigan, A., Upson, D. and Constable, P. (1991) Ruminant pharmacology. *Veterinary Clinics of North America: Food Animal Practice*, **7**, 633–649.
14. Fowler, M. (2010) Digestive system, in *Medicine and Surgery of Camelids*, 3rd edn (ed M. Fowler), Wiley-Blackwell, Ames, pp. 351–402.
15. Somers, M. (1958) Comparison of the salivary secretion of both parotid glands in a sheep. *Nature*, **182**, 400.
16. Kay, R. (1960) The rate of flow and composition of various salivary secretion in sheep and calves. *The Journal of Physiology*, **150**, 515–537.
17. Weaver, A. (1971) Complications in halothane anesthesia of cattle. *Zentralbl Veterinarmed A*, **18**, 409–416.
18. Thurmon, J. and Benson, G. (1981) Anesthesia in ruminants and swine, in *Current Veterinary Therapy: Food Animal Practice* (ed J. Howard), WB Saunders, Philadelphia, pp. 58–81.
19. Fujii, J., Otsu, K., Zorzato, F. *et al.* (1991) Identification of a mutation in porcine ryanodine receptor associated with malignant hyperthermia. *Science*, **253**, 448–451.
20. Geers, R., Decanniere, C., Ville, H. *et al.* (1992) Identification of halothane gene carriers by use of an in vivo 3IP nuclear magnetic resonance spectroscopy in pigs. *American Journal of Veterinary Research 0002-9645 (P)*, **53**, 1711–1714.
21. Houde, A., Pomnier, S. and Roy, R. (1993) Detection of the ryanodine receptor mutation associated with malignant hyperthermia in purebred swine populations. *Journal of Animal Science*, **71**, 1414–1418.
22. Fraser, C. (1991) Hearty disease, in *The Merck Veterinary Manual*, 7th edn (ed C. Fraser), Merck, Rahway, pp. 3–50.
23. Thurmon, J. and Benson, G. (1987) Special anesthesia considerations of swine, in *Principles & Practice: Veterinary Anesthesia* (ed C. Short), Baltimore, Williams & Wilkins, pp. 308–322.
24. Hildebrand, S. (1987) Hyperthermia, malignant hyperthermia, and myopathy, in *Principle & Practice of Veterinary Anesthesia* (ed C. Short), Williams & Wilkins, Baltimore, pp. 517–532.
25. Stoelting, R. and Hillier, S. (2006) Inhaled anesthetics, in *Pharmacology & Physiology in Anesthetic Practice*, 4th edn (eds R. Stoelting and S. Hillier), Lippincott Williams & Wilkins, A Wolters Kluwer Company, Philadelphia, pp. 42–86.
26. Hopkins, P. (2011) Malignant hyperthermia: Pharmacology of triggering. *British Journal of Anaesthesia*, **107**, 48–56.
27. Reed, S. and Strobel, G. (1978) An in-vitro model of malignant hyperthermia: differential effects of inhalation anesthetics on caffeine-induced muscle contractures. *Anesthesiology*, **48**, 254–259.

28. Wedel, D., Gammel, S., Milde, J. and Iaizzo, P. (1993) Delayed onset of malignant hyperthermia induced by isoflurane and desflurane compared with halothane in susceptible swine. *Anesthesiology*, **78**, 1138–1144.
29. Claxton-Gill, M., Cornick-Seahorn, J., Gamboa, J. and Boatright, B. (1993) Suspected malignant hyperthermia syndrome in a miniature pot-bellied pig anesthetized with isoflurane. *Journal of the American Veterinary Medical Association*, **203**, 1434–1436.
30. Shulman, M., Braverman, B., Ivankovich, A. and Gronert, G. (1981) Sevoflurane triggers malignant hyperthermia in swine. *Anesthesiology*, **54**, 259–260.
31. Bonome-Gonzales, C., Alvarez-Refojo, F., Fernandez-Goti, C. *et al.* (2001) Malignant hyperthermia in a pig anesthetized with desflurane. *Revista Espanola de Anestesiologia y Reanimacion*, **48**, 81–84.
32. McGrath, C., Rempel, W., Addis, P. and Crimi, A. (1981) Acepromazine and droperidol inhibition of halothane-induced malignant hyperthermia (porcine stress syndrome) in swine. *American Journal of Veterinary Research*, **42**, 195–198.
33. Greene, S. and Thurmon, J. (1988) Xylazine – a review of its pharmacology and use in veterinary medicine. *Journal of Veterinary Pharmacology and Therapeutics*, **11**, 295–313.
34. Raptopoulos, D. and Weaver, B. (1984) Observation following intravenous xylazine administration in steers. *The Veterinary Record*, **114**, 567–569.
35. Trim, C. (1987) Special anesthesia considerations in the ruminant, in *Principles and Practice of Veterinary Anesthesia* (ed C. Short), Williams & Wilkins, Baltimore, pp. 285–300.
36. LeBlanc, M., Hubbell, J. and Smith, H. (1984) The effect of xylazine hydrochloride on intrauterine pressure in the cow. *Theriogenology*, **21**, 681–690.
37. Jansen, C., Lowe, K. and Nathanielsz, P. (1984) The effects of xylazine on uterine activity, fetal and maternal oxygenation, cardiovascular function, and fetal breathing. *American Journal of Obstetrics and Gynecology*, **148**, 386–390.
38. Hodgson, D., Dunlop, C., Chapman, P. and Smith, J. (2002) Cardiopulmonary effects of xylazine and acepromazine in pregnant cows in late gestation. *American Journal of Veterinary Research*, **63**, 1695–1699.
39. Fayed, A., Abdalla, E., Anderson, R. *et al.* (1989) Effect of xylazine in heifers under thermoneutral or heat stress conditions. *American Journal of Veterinary Research*, **50**, 151–153.
40. Steffey, E., Baggot, J., Eisele, J. *et al.* (1994) Morphine-isoflurane interaction in dogs, swine, and rhesus monkeys. *Journal of Veterinary Pharmacology and Therapeutics*, **17**, 202–210.
41. Moon, P., Scarlett, J., Ludders, J. *et al.* (1995) Effect of fentanyl on the minimum alveolar concentration of isoflurane in swine. *Anesthesiology*, **83**, 535–542.
42. Ko, J., Thurmon, J., Tranquilli, W. *et al.* (1993) Problems encountered when anesthetizing potbellied pigs. *Veterinary Medicine*, **88**, 435–440.
43. Read, M., Duke, T. and Toews, A. (2000) Suspected tolazoline toxicosis in a llama. *Journal of the American Veterinary Medical Association*, **216**, 227–229.
44. Lin, H. and Riddell, M. (2008) Tolazoline: dose responses and side effects in non-sedated Holstein calves. *The Bovine Practitioner*, **42**, 86–96.
45. Anderson, D. (2011) New methods for chemical restraint and field anesthesia in cattle. *North American Veterinary Community Conference*, pp. 6–11.
46. pigs4ever (2009). http://www.pigs4ever.com/pot_belly_pig-information; http://wwwpigs4evercom/pot_belly_pig-information (accessed January 21, 2014).
47. Lin, H., Thurmon, J., Benson, G. *et al.* (1993) Telazol – a review of its pharmacology and use in veterinary medicine. *Journal of Veterinary Pharmacology and Therapeutics*, **16**, 383–418.
48. Lin, H., Thurmon, J., Benson, G. *et al.* (1989) The hemodynamic response of calves to tiletamine-zolazepam anesthesia. *Veterinary Surgery*, **18**, 328–334.

49. Kumar, A., Mann, H. and Remmel, R. (2006) Pharmacokinetics of tiletamine and zolazepam (Telazol) in anesthetized pigs. *Journal of Veterinary Pharmacology and Therapeutics*, **29**, 587–589.
50. Swindle, M. (1998) Anesthesia and analgesia, in *Surgery, Anesthesia, and Experimental Techniques in Swine* (ed M. Swindle), Iowa State University Press, Ames, pp. 33–63.
51. Snyder, J. and Wolff, P. (2009) Small ruminant tips for small animal practitioners. *North American Veterinary Community Conference*, pp. 331–337.
52. Fowler, M. (1983) The jugular vein (Lama peruana): a clinical note. *Journal of Zoo and Animal Medicine*, **14**, 77–78.
53. Fowler, M. (1984) Anatomy information. *Camelid Medicine Workshop*, pp. 5–16.
54. Amsel, S., Kainer, R. and Johnson, L. (1987) Choosing the best site to perform venipuncture in a llama. *Veterinary Medicine*, **82**, 535–536.
55. Riebold, T., Kaneps, A. and Schmotzer, W. (1989) Anesthesia in the llama. *Veterinary Surgery*, **18**, 400–404.
56. Pugh, D., Navarre, C., Ruffin, D. and Belknap, E. (1999) A review of diagnostic procedures in llamas and alpacas. *Veterinary Medicine*, **94**, 654–659.
57. Heath, R. (1989) Llama anesthetic programs. *Veterinary Clinics of North America: Llama Medicine*, **5**, 71–80.
58. Wilbers, A. (2009) Routine veterinary care of pot-bellied pigs. *North American Veterinary Community Conference*, pp. 410–412.

Chapter 2

Commonly used preanesthetics

HuiChu Lin

Department of Clinical Sciences, College of Veterinary Medicine, Auburn University, USA

Preanesthetic tranquilization or sedation is rarely necessary in ruminants, but on occasion, its use may be required to calm intractable animals for the safety of the animals and also for the safety of the personnel handling the animals. The choice of whether a tranquilizer/sedative is needed for a particular animal is based on that animal's temperament and physical condition. However, a complete physical examination prior to anesthesia in large ruminants often is not feasible because some of these animals are not accustomed to being handled and restrained, particularly free-ranging animals. In addition to relocation to unfamiliar surroundings for the intended procedure, special equipment like a head catch or restraining chute that may be used for proper restraint of an intractable animal can add another level of stress to the patient. In large aggressive animals, the use of a tranquilizer/sedative will minimize the stress from forceful restraint, ease of the anesthetic induction process, and decrease the dose of general anesthetic required, thus preventing the possibility of disastrous hypotension due to the use of large doses of an anesthetic. Camelids and swine are less tolerant of physical restraint; consequently, deep sedation or general anesthesia is often needed to perform even minor surgical procedures. Oral administration of a tranquilizer/sedative may be used to reduce stress associated with physical restraint in free-ranging animals under field conditions or for animals intolerant of physical restraint. Drugs used for tranquilization and sedation are also used to produce chemical restraint. In ruminants and camelids, oral medication has to pass through the rumen or rumen-like C1 compartment, respectively. Thus, the absorption and distribution of the drug will be affected by forestomach motility and the pH of the contained fluid [1]. Reticuloruminal motility is controlled by the medullary gastric center of the brain. Physical conditions affecting the patient, such as depression, pain, fear, excitement, and extreme distension of the ruminal wall (e.g., bloating), or administration of analgesics like opioids, α_2 agonists, or anesthetics (e.g., thiopental and propofol) have been reported to decrease gastric motility resulting in prolonged gastric emptying time and increased absorption of a drug [1].

Farm Animal Anesthesia: Cattle, Small Ruminants, Camelids, and Pigs, First Edition.
Edited by HuiChu Lin and Paul Walz.

The difference in pH between saliva (8.2), plasma (7.4), and ruminal content (5.5–6.5) also affects the absorption and distribution of the drug by its effect on the degree of ionization of the drug. Nonionized drugs have higher lipid solubility and easily diffuse across cell membranes, whereas ionized drugs have lower lipid solubility and are, hence, less capable of diffusion across cell membranes. Weak acidic drugs ionize and accumulate in the alkalinized saliva and thus allow the delivery of large quantities of the drug into the rumen with the flow of saliva. Once in the more acidic environment of the rumen, ionized drugs become nonionized and diffuse across the rumen membrane into the local blood circulation. On the contrary, drugs that are weak bases become ionized and accumulate in the rumen. The degree of ionization and the diffusion of the drug between saliva, ruminal content, and plasma is constantly changing, which increases the difficulty in predicting the bioavailability, distribution, and calming effect of an orally administered tranquilizer/sedative [1]. Drugs administered intramuscularly or intravenously usually produce more predictable and reliable calming effects in ruminants and camelids and are the preferred routes for administering a tranquilizer/sedative when possible. For monogastric animals like pigs, the pH in the stomach is acidic (1.5–2.5) [2]. Therefore, orally administered acidic drugs will present with a greater percentage in nonionized form and, therefore, better and faster absorption from the stomach and greater bioavailability of the drug. Basic drugs tend to have lower bioavailability due to a higher degree of ionization of the drugs in the stomach.

Acepromazine (phenothiazine derivatives)

Cattle

Acepromazine produces mild tranquilization without analgesia in animal species. Acepromazine produces calming effect by blocking dopaminergic receptors at the basal ganglia in the brain [3]. The drug has minimal effects on heart rate and respiratory function. Vasodilation and subsequent hypotension often observed with the administration of acepromazine are the result of its effect on blocking α_1 adrenoceptors located at the peripheral vasculature [3, 4]. In addition to a calming effect, acepromazine produces beneficial effects such as antiarrhythmic and antiemetic effects. Acepromazine may cause relaxation of the esophagus and cardia which increases the risk of regurgitation in ruminants [4, 5]. Thus, special measures to protect the airway should be taken if the animal is to be placed in lateral or dorsal recumbency during the procedure. Avoid using the coccygeal vein for intravenous (IV) injection when administering acepromazine because of its close proximity to the coccygeal artery [3]. Prolapse of the penis with potential subsequent trauma following the administration of acepromazine as reported in horses may occur in ruminants as well. The IV and intramuscular (IM) doses of acepromazine recommended for ruminants are 0.01–0.02 mg/kg and 0.03–0.1 mg/kg, respectively [6]. The duration of tranquilization of acepromazine usually lasts 2–4 hours when administered at recommended dosages, but effects of 4–8 hours have been reported [7]. The use of acepromazine is contraindicated in debilitated or hypovolemic animals due to its hypotensive effect [3]. In addition, acepromazine depresses the thermoregulatory center, resulting in significant hypothermia and prolonged recovery in anesthetized newborns and neonatal animals. Acepromazine (0.03 mg/kg IM) has been administered occasionally to calm fractious bulls prior to induction of anesthesia with IV xylazine and ketamine.

Small ruminants and camelids

Acepromazine, though rarely used in small ruminants, can be administered at 0.05–0.1 mg/kg to produce mild tranquilization [8]. The drug has been used as an alternative for xylazine in goats with urethral obstruction where increased urine output associated with α_2 agonists is contraindicated. Doses from 0.05 to 0.2 mg/kg can be administered IM or IV to produce tranquilization in sheep and goats [9]. In camelids, 0.033 mg/kg has been used to produce some calming effect in a female guanaco for eye examination [10]. However, a dose of up to 0.15 mg/kg was needed to quiet an aggressive male llama prior to induction of anesthesia with halothane [11].

Swine

Acepromazine is not an effective tranquilizer in pigs, for though tranquilized, they can still resist and fight the imposing restraint viciously. The doses of acepromazine recommended for pigs are 0.11–0.44 mg/kg IV or IM with a maximum total dose of 15 mg [6]. Large doses of acepromazine have been administered in addition to local anesthesia to sows undergoing cesarean section surgery, resulting in severe hypotensive shock. Several sows did not recover following the surgery [12]. IM doses of 0.05–0.5 mg/kg have been given to Vietnamese potbellied pigs with unreliable calming effect even with high doses [13]. Acepromazine is frequently used in combination with ketamine or Telazol (tiletamine/zolazapam) to produce excellent sedation and muscle relaxation [14]. In pigs susceptible to malignant hyperthermia, acepromazine at 1.1 and 1.65 mg/kg IM has been reported to reduce the incidence of malignant hyperthermia by 40% and 73%, respectively. A lower dose of 0.55 mg/kg IM only delayed but did not prevent the onset of the episode [15].

Droperidol and azaperone (butyrophenone derivatives)

Butyrophenone derivatives like droperidol and azaperone have pharmacological effects very similar to acepromazine (phenothiazine derivatives). Droperidol alone has been administered to pigs at 0.3 mg/kg IM to produce sedation for 2 hours [16]. However, droperidol is seldom administered alone to animals; it is manufactured as a proprietary combination of droperidol (20 mg/ml) and fentanyl (0.4 mg/ml) and marketed as **Innovar-Vet** for veterinary use. **Innovar-Vet** is a neuroleptanalgesic combination which consists of a tranquilizer (droperidol) and an analgesic (fentanyl). The combination of two drugs not only potentiates the CNS-depressing effect and the analgesic effect of each drug but also reduces the dose requirement for each drug, which decreases the side effects of each drug. **Innovar-Vet** is often used to calm intractable or vicious animals but is rarely used in ruminants. When given at 0.19, 0.25, or 0.3 ml/kg to sheep, **Innovar-Vet** was reported to produce adequate analgesia and smooth induction and recovery [17]. **Innovar-Vet** had been shown to produce satisfactory calming effect in pigs (1 ml/12–25 kg (26.4–55 lb) IM). However, pigs often sneezed and became more excited if stimulated while under the influence of **Innovar-Vet** [18]. Variable responses ranging from light sedation to pronounced relaxation and analgesia have been reported when 1 ml/10 kg (22 lb) of **Innovar-Vet** was administered to young pigs [19]. Better and more reliable sedation was observed when xylazine was administered with **Innovar-Vet** [12]. When administered to miniature pigs, **Innovar-Vet** induced CNS stimulation rather than sedation [20]. Contrary to the previous report, Piermattei and Swan [21] showed that 1 ml/14 kg (30.8 lb) of **Innovar-Vet** IM produced good sedation prior to halothane anesthesia.

Azaperone, another butyrophenone derivative, has pharmacologic effects similar to acepromazine and droperidol. Hughes et al. (1977) [22] compared the effects of azaperone and acepromazine in free-ranging sheep. At 1 mg/kg, azaperone produced a calming effect and reduced the stress response as evidenced by calmer behavior and a greater comfort level of the animals studied. In this study, azaperone appeared to be more effective in reducing the stress response than acepromazine [22]. Madsen et al. (1980) [23] observed greater disorientation for a longer duration with azaperone. Interestingly, sheep tended to disperse with acepromazine but they tended to congregate with azaperone.

In pigs, azaperone has been shown to be the most effective tranquilizer. Azaperone has been used for the prevention of aggressiveness and savaging of newborn pigs by sows, for the treatment of stress, and for the completion of minor surgical procedures. At 2.2 mg/kg IM, azaperone was effective in reducing fighting following intermingling [24]. Approximately 20 minutes of deep sedation sufficient for minor surgeries was produced by 4–8 mg/kg of azaperone IM. Excessive salivation during deep sedation has been observed [24–29]. Practitioners should keep in mind that tranquilizers like acepromazine, droperidol, azaperone, diazepam, and midazolam do not possess analgesic effect. Therefore, a tranquilizer may render the animal unresponsive to painful manipulations, but the physiological stress response resulting from painful stimulations still exists. Similar to acepromazine, azaperone is effective in preventing malignant hyperthermia episodes due to halothane in susceptible pigs. Doses of 0.5–2.0 mg/kg IM, azaperone offered 100% protection against malignant hyperthermia in susceptible Pietrain pigs [30].

Detomidine, medetomidine, romifidine, and xylazine (α_2 agonists)

The α_2 agonists (e.g., xylazine, detomidine, medetomidine, dexmedetomidine, and romifidine) are classified as sedatives/analgesics. In addition to effective sedation, these drugs produce profound analgesia and good central muscle relaxation. The α_2 agonists produce their pharmacologic effects by their actions on both the central and peripheral α_2 adrenoceptors. Stimulation of central (presynaptic) α_2 adrenoceptors inhibits the release of catecholamines, thus reducing the response to excitatory input, and as a result, sedation occurs.

Peripheral (postsynaptic) α_2 receptors are found in the vasculature, pancreatic islet cells, and uterine muscles. As a result, transient hypertension, hypoinsulinemia, hyperglycemia, and oxytocin-like effect are often associated with the administration of an α_2 agonist [31]. Other side effects associated with the administration of α_2 agonists include direct myocardial depression and augmentation of parasympathetic stimulation resulting in a decrease in cardiac output, bradycardia, and hypotension. Up to a sixfold increase in urine output subsequent to a decrease in secretion of antidiuretic hormone is a common side effect of α_2 agonists. The central muscle-relaxing effect produced by α_2 agonists is believed to be mediated through the inhibition of nerve impulse transmission at the internuncial neurons of the spinal cord, brain stem, and subcortical level of the brain [32]. Because of this, α_2 agonists are often given in combination with anesthetics that do not provide adequate muscle relaxation for surgical procedures. For example, when ketamine is administered alone, it is often associated with muscle tremors, jerking activity, and rigidity; xylazine is administered concurrently to improve the muscle relaxation during ketamine anesthesia. All α_2 agonists, though considered as pure α_2 agonists, also have affinity for α_1 receptors. The α_2:α_1 selectivity ratios for xylazine, detomidine, romifidine, and medetomidine/dexmedetomidine are 160:1, 260:1, 340:1, and 1,620:1, respectively [33, 34].

Cattle

Xylazine

Xylazine is the most popular sedative in large animal practice today. Cattle are much more sensitive to xylazine than horses and require only one-tenth of the dose needed for horses to produce the same degree of sedation [31]. The degree of sensitivity to xylazine varies within breeds, and Brahmans appear to be the most sensitive, Herefords intermediate, and Holsteins are the least sensitive [35]. Xylazine produces potent sedation, profound analgesia, and good muscle relaxation. It is frequently used for chemical restraint or anesthetic adjunct in ruminants. Xylazine alone produces dose-dependent CNS depression from standing sedation (0.015–0.025 mg/kg IV or IM) [19, 36] to recumbency and immobilization (0.1 mg/kg IV or 0.2 mg/kg IM) [37]. Administration of xylazine to ruminants in the final trimester of pregnancy may cause premature parturition and retention of fetal membranes [38, 39]. In pregnant dairy cows during late gestation, administration of xylazine (0.04 mg/kg IV) resulted in a significant increase in uterine vascular resistance (118–156%) and a decrease in uterine blood flow (25–59%) accompanied by a drastic decrease in fetal O_2 delivery (59%) [40]. Due to these detrimental effects on the fetus, the use of xylazine during late gestation in pregnant cows is not recommended. Fayed et al. [41] observed pronounced and prolonged drug effects when xylazine was administered to cattle under high ambient temperature. Xylazine should be used with extreme caution in animals with preexisting cardiopulmonary disease or urinary tract obstruction due to its adverse effects on the myocardium and urine output [31]. Higher dose of xylazine (single average dose, 0.55 ± 0.18 mg/kg) delivered by tranquilizer gun has been used to produce complete immobilization to capture free-ranging cattle [42]. Xylazine is often used with butorphanol to produce neuroleptanalgesia. Enhanced sedation and analgesia develop when these two drugs are administered concurrently.

Administration of high doses of butorphanol alone to nonpainful cattle may induce slight CNS stimulation and behavioral changes. Thus, when used in combination with xylazine, it is recommended the dose of butorphanol be maintained below 0.05 mg/kg to avoid butorphanol-induced CNS excitation offsetting the sedative effect of xylazine [43]. Detailed discussion of chemical restraint techniques using xylazine combinations is described in Chapter 3.

Epidural administration of xylazine to standing cattle produced effective perineal analgesia for 2.5–4 hours. Compared to epidural lidocaine, xylazine produced less disruption of hind limb motor function and provides a longer duration of perineal analgesia [44, 45]. Systemic effects like mild to moderate sedation and slight ataxia sometimes occur following caudal epidural administration of xylazine, which is a result of absorption of the drug into blood circulation from the injection site and/or diffusion of the drug into cerebrospinal fluid (CSF) with subsequent cranial migration of the drug into the CNS. Similarly, studies in humans [46] and dogs [47] showed that diffusion of epidurally administered morphine into the CSF and the subsequent migration of the drug up the spinal cord, rather than the total injected drug volume, were the primary factors responsible for the widespread analgesia of epidural morphine. IV administration of an α_2 antagonist such as tolazoline reversed the systemic effects (sedation and ataxia) but did not affect the caudal epidural analgesia of xylazine [48]. It is believed that the epidural analgesia of xylazine is the result of the binding of xylazine to the α_2 adrenoceptors located in the dorsal horn of the spinal cord, not the effect of xylazine on the central α_2 adrenoceptors in the CNS [49, 50]. Therefore, IV or IM administration of an α_2 antagonist does not affect the binding of an α_2 agonist to the receptors in the epidural space due to low concentration of the α_2 antagonist in the epidural space.

Detomidine

Detomidine has pharmacologic effects that are very similar to xylazine. Interestingly, ruminants appear to be less sensitive to detomidine than they are to xylazine. The dose of detomidine required to produce standing sedation is similar to the dose required for horses. When administered at 0.05 mg/kg IV or IM to adult cattle, detomidine produced effective sedation, though the analgesic effect appeared to be more intense when the drug was administered intravenously [51]. Standing sedation of 30–60 minutes was evident with 0.025–0.01 mg/kg IV of detomidine [36, 52, 53]. Unlike xylazine, detomidine does not produce an oxytocin-like effect on the uterus in gravid cattle at IV doses less than 0.04 mg/kg. However, doses greater than 0.04 mg/kg were observed to cause increased electrical activity of the uterine muscle without inducing synchronizing burst potentials characteristics of parturition [54, 55]. This indicates that detomidine is less likely to induce premature parturition in pregnant ruminants at recommended doses and thus may make it safer for use in pregnant ruminants. Slight sedation without analgesic effect was observed when 0.01 mg/kg of IM detomidine was given to Lanka buffaloes. Moderate sedation with analgesia was observed at 0.02 mg/kg, while deep sedation with excellent analgesia occurred with 0.04 mg/kg. However, 50% of the animals receiving 0.04 mg/kg became recumbent. When increasing the dose to 0.08 mg/kg, detomidine induced recumbency and complete immobilization in these buffaloes. The author of the study concluded that 0.02 and 0.04 mg/kg of detomidine induced adequate sedation and analgesia that suffices most clinical and practical purposes [56]. At higher doses (0.08–0.1 mg/kg IM), detomidine induced complete immobilization and excellent muscle relaxation, but regurgitation and subsequent aspiration pneumonia could be a risk if the animal's airway is not protected [56, 57]. In dairy cattle, IV detomidine alone (0.1 mg/kg) induced moderate sedation with significant decreased heart rate and respiratory rate for 39–55 minutes. Similar to xylazine and butorphanol administered to Holstein cows as mentioned previously, CNS excitation produced by butorphanol (0.05 mg/kg IV) seemed to offset the sedative effect of detomidine (0.1 mg/kg IV) when the two drugs were administered concurrently [43].

Caudal epidural administration of detomidine (0.04 mg/kg) induced perineal analgesia within 5 minutes following administration and lasted for 175 minutes [58]. In horses, caudal epidural detomidine has a slightly faster onset and shorter duration of perineal analgesia than xylazine, 12.5 ± 2.7 and 160 ± 8 minutes versus 13.1 ± 3.7 and greater than 165–180 minutes, respectively [59]. Recently, sublingual detomidine gel with a concentration of 7.6 mg/ml in a 3-ml syringe is available for horses to be used in the field or on the farm. The oral bioavailability of this application was 22% in horses, and the peak plasma concentration was approximately 40% of the plasma concentration following IM administration. A mild to moderate degree of sedation occurred within 30–40 minutes and lasted for 90–180 minutes [60, 61]. Minor procedures like grooming or examination can be accomplished with this application [62]. The pharmacokinetic results showed a 48-hour and 3-day withdrawal time of detomidine from blood and urine samples [61, 63]. However, the pH difference between a monogastric (2.0) [2] and a ruminant (5.5–6.5) [1] may greatly affect the bioavailability of detomidine gel in ruminants. When administered IV or IM at 0.08 mg/kg to six cows, the concentration of detomidine measured in milk was below 0.4 ng/g at 11 hours, and no detectable concentration was measured at 23 hours post administration. Drug residue was detected in the liver of three cows (0.3–3.9 µg/kg tissue weight) and in the lung (2.3 µg/kg), kidney (0.3 µg/kg), and muscle of the injection site (0.5 µg/kg) of one cow, respectively. Only minute concentrations of 0.4 and 2.5 ng/g in the lungs and 0.7 and 0.8 ng/g in the muscle sample from the injection site were detected in two cows at 48 hours post administration [64]. These residual concentrations of detomidine in different tissues would affect the withdrawal time in food-producing animals.

Medetomidine

IV administration of medetomidine (0.005 mg/kg) to domestic ruminants produced a short duration of standing sedation with minimal analgesia [52]. However, IM administration of 0.03 mg/kg in domestic calves resulted in lateral recumbency with analgesia lasting for 60–75 minutes [65]. Higher doses of medetomidine (0.04 mg/kg in heifers, 0.08 mg/kg in cows) delivered by tranquilizer gun have been used successfully to produce immobilization for the capture of free-ranging cattle. In both studies, atipamezole was used effectively to reverse medetomidine's effect [66, 67]. In one study, two cows were in the last month of pregnancy and both calved normally at full term [67]. Caudal epidural injection of medetomidine (0.015 mg/kg) has been reported to induce rapid onset of perineal analgesia, similar to that of lidocaine, but with a significantly longer duration (4–9.5 hours). Moderate sedation and ataxia were observed in these cows.

Two cows became recumbent at 20 and 40 minutes following drug administration, but both were easily coaxed to stand. It was believed that the recumbency in these two cows was caused by the nature of the ruminants during deep sedation, not the result of motor nerve function disruption due to caudal epidural medetomidine [68].

Romifidine

When administered at 0.02 mg/kg IM to cattle, romifidine produced deep sedation with recumbency at 14.8 ± 3.4 minutes after injection. The duration of immobilization was 45.2 ± 3.4 minutes, and standing recovery occurred at 78.7 ± 17.7 minutes. The degree of analgesia produced by romifidine at this dose was similar to that produced by 0.2 mg/kg of IM xylazine. Similar to other α_2 agonists, romifidine caused bradycardia, and the heart rate was significantly lower with romifidine. Other side effects of romifidine observed included bradypnea, decreased hematocrit, and ruminal tympany [69]. Romifidine (0.05 mg/kg) and morphine (0.1 mg/kg) have been combined and diluted in saline to a total volume of 30 ml and administered through a caudal epidural to Holstein–Friesian cows. Significant perineal analgesia with moderate sedation lasted 6 hours, but on occasion, analgesia lasted up to 12 hours. Cows in this study had a tendency to sit down and assume a recumbent position. The authors were not clear whether the recumbency was due to the deep sedation and ataxia from systemic absorption of romifidine and morphine into blood circulation or the natural instinct of the cattle to sit down during sedation. One cow developed hind limb paresis and became recumbent 24 hours after drug administration. The cow showed no improvement 72 hours later and was humanely euthanized. Postmortem examination did not reveal any pathological changes like necrosis, inflammation, or degenerative lesions in the spinal cord to explain the hind limb paresis. However, the cow did have severe muscle necrosis of the adductor muscles, mild hepatic lipidosis, and moderate acute abomasal ulceration [70].

Small ruminants and camelids

Xylazine

Similar to cattle, small ruminants (e.g., sheep and goats) are very sensitive to xylazine, and goats are more sensitive than sheep [4]. Camelids (e.g., alpacas, llamas), though more sensitive to xylazine than horses, are not as sensitive as cattle and small ruminants. Therefore, the dose of xylazine required to produce a similar degree of sedation in goats is equal to or slightly less than that of cattle, whereas a slightly higher dose is required in camelids than in cattle and small ruminants. Compared to llamas, alpacas require dosages 10–15% higher than the recommended dose for llamas. Xylazine alone produces dose-dependent CNS depression ranging from standing sedation to recumbency and immobilization in small ruminants and camelids. Extreme caution should be practiced when xylazine is used in animals with preexisting cardiopulmonary disease and urinary tract obstruction or in late pregnancy [31, 38, 71]. Severe hypoxemia and pulmonary edema have been implicated as the cause of death in sheep under xylazine sedation/anesthesia [72–75]. Lateral recumbency in conscious sheep has been reported to induce a significant decrease in $Pa{O_2}$ [76]. Xylazine has been reported to cause hypoxemia in xylazine-sedated standing sheep [77, 78]. Apparently, all α_2 agonists cause similar and significant decrease in PaO_2 in sheep without affecting the $PaCO_2$ [79]. Nolan et al. (1986) [80] had demonstrated that xylazine-induced increased airway pressure (from 13.7 to 35 mm of Hg) in sheep was a result of dose-dependent stimulation of peripheral (postsynaptic) α_2 adrenoceptors located in the airway smooth muscles (0.002–0.02 mg/kg). The effect of xylazine on the airway smooth muscles occurred within 5 minutes following IV administration and lasted longer than 60 minutes, long after the measured cardiovascular variables had returned to baseline values [80]. Furthermore, severe pulmonary parenchymal damage was seen with substantial morphological changes, such as extensive damages to capillary endothelium and alveolar type I cells, intra-alveolar hemorrhage, and interstitial and alveolar edema. Such changes occurred almost immediately following IV administration of 0.15 mg/kg of xylazine [81]. Bronchospasm and venospasm due to direct action of α_2 adrenoceptors on the vascular and bronchial smooth muscles, transient α_2-induced platelet aggregation with pulmonary microembolism, and release of cytokines and other inflammatory mediators subsequent to α_2-induced pulmonary intravascular macrophage activation have been suggested as the contributing factors for the development of hypoxemia in sheep [82].

Caudal epidural administration of xylazine (0.07–0.1 mg/kg), with or without lidocaine, induced long-lasting somatic analgesia for open castration in rams (8 hours, without lidocaine) and correction of vaginal prolapse in ewes (24 hours, with 0.5 mg/kg of lidocaine) [83, 84]. However, visceral analgesia induced by epidural xylazine alone may not be sufficient for ligation of the spermatic cord [83].

Detomidine

At 0.02 mg/kg IV, detomidine produced sedation which is comparable to that of 0.04 mg/kg of xylazine [85]. Increasing the dose to 0.03 mg/kg, detomidine induced recumbency in sheep with sedation that was equivalent to 0.15 mg/kg of xylazine and 0.01 mg/kg of medetomidine [86]. Effective sedation and significant but transient hypotension and bradycardia followed by tachycardia and hypoxemia were reported during sedation with 0.091 ± 0.004 mg/kg of IV detomidine. Cardiac arrhythmias (e.g., atrioventricular block, ST elevation, and premature ventricular contraction) were also observed in this study [87]. Deep sedation with hypotension of 108 ± 9.1 minutes occurred when detomidine (0.092 ± 0.006 mg/kg IV) was combined with diazepam (0.7 ± 0.2 mg/kg IV). Cardiac arrhythmias, but not hypoxemia or hypercapnia, were observed when diazepam was administered with detomidine [88]. Obviously, hypoxemia and pulmonary edema can occur with any of the α_2 agonists, but the severity of hypoxemia was reported to be less with detomidine [82]. IV administration of α_2 agonists normally induces a characteristic biphasic blood pressure response characterized by, transient hypertension followed by longer-lasting hypotension. The initial hypertension is the result of vasoconstriction from stimulation of peripheral (postsynaptic) α_2 adrenoceptors, and the subsequent hypotension is due to activation of central (presynaptic) α_2 adrenoceptors resulting in decreased sympathetic outflow and catecholamines release [31]. Celly et al. [79] reported a longer-lasting hypertension was observed following IV administration of detomidine (0.03 mg/kg). Interestingly, in that study, mean arterial blood pressure showed the characteristic biphasic patterns for all four α_2 agonists (xylazine, detomidine, medetomidine, and romifidine), but all the values were within or above normal values. In other words, hypotension, defined as below-normal arterial blood pressure values, was not observed with any of the α_2 agonists in this study [79]. Unlike xylazine, detomidine at IV doses less than 0.04 mg/kg did not produce oxytocin-like effect on the uterus in gravid cattle. Doses higher than 0.04 mg/kg may increase the electrical activity of the uterine muscles, but it did not induce the synchronization of the bursts of potentials that is characteristic of parturition. Therefore, detomidine at the therapeutic dose is unlikely to induce premature parturition in pregnant ruminants [54, 55].

Medetomidine

Medetomidine induced dose-dependent sedation and analgesia in sheep at doses of 0.001–0.007 mg/kg IV, with the level of analgesia produced by 0.005 mg/kg comparable to that of 0.015 mg/kg of fentanyl [89]. At 0.04 mg/kg IM, medetomidine induced 30–45 minutes of good analgesia and marked muscle relaxation and 58 minutes of recumbency. Full recovery usually occurred within 1½–2 hours after regaining the righting reflex [90]. When used as a preanesthetic administered 30 minutes prior to induction with propofol and maintenance with isoflurane, medetomidine (0.005 or 0.01 mg/kg IM) decreased heart rate and respiratory rate. Mean arterial blood pressure values were significantly higher following a high dose (0.01 mg/kg IM) as compared to those without preanesthetic medetomidine or those administered at a lower dose (0.005 mg/kg IM). In general, the administration of medetomidine reduced the dose requirement of propofol for induction and isoflurane for maintenance of anesthesia during surgery [91]. In sheep breathing room air that are anesthetized with medetomidine (0.02 mg/kg IV) and ketamine (2 mg/kg IV), PaO_2, arterial pH, and arterial O_2 saturation (SaO_2) decreased and $PaCO_2$ increased significantly. Supplementation of 100% O_2 improved PaO_2 and SaO_2 [92]. Similar to all other α_2 agonist drugs, medetomidine (0.01 mg/kg IV) caused characteristic hypoxemia in sheep breathing room air during sedation [79].

When given to produce lumbosacral analgesia in goats, medetomidine at doses of 0.01, 0.02, and 0.03 mg/kg diluted in sterile water to a total volume of 5 ml produced satisfactory analgesia in the perineum and flank regions, and the analgesia extended to the thorax, forelimbs, neck, and head for a period of at least 3 hours. Ten goats receiving 0.02 mg/kg underwent laparotomy surgery; adequate analgesia was apparent in all tissue layers (from skin to external and internal oblique muscles and transverse muscles). All ten goats recovered uneventfully from surgery. Lateral recumbency and characteristic side effects of other α_2 agonists were observed during the study, particularly with higher doses (0.02 and 0.03 mg/kg). One goat receiving 0.01 mg/kg was paralyzed following lumbosacral injection and was humanely euthanized. Because of the caudal extension of the spinal cord into the cauda equina in goats, it was speculated that the trauma to the conus medullaris and/or cauda equina resulting from struggling of the animal at the time of spinal needle insertion was responsible for the paralysis observed in this goat [93].

IM administration of medetomidine (0.01–0.03 mg/kg IM) has also been used in llamas. Sternal recumbency (5.3 ± 4.7 minutes) and mild to moderate sedation (37.3 ± 9.5 minutes) without analgesia were observed in two of three llamas receiving 0.01 mg/kg of the drug.

All llamas receiving 0.02 mg/kg assumed sternal recumbency but with only slightly more profound sedation (58 ± 12.1 minutes) and analgesia (30 minutes) than that of 0.01 mg/kg. When the dose was increased to 0.03 mg/kg, medetomidine induced immobilization (91.5 ± 24.7 minutes) with profound analgesia (61.7 ± 2.9 minutes) and muscle relaxation. The only side effect observed during the period of immobilization was a significant decrease in heart rate. Atipamezole (0.125 mg/kg IM) effectively reversed the effect of medetomidine (0.03 mg/kg IM), and standing recovery occurred within 5.8 ± 3.3 minutes [94].

Romifidine

In foals, romifidine was reported to produce sedation and analgesia with greater intensity and longer duration than xylazine [95]. Celly et al. [79] reported that romifidine at 0.05 mg/kg IV produced a similar degree of hypoxemia but a significantly longer duration of initial hypertension than other α_2 agonists. When xylazine (0.15 mg/kg IV), detomidine (0.03 mg/kg IV), romifidine (0.05 mg/kg IV), and medetomidine (0.01 mg/kg IV) were administered to sheep at quasiequipotent doses, similar decreases in PaO_2 and increases in respiratory rate and maximum changes in transpulmonary pressure (ΔP_{pl}) were observed with all four drugs except the duration of increase in respiratory rate, and ΔP_{pl} were longest with romifidine [79].

When romifidine (0.05 mg/kg) was administered by lumbosacral epidural injection, it produced moderate to complete analgesia of the perineum, flank, and abdominal regions. Increasing the dose to 0.075 mg/kg did not enhance the degree of analgesia but only prolonged the duration. Amarpal et al. (2002) [96] indicated that higher doses of romifidine (0.075 mg/kg) produced a wider region of analgesia from the tail regions to the thorax. This may be the result of a higher concentration of the injected drug solution with 0.075 mg/kg than 0.05 mg/kg since the total volume of the injected solution was maintained at the same 4 ml for both dosages in this study. Side effects resulting from spinally administered romifidine included dose-dependent ataxia and decreased heart rate, respiratory rate, and mean arterial blood pressures [96].

In camels, the sedative and analgesic effects of romifidine were assessed at three different doses (0.04, 0.08, and 0.12 mg/kg IV). Both the sedative and analgesic effects were dose dependent with the duration of sedation (37, 51, and 65 minutes, respectively) lasting longer than the analgesic effect (21, 34, and 46 minutes, respectively). Bradycardia, ruminal tympany, increased urine output, and hyperglycemia are commonly observed side effects during romifidine sedation. Camels may not represent domestic camelids like llamas and alpacas, and they have been reported to require higher doses of xylazine to produce a similar degree of sedation. Thus, llamas and alpacas may require a lower dose of romifidine to produce desirable sedation and analgesia [97].

Swine

Xylazine

Compared to other domestic species, pigs are the least sensitive to xylazine. A higher dose (1.65 mg/kg IV, 2.2 mg/kg IM) is required to produce mild to moderate sedation, but still, the pigs are easily aroused and able to flee when approached [6, 12]. Vomiting and bloating have been observed in pigs that were not fasted prior to anesthesia [14, 19]. When tested at doses of 1, 2, 4, 8, and 16 mg/kg IV in young pigs, xylazine alone did not produce effective sedation and analgesia. Xylazine induced a significant decrease in mean arterial blood pressure, but it gradually returned to baseline values 10 minutes after administration [98].

Detomidine

In pigs, doses of detomidine at 0.04 mg/kg IV or 0.08 mg/kg IM have been used in combination with ketamine to produce short-term anesthesia [99]. Analgesia following lumbosacral epidural administration of detomidine was not as profound as xylazine in pigs [100]. In addition, detomidine- or xylazine-induced epidural analgesia may be mediated through a different mechanism of action in that IV administration of an antagonist was capable of antagonizing epidural detomidine-induced sedation, analgesia, and immobilization but was only able to antagonize the sedation induced by epidural xylazine but not the analgesia and immobilization [100]. This observation is supported by reports in horses and cattle [101–103]. Perhaps the difference of response to the IV administration of an antagonist lies in the fact that xylazine itself has local anesthetic effect and detomidine does not [104].

Medetomidine

In pigs, medetomidine at IM doses of 0.03–0.08 mg/kg induced dose-dependent sedation and muscle relaxation. Increasing the dose to greater than 0.1 mg/kg did not increase the degree of sedation or muscle relaxation but did prolonge the duration of activity. Compared to 2 mg/kg of xylazine, enhanced sedation, better muscle relaxation, and greater analgesia were observed with 0.03 mg/kg of medetomidine [105]. Medetomidine has been used in combination with butorphanol (0.2 mg/kg IM) and ketamine (10 mg/kg IM) (**MBK**) to produce anesthesia for 98.8 ± 22.5 minutes, which is significantly longer that of xylazine (2 mg/kg IM)–butorphanol (0.2 mg/kg IM)–ketamine (10 mg/kg IM) combination (47.5 ± 16.5 minutes). The muscle relaxation was adequate for tracheal intubation, but moderate cardiovascular depression was observed during MBK anesthesia [106]. Atipamezole effectively reversed the effects produced by 0.16–0.32 mg/kg IM of medetomidine [99].

Atipamezole, tolazoline, and yohimbine (α_2 antagonists)

The pharmacologic effects induced by any one of the α_2 agonists can be antagonized effectively with an α_2 antagonist, such as yohimbine, tolazoline, or atipamezole. These antagonists can be used to shorten the time of recovery to standing, to treat severe α_2 agonist-induced bradycardia, and to minimize adverse effects associated with accidental overdose. The α_2 agonists are known to cause bloating and ruminal tympany by decreasing GI motility. Administration of any of the α_2 antagonists effectively reversed the decrease in GI motility [85, 107]. However, administration of these antagonists is not without risk. Sudden awareness of pain, significant peripheral vasodilation, and CNS excitement have occurred following rapid IV administration of an antagonist. The death of a sheep after administration of a large dose of yohimbine (0.8 mg/kg IV) has been reported [72]. Rapid IV injection of tolazoline has also been reported to cause significant cardiac stimulation, tachycardia, increased cardiac output, vasodilation, and GI distress [108]. Ruminants and camelids are more sensitive to tolazoline than other species, and death has been reported after its use [109, 110]. When administered alone at 1.5 mg/kg IV to Holstein calves, tolazoline caused coughing, an increased frequency of defecation, and a mild increase in breathing effort. At higher doses (2–10 mg/kg IV), adverse effects including bright red conjunctival mucous membranes, coughing, nasal discharge, salivation, labored breathing, CNS depression, signs of abdominal pain, straining, head pressing, restlessness, and severe diarrhea were observed. All calves in the study recovered uneventfully [110]. Currently, lower doses of tolazoline (0.5–1.5 mg/kg IV) are recommended for use in all ruminants including camelids. Others have suggested that, except in emergency situations, IV administration of tolazoline should be avoided to prevent adverse effects such as cardiac asystole [111]. When atipamezole (0.1 mg/kg IV) was administered to six goats to antagonize medetomidine (0.02 mg/kg IV)-induced sedation and recumbency, all goats stood within 2 minutes. Four goats developed piloerection and all appeared to be agitated and vocalized [112]. When given to reverse IM xylazine- or medetomidine-induced sedation in free-ranging cattle, atipamezole (0.04–0.09 mg/kg) induced a brief period of excitement following IV administration. Relapse into medetomidine (0.04 mg/kg IV)-induced sedation 1–2 hours after the administration of atipamezole (0.2 mg/kg IV) as a result of the shorter half-life of the drug has been observed in dairy calves. In free-ranging cattle, atipamezole (0.057 ± 0.017 mg/kg IV) has been administered to reverse xylazine-induced immobilization. Eight cows receiving xylazine in this report were in the last 2 months of pregnancy and all cows calved normally and no premature parturition occurred [67]. Administration of a reversal agent (atipamezole) may have shortened the duration of xylazine-induced increases in uterine contraction, thus preventing the adverse effect of xylazine on pregnant cows. Slow injection is recommended when administering an antagonist, to avoid sudden awareness of pain and excitement. The undesirable effects of α_2 antagonists are extremely rare in healthy animals when the drugs are administered at appropriate dosages and by slow IV injection.

Diazepam and midazolam (benzodiazepine derivatives)

Benzodiazepine derivatives like diazepam and midazolam are classified as minor tranquilizers. These drugs are used for their anxiolytic, anticonvulsant, and central muscle-relaxing effects. Benzodiazepines produce little or no analgesic effect, but they can reduce the dose requirement of the concurrently administered general anesthetics [20]. Benzodiazepines produce minimal cardiovascular depression. It is the reason that these drugs are favorable for use in animals with increased anesthetic risk. Benzodiazepines can be used as alternatives to α_2 agonists to produce tranquilization when adverse effects associated with α_2 agonists (e.g., hypoxemia, pulmonary edema, or increased airway pressure) become undesirable. Diazepam and midazolam are the two most commonly used benzodiazepines in clinical veterinary practice. Diazepam is insoluble in water; its injectable solution contains 40% propylene glycol as solvent. IV propylene glycol administered rapidly sometimes results in hypotension and vascular irritation. Dilution, mixture of the injectable solution of diazepam with water, or a water-soluble drug solution may cause cloudiness of the mixture which does not affect the potency of the drug. Midazolam is two to three times more potent than diazepam. Its injectable solution is water soluble. Thus, IM administration of midazolam will not cause tissue irritation [113]. Diazepam can be used as a preanesthetic for its anxiolytic and muscle-relaxing effect, or it can be used with ketamine to improve muscle relaxation during anesthesia [114]. Other benzodiazepines including flurazepam (2 mg/kg IV) [115], lorazepam (0.1 mg/kg IV) [116], and brotizolam (1–10 mg/kg PO) [117] have been used in pigs.

Cattle, small ruminants, and camelids

Diazepam can be administered alone to produce dose-dependent CNS depression, from mild sedation to recumbency for 15–30 minutes. The tranquilizing effects of diazepam in healthy animals tend to be variable and somewhat unreliable [8]. Doses from 0.55 to 1.1 mg/kg IM had been recommended for use in ruminants and swine [118]. Diazepam at 0.2 mg/kg IV has been used to produce mild tranquilization for performing a transdermal tracheal wash [8]. Diazepam (0.1 mg/kg IV) has been administered with xylazine (0.2 mg/kg IV) to a bull to produce immobilization for wire placement during mandibular fracture repair. No additional local anesthetic was needed during the wiring process. The duration of deep sedation was 30 minutes and the bull stood within an hour after administration of the drugs [119]. Diazepam (0.1 mg/kg IV) and butorphanol (0.1 mg/kg IV) induce recumbency for a short period of time in camelids [120].

Midazolam (0.2 mg/kg IV) was able to decrease the response of sheep to painful mechanical stimulation [121]. In goats, IM midazolam (0.6 mg/kg) induced 20 minutes of sedation. Hypnosis with recumbency occurred and lasted for 10–20 minutes when midazolam was administered intravenously at 0.6 and 1.2 mg/kg. Increasing the dose to 1.2 mg/kg enhanced the degree of reflex suppression, and the animals appeared to be in a light plane of anesthesia as indicated by the lack of response to mechanical stimulation applied using the tail base clamp [122]. In goats with urethral obstruction, when the effect of increasing urine output of xylazine is contraindicated, diazepam or midazolam can be given alone or with other anesthetics to induce anesthesia. Flumazenil, a benzodiazepine antagonist, can be administered at 0.02 mg/kg IV or a 1:13 ratio (1 part of flumazenil to 13 parts of diazepam) to antagonize the CNS-depressing or CNS-tranquilizing effects of diazepam and midazolam [8].

Swine

Diazepam has been given to miniature pigs at doses from 5.5 to 8.5 mg/kg IM with maximal sedation occurring within 30 minutes following administration [20]. Prolonged recovery has occurred when large doses of diazepam are given intramuscularly to older sows and boars. A continuous rate infusion (CRI) of diazepam (CRI: 1 mg/kg/hour IV, following 0.5–10 mg/kg IM and 0.44–2 mg/kg IV) has been used in pigs to maintain long-term hypnosis and sedation for up to 6 hours in a research setting [123, 124]. Satisfactory sedation with 0.1–0.5 mg/kg of midazolam IM has been reported [16], whereas calming effect and sedation occur within 3–4 minutes following intranasal administration of 0.2–0.4 mg/kg of the drug [125]. In piglets and adult swine, midazolam administered either intramuscularlly or intranasally at 0.1–0.2 mg/kg produced effective tranquilization [125, 126]. Midazolam (1 mg/kg IM) has been combined with azaperone (4 mg/kg IM) to produce preanesthetic tranquilization prior to induction with propofol [127]. Midazolam in general has minimal cardiopulmonary effects. However, it has been shown to cause a 20% decrease in heart rate and 50% decrease in respiratory rate in pigs receiving 0.1 mg/kg IM of midazolam [126].

Chloral hydrate

Chloral hydrate was one of the first general anesthetics used in large animal practice. Chloral hydrate itself does not have a CNS-depressing effect; it depends on its metabolite, trichloroethanol, to produce sedative and anesthetic effects. This latency of action as well as the narrow margin of safety of the drug makes it an undesirable anesthetic for use in clinical practice. Nonetheless, chloral hydrate is a very reliable sedative. In horses, chloral hydrate is often administered as an alternative when other tranquilizers or sedatives fail to produce the desired calming effect. Chloral hydrate does not have an analgesic effect; thus, an additional analgesic is required if the animal is in pain or the procedure being performed is painful. Chloral hydrate is very irritating to the tissue. Therefore, IV injection of the drug is better via an IV catheter to prevent accidental perivascular injection and the consequential severe tissue damage. Chloral hydrate has been used to sedate unapproachable but confined cattle via oral administration. Withhold water for 24–36 hours prior to offering the animal diluted chloral hydrate drinking solution to ensure complete consumption of the drug. The dose recommended for oral administration is 100–150 gm in 8–12 L of water per animal for sedation and 5–7 g per 100 kg (220 lb) for light to moderate narcosis [128].

In pigs, oral chloral hydrate (13 g/50 kg [110 lb]) produced sedation within 20–30 minutes following the administration via a stomach tube [129]. Though intraperitoneal administration (4–6 ml of 5% solution/kg) has been reported in the pig, the technique is not recommended as peritonitis is a common complication [130]. However, Jennings reported intraperitoneal chloral hydrate (0.3 mg/kg in 5% solution) administration produced sedation within 30 minutes with a duration of 60 minutes. No tissue irritation or signs of peritonitis were observed [128]. Chloral hydrate (1–4 ml of 5% solution) has been used in combination with azaperone (4 mg/kg IM) in 500 pigs to produce general anesthesia for 2 hours with complete recovery to standing within 4–5 hours [131].

References

1. Hinchcliff, K., Jernigan, A., Upson, D. and Constable, P. (1991) Ruminant pharmacology. *Veterinary Clinics of North America: Food Animal Practice*, **7**, 633–649.
2. DeRouchey, J., Goodband, B., Tokach, M. *et al.* (2009) Digestive system of the pig-anatomy and function. *North American Veterinary Community Conference,* 375–376.

3. Gross, M. and Booth, N. (1995) Tranquilizers, α2-adrenergic agonists, and related agents, in *Veterinary Pharmacology and Therapeutics*, 7th edn (ed H. Adams), Iowa State University Press, Ames, pp. 311–357.
4. Taylor, P. (1991) Anesthesia in sheep and goats. *In Practice*, **13**, 31–36.
5. Jones, R. (1972) A review of tranquilizers and sedation in large animals. *The Veterinary Record*, **90**, 613–617.
6. Riebold, T., Geiser, D. and Goble, D. (1995) Anesthetic agents and ancillary drugs, in *Large Animal Anesthesia: Principles and Techniques*, 2nd edn (eds T. Riebold, D. Geiser and D. Goble), Iowa State University Press, Ames, pp. 11–64.
7. Tranquilli, W. and Grimm, K. (1996) Pharmacology of drugs used for anesthesia and sedation. *Veterinary Clinics of North America: Food Animal Practice*, **12**, 501–529.
8. Hall, L., Clarke, K. and Trim, C. (2001) Anaesthesia of sheep, goats, and other herbivores, in *Veterinary Anaesthesia*, 10th edn (eds L. Hall, K. Clarke and C. Trim), WB Saunders, London, pp. 341–366.
9. Lin, H., Caldwell, F. and Pugh, D. (2012) Anesthetic management, in *Sheep and Goat Medicine*, 2nd edn (eds D. Pugh and A. Baird), Elsevier, Maryland Height, pp. 517–538.
10. Barrie, K., Jacobson, E. and Peiffer, R. (1978) Unilateral cataract with lens coloboma and bilateral corneal edema in guanaco. *Journal of the American Veterinary Medical Association*, **173**, 1251–1252.
11. Fowler, M. (1998) Anesthesia, in *Medicine and Surgery of South American Camelids*, 2nd edn (ed M. Fowler), Iowa State University Press, Ames, pp. 89–107.
12. Thurmon, J. and Smith, G. (2007) Swine, in *Lumb & Jones' Veterinary Anesthesia and Analgesia*, 4th edn (eds W. Tranquilli, J. Thurmon and K. Grimm), Blackwell Publishing, Ames, pp. 747–763.
13. Gleed, R. (1994) Anesthesia for parlor pigs (Vietnamese potbellied pigs). *North American Veterinary Community Conference,* pp. 647.
14. Moon, P. and Smith, L. (1996) General anesthetic techniques in swine. *Veterinary Clinics of North America: Food Animal Practice*, **12**, 663–691.
15. McGrath, C., Rempel, W., Addis, P. and Crimi, A. (1981) Acepromazine and droperidol inhibition of halothane-induced malignant hyperthermia (porcine stress syndrome) in swine. *American Journal of Veterinary Research*, **42**, 195–198.
16. Bustamante, R. and Valverde, A. (1997) Determination of a sedative dose and influence of droperidol and midazolam on cardiovascular function in pigs *Canadian Journal of Veterinary Research*, pp. **61**:246–250.
17. Mascarenhas, R., Raiser, H., Sturion, D. and Susko, I. (1980) Neuroleptanalgesia by droperidol in sheep. *Revista do Centro de Ciencias Rurais*, **10**, 387–393.
18. Thurmon, J. and Benson, G. (1993) Anesthesia in ruminants and swine, in *Current Veterinary Therapy: Food Animal Practice*, 3rd edn (ed J. Howard), WB Saunders, Philadelphia, pp. 58–76.
19. Short, C. (1986) Preanesthetic medications in ruminants and swine. *Veterinary Clinics of North America: Food Animal Practice*, **2**, 553–566.
20. Regan, H. and Gillis, M. (1975) Restraint, venipuncture, endotracheal intubation, and anesthesia of miniature swine. *Laboratory Animal Science*, **25**, 409–419.
21. Piermattei, D. and Swan, H. (1970) Techniques for general anesthesia in miniature pigs. *The Journal of Surgical Research*, **10**, 587–592.
22. Hughes, R., Syme, L. and Syme, G. (1977) Open-field behavior in sheep following treatment with neuroleptics azaperone and acetylpromazine. *Psychopharmacology*, **52**, 107–109.
23. Madsen, B., Syme, G. and Syme, L. (1980) Effects of azaperone and acetylpromazine on social and environmental behavior in sheep. *British Journal of Pharmacology*, **69**, 179–183.

24. Thurmon, J. and Benson, G. (1981) Anesthesia in ruminants and swine, in *Current Veterinary Therapy: Food Animal Practice* (ed J. Howard), WB Saunders, Philadelphia, pp. 58–81.
25. Callear, J. (1971) An analysis of the results of field experiments in pigs in the U.K. and Ireland with the sedative neuroleptic azaperone. *The Veterinary Record*, **89**, 453–458.
26. Symoens, J., vanGestel, J. and Marsboom, R. (1973) Clinical trial of a new sedative for pigs, azaperone. *Tierarztliche Umschau*, **28**, 232–240.
27. Anderson, I. (1977) Anesthesia of swine. *New Zealand Veterinary Journal*, **25**, 319–321.
28. Portier, D. and Slusser, C. (1985) Azaperone: A review of a new neuroleptic agent for swine. *Journal of Veterinary Medicine*, **80**, 88–92.
29. Boldrick, L. and Blackburn, A. (1993) Anesthesia. *Veterinary Care of Pot-bellied Pigs*. Orange: All Publishing Co, pp. 104–110.
30. McGrath, C., Lee, J. and Ashen, M. (1984) Azaperone (Stresnil) in malignant hyperthermia (MH) susceptible swine: determination of protective effects to halothane challenge and toxicity [Abstract]. *Veterinary Surgeons*, **14**, 75.
31. Greene, S. and Thurmon, J. (1988) Xylazine – A review of its pharmacology and use in veterinary medicine. *Journal of Veterinary Pharmacology and Therapeutics*, **11**, 295–313.
32. Booth, N. (1988) Intravenous and other parenteral anesthetics, in *Veterinary Pharmacology and Therapeutics*, 6th edn (eds N. Booth and L. McDonald), Iowa State University Press, Ames, pp. 212–274.
33. Virtanen, R. (1989) Pharmacological profiles of medetomidine and its antagonist, atipamezole. *Acta Veterinaria Scandinavica Supplementum*, **85**, 29–37.
34. Moens, Y., Lanz, F., Doherr, M. and Schatzmann, U. (2003) A comparison of the antinociceptive effects of xylazine, detomidine, and romifidine on experimental pain in horses. *Veterinary Anaesthesia and Analgesia*, **30**, 183–190.
35. Raptopoulos, D. and Weaver, B. (1984) Observation following intravenous xylazine administration in steers. *The Veterinary Record*, **114**, 567–569.
36. Carroll, G. and Hartsfield, S. (1996) General anesthetic techniques in ruminants. *Veterinary Clinics of North America: Food Animal Practice*, **12**, 627–661.
37. Trim, C. (1987) Special anesthesia considerations in the ruminant, in *Principles and Practice of Veterinary Anesthesia* (ed C. Short), Williams & Wilkins, Baltimore, pp. 285–300.
38. LeBlanc, M., Hubbell, J. and Smith, H. (1984) The effect of xylazine hydrochloride on intrauterine pressure in the cow. *Theriogenology*, **21**, 681–690.
39. Jansen, C., Lowe, K. and Nathanielsz, P. (1984) The effects of xylazine on uterine activity, fetal and maternal oxygenation, cardiovascular function, and fetal breathing. *American Journal of Obstetrics and Gynecology*, **148**, 386–390.
40. Hodgson, D., Dunlop, C., Chapman, P. and Smith, J. (2002) Cardiopulmonary effects of xylazine and acepromazine in pregnant cows in late gestation. *American Journal of Veterinary Research*, **63**, 1695–1699.
41. Fayed, A., Abdalla, E., Anderson, R. *et al.* (1989) Effect of xylazine in heifers under thermoneutral or heat stress conditions. *American Journal of Veterinary Research*, **50**, 151–153.
42. Stewart, J. (1972) Observations on the restraint and immobilization of uncontrollable cattle with Rompun. *Veterinary Medical Review*, **3**, 197–204.
43. Lin, H. and Riddell, M. (2003) Preliminary study of the effects of xylazine or detomidine with or without butorphanol for standing sedation in dairy cattle. *Veterinary Therapy*, **4**, 285–291.
44. Caron, J. and LeBlanc, P. (1989) Caudal epidural analgesia in cattle using xylazine. *Canadian Journal of Veterinary Research*, **53**, 486–489.
45. StJean, G., Skarda, R., Muir, W. and Hoffsis, G. (1990) Caudal epidural analgesia induced by xylazine administration in cows. *American Journal of Veterinary Research*, **51**, 1232–1236.

46. Angst, M., Ramaswamy, B., Riley, E. and Stanski, D. (2000) Lumbar epidural morphine in humans and supraspinal analgesia to experimental heat pain. *Anesthesiology*, **92**, 312–324.
47. Valverde, A., Conlon, P., Dyson, D. and Burger, J. (1992) Cisternal CSF and serum concentrations of morphine following epidural administration in the dog. *Journal of Veterinary Pharmacology and Therapeutics*, **15**, 91–95.
48. Skarda, R., StJean, G. and Muir, W. (1990) Influence of tolazoline on caudal epidural administration of xylazine in cattle. *American Journal of Veterinary Research*, **51**, 556–560.
49. Bouchenafa, O. and Livingston, A. (1987) Autoradiographic localisation of alpha 2 adrenoreceptor binding sites in the spinal cord of the sheep. *Research in Veterinary Science*, **42**, 382–386.
50. Lawhead, R., Blaxall, H. and Bylund, D. (1992) A2A is the predominant α-2 adrenergic receptor subtype in human spinal cord. *Anesthesiology*, **77**, 983–991.
51. Natalini, C. (1991) Detomidine sedative and analgesic effects in bovine. *International Congress Veterinary Anaesthesia*, pp. 375–376.
52. Greene, S. (2003) Protocols for anesthesia of cattle. *Veterinary Clinics of North America: Food Animal Practice*, **19**, 679–693.
53. Hendrickson, D. (2007) Anesthesia and fluid therapy, in *Techniques in Large Animal Surgery*, 3rd edn (ed D. Hendrickson), Blackwell Publishing, Ames, pp. 7–32.
54. Pyrörälä, E., Koppinen, J., Vainio, O. and Alanko, M. (1986) Detomidine to pregnant cows. *Nordisk Veterinaermedicin*, **38**, 237–240.
55. Jedruch, J. and Gajewski, Z. (1986) The effect of detomidine hydrochloride (Domosedan) on the electrical activity of the uterus in cows. *Acta Veterinaria Scandinavica*, **82**, 189–192.
56. deSilva, D. (1991) Sedative analgesic effects of detomidine HCL (Domosedan) in Lanka buffaloes. *International Congress Veterinary Anaesthesia*, pp. 211–213.
57. Krogh, K. (2000) Immobilisation of wild heifers with detomidine and detomidine combinations. *International Congress Veterinary Anaesthesia*, p. 105.
58. Prado, M., Streeter, R., Mandsager, R. *et al.* (1999) Pharmacologic effects of epidural versus intramuscular administration of detomidine in cattle. *American Journal of Veterinary Research*, **60**, 1242–1247.
59. Skarda, R. and Muir, W. (1996) Comparison of antinociceptive, cardiovascular, and respiratory effects, head ptosis, and position of pelvic limbs in mares after caudal epidural administration of xylazine and detomidine hydrochloride solution. *American Journal of Veterinary Research*, **57**, 1338–1345.
60. Kaukinen, H., Aspergén, J., Hyyppä, S. *et al.* (2011) Bioavailability of detomidine administered sublingually to horses as an oromucosal gel. *Journal of Veterinary Pharmacology and Therapeutics*, **34**, 76–81.
61. Dimaio-Knych, H. and Stanley, S. (2011) Pharmacokinetics and pharmacodynamics of detomidine following sublingual administration to horses. *American Journal of Veterinary Research*, **72**, 1378–1385.
62. Gardner, R., White, G., Ramsey, D. *et al.* (2010) Efficacy of sublingual administration of detomidine gel for sedation of horses undergoing veterinary and husbancy procedures under field conditions. *Journal of the American Veterinary Medical Association*, **237**, 1459–1464.
63. I'ami, J., Vermunt, L., vanLoon, J. *et al.* (2012) Sublingual administration of detomidine in horses: sedative effect, analgesia and detection time. *Veterinary Journal*. http://dx.doi.org/10.106/j.tvjl.2012.08.016 (accessed January 21, 2014).
64. Salonen, J., Vähä-Vahe, T., Vainio, O. and Vakkuri, O. (1989) Single-dose pharmacokinetics of detomidine in the horse and cow. *Journal of Veterinary Pharmacology and Therapeutics*, **12**, 65–72.

65. Sharma, S., Nigam J., Kumar, A. *et al.* (1994) Preliminary studies on the use of medetomidine in calves and its reversal by atipamezole. *International Congress Veterinary Anaesthesia*, p. 121.
66. Arnemo, J. and Søli, N. (1993) Chemical capture of free-ranging cattle: immobilization with xylazine or medetomidine, and reversal with atipamezole. *Veterinary Research Communications*, **17**, 469–477.
67. Arnemo, J. and Søli, N. (1995) Immobilization of free-ranging cattle with medetomidine and its reversal by atipamezole. *Veterinary Research Communications*, **19**, 59–62.
68. Lin, H., Trachte, E., DeGraves, F. *et al.* (1998) Evaluation of analgesia induced by epidural administration of medetomidine to cows. *American Journal of Veterinary Research*, **59**, 162–167.
69. Massone, F., Luna, S., Castro, G. *et al.* (1993) Sedation with romifidine or xylazine in cattle, is it the same? *Journal of the Association of Veterinary Anaesthetists*, **20**, 55.
70. Fierheller, E., Caulkett, N. and Bailey, J. (2004) A romifidine and morphine combination for epidural analgesia of the flank in cattle. *The Canadian Veterinary Journal*, **45**, 917–923.
71. Rosenberger, G., Hempel, E. and Baumeister, M. (1968) Contributions to the effect and use of Rompun in cattle. *Deutsche tierarztliche Wochenschrift*, **75**, 572–578.
72. Hsu, W., Schaffer, D. and Hanson, C. (1987) Effects of tolazoline and yohimbine on xylazine-induced central nervous system depression, bradycardia, and tachypnea in sheep. *Journal of the American Veterinary Medical Association*, **190**, 423–426.
73. Hsu, W., Hanson, C., Hembrough, F. and Schaffer, D. (1989) Effects of idazoxan, tolazoline, and yohimbine on xylazine-induced respiratory changes and central nervous system depression in ewes. *American Journal of Veterinary Research*, **50**, 1570–1573.
74. Lin, H., Thurmon, J., Benson, G. *et al.* (1989) The hemodynamic response of calves to tiletamine-zolazepam anesthesia. *Veterinary Surgeons*, **18**, 328–334.
75. Lin, H., Tyler, J., Welles, E. *et al.* (1993) Effects of anesthesia induced and maintained by continuous intravenous administration of guaifenesin, ketamine, and xylazine in spontaneously breathing sheep. *American Journal of Veterinary Research*, **54**, 1913–1916.
76. Mitchell, B. and Williams, J. (1976–1977) Respiratory function changes in sheep associated with lying in lateral recumbency and with sedation by xylazine. Great Britain and Ireland Association of Veterinary Anaesthetists, 30.
77. Doherty, T., Ballinger, J., McDonnell, W. *et al.* (1987) Antagonism of xylazine-induced sedation by idazoxan in calves. *Canadian Journal of Veterinary Research*, **51**, 244–248.
78. Waterman, A., Nolan, A. and Livingston, A. (1987) Influence of idazoxan on the respiratory blood gas changes induced by alpha 2-adrenoceptor agonist drugs in conscious sheep. *The Veterinary Record*, **121**, 105–107.
79. Celly, C., McDonnell, W., Young, S. and Black, W. (1997) The comparative hypoxaemic effects of four α-2 adrenoceptor agonists (xylazine, romifidine, detomidine, and medetomidine) in sheep. *Journal of Veterinary Pharmacology and Therapeutics*, **20**, 464–471.
80. Nolan, A., Livingston, A. and Waterman, A. (1986) The effects of alpha2 adrenoceptor agonists on airway pressure in anaesthetized sheep. *Journal of Veterinary Pharmacology and Therapeutics*, **9**, 157–163.
81. Celly, C., Atwal, O., McDonell, W. and Black, W. (1999) Histopathologic alterations induced in the lungs of sheep by use of α2-adrenergic receptors agonists. *American Journal of Veterinary Research*, **60**, 154–161.
82. Kästner, S. (2006) α2-agonists in sheep: a review. *Veterinary Anaesthesia and Analgesia*, **33**, 79–96.
83. Scott, P., Henshaw, C., Sargison, N. *et al.* (1994) Assessment of xylazine hydrochloride epidural analgesia for open castration of rams. *Theriogenology*, **42**, 1029–1034.

84. Scott, P. and Gessert, M. (1997) Management of post-partum cervical uterine or rectal prolapses in ewes using caudal epidural xylazine and lignocaine injection. *Veterinary Journal*, **153**, 115–116.
85. Ruckebusch, Y. and Allal, C. (1987) Depression of reticulo-ruminal motor functions through the stimulation of alpha 2-adrenoceptors. *Journal of Veterinary Pharmacology and Therapeutics*, **10**, 1–10.
86. Celly C, McDonnell W, Black W, *et al.* Comparative cardiopulmonary effects of four α-2 adrenoceptor agonists in sheep. *International Congress Veterinary Anaesthesia* 1994; 117.
87. Kariman, A., Sharifi, D., Teshfam, M. *et al.* (1994) The effects of detomidine hydrochloride on cardiovascular and hemodynamics in sheep. *International Congress Veterinary Anaesthesia*, p. 119.
88. Sharifi, D., Kariman, A., Teshfam, M. *et al.* (1994) The effects of detomidine hydrochloride and diazepam on cardiovascular and haemodynamics in sheep. *International Congress Veterinary Anaesthesia*, p. 83.
89. Muge, D., Chambers, J., Livingston, A. and Waterman, A. (1994) Analgesic effects of medetomidine in sheep. *The Veterinary Record*, **135**, 43–44.
90. Mohammad, F., Zangana, I. and Abdul-Latif, A. (1993) Medetomidine sedation in sheep. *Zentralblatt fur Veterinarmedizin. Reihe A*, **40**, 328–331.
91. Kästner, S., Kutter, A., vonRechenberg, B., and Bettschart-Wolfensberger, R. (2006) Comparison of two pre-anesthetic medetomidine doses in isoflurane anesthetized sheep. *Veterinary Anaesthesia and Analgesia*, **33**, 8–16.
92. Tulamo, R.-M., Raekallio, M. and Ekblad, A. (1995) Cardiovascular effects of medetomidine-ketamine anaesthesia in sheep, with and without 100% oxygen and its reversal with atipamezole. *Journal of Veterinary Anaesthesia*, **22**, 9–14.
93. Mpanduji, D., Bittegeko, S., Mgasa, M. and Batamuzi, E. (2000) Analgesic, behavioural and cardiopulmonary effects of epidurally injected medetomidine (Domitor) in goats. *Journal of Veterinary Medicine. A, Environmental Child Health radiology: JVIR Physiology, Pathology, Clinical Medicine*, **47**, 65–72.
94. Waldridge, B., Lin, H., DeGraves, F. and Pugh, D. (1997) Sedative effects of medetomidine and its reversal by atipamezole in llamas. *Journal of the American Veterinary Medical Association*, **211**, 1562–1565.
95. Naylor, J., Gasven, E. and Fraser, L. (1997) A c omparison of romifidine and xylazine in foals. The effects on sedation and analgesia. *Equine Veterinary Education*, **9**, 329–334.
96. Khattri, S., Kinjavdekar, P., Amarpal *et al.* (2002) Analgesic, sedative and hemodynamic effects of spinally administered romifidine in female goats. *Journal ofVeterinary Medicine. A, Environmental Child Healthradiology: JVIR Physiology, Pathology, Clinical Medicine*, 49, 3–8.
97. Marzok, M. and El-Khodery, S. (2009) Sedative and analgesic effects of romifidine in camels (Camelus dromedaries). *Veterinary Anaesthesia and Analgesia*, **36**, 352–360.
98. deSegura, I., Tendillo, F., Mascías, A. *et al.* (1997) Actions of xylazine in young swine. *American Journal of Veterinary Research*, **58**, 99–102.
99. Nishimura, R., Kim, H., Matsunaga, S. *et al.* (1992) Antagonism of medetomidine sedation by atipamezole in pigs. *Journal of Veterinary Medical Science*, **54**, 1237–1240.
100. Ko, J., Thurmon, J., Benson, G. and Tranquilli, W. (1992) Evaluation of analgesia induced by epidural injection of detomidine or xylazine in swine. *Veterinary Anaesthesia and Analgesia*, **19**, 56–60.
101. LeBlanc, P., Caron, J., Patterson, J. *et al.* (1988) Epidural injection of xylazine for perineal analgesia in horses. *Journal of the American Veterinary Medical Association*, **193**, 1405–1408.
102. Fikes, L., Lin, H. and Thurmon, J. (1989) A preliminary comparison of lidocaine and xylazine as epidural analgesics in ponies. *Veterinary Surgery & Anesthesia*, **18**, 85–86.

103. Ko, J., Althouse, G., Hopkins, S. *et al.* (1989) Effects of epidural administration of xylazine or lidocaine on bovine uterine motility and perineal analgesia. *Theriogenology*, **32**, 779–786.
104. Aziz, M. and Martin, R. (1978) Alpha agonist and local anaesthetic properties of xylazine. *Zentralblatt fur Veterinarmedizin. Reihe A*, **25**, 181–188.
105. Sakaguchi, M., Nishimura, R., Sasaki, N. *et al.* (1992) Sedative effects of medetomidine in pigs. *The Journal of Veterinary Medical Science*, **54**, 643–647.
106. Sakaguchi, M., Nishimura, R., Sasaki, N. *et al.* (1996) Anesthesia induced in pigs by use of a combination of medetomidine, butorphanol and ketamine and its reversal by administration of atipamezole. *American Journal of Veterinary Research*, **57**, 529–534.
107. vanMiert, A., Faghihi, S. and vanDuin, C. (1994) Food intake and rumen motility in dwarf goats. Effects of atipamezole on the inhibitory effects induced by detomidine, medetomidine, and romifidine. *Veterinary Research Communications*, **18**, 457–469.
108. Yellin, T., Sperow, J. and Buck, S. (1975) Antagonism of tolazoline by histamine H2-receptor blockers. *Nature*, **253**, 561–563.
109. Read, M., Duke, T. and Toews, A. (2000) Suspected tolazoline toxicosis in a llama. *Journal of the American Veterinary Medical Association*, **216**, 227–229.
110. Lin, H. and Riddell, M. (2008) Tolazoline: dose responses and side effects in non-sedated Holstein calves. *The Bovine Practitioner*, **42**, 86–96.
111. Anderson, D. (2011) New methods for chemical restraint and field anesthesia in cattle. *North American Veterinary Community Conference*, pp. 6–11.
112. Carroll, G., Hartsfield, S., Champney, T. *et al.* (2005) Effect of medetomidine and its antagonism with atipamezole on stress-related hormone, metabolites, physiologic responses, sedation, and mechanical threshold in goats. *Veterinary Anaesthesia and Analgesia*, **32**, 147–157.
113. Stoelting, R. and Hillier, S. (2006) Benzodiazepines, in *Pharmacology and Physiology in Anesthetic Practice*, 4th edn, Lippincott Willimas & Wilkins, A Wolters Kluwer Company, Philadelphia, pp. 140–154.
114. Gray, P. and McDonell, W. (1986) Anesthesia in goats and sheep, Part II: general anesthesia. *Compendium on Continuing Education*, **8**, S127–S135.
115. Ochs, H., Greenblatt, D., Eichelkraut, W. *et al.* (1987) Hepatic vs gastrointestinal presystemic extraction of oral midazolam and flurazepam. *The Journal of Pharmacology and Experimental Therapeutics*, **243**, 852–856.
116. Penders, K., Pollack, C., Woodall, B. and Parks, B. (1991) Intraoesseous administration of lorazepam: same-dose comparison with intravenous administration in the weanling pig. *Journal of the Mississippi State Medical Association*, **32** (10), 365–368.
117. Danneberg, P., Bauer, R., Boke-Kuhn, K. *et al.* (1986) General pharmacology of brotizolam in animals. *Arzneimittel-Forschung*, **36**, 540–551.
118. Lumb, W. and Jones, E. (1973) Preanesthetic agents, in *Veterinary Anesthesia* (eds W. Lumb and E. Jones), Lea & Fabiger, Philadelphia, pp. 179–208.
119. Lin, H. (2012) Large ruminant anesthesia: review and update. Western Veterinary Conference, FA#1.
120. Abrahamsen, E. (2009) Chemical restraint, anesthesia, and analgesia for camelids. *Veterinary Clinics of North America: Food Animal Practice*, **25**, 455–494.
121. Kyles, A., Waterman, A. and Livingston, A. (1995) Antinociceptive activity of midazolam in sheep. *Journal of Veterinary Pharmacology and Therapeutics*, **18**, 54–60.
122. Stegmann, G. and Bester, L. (2001) Sedative-hypnotic effects of midazolam in goats after intravenous and intramuscular administration. *Veterinary Anaesthesia and Analgesia*, **28**, 49–55.
123. Benson, G. and Thurmon, J. (1979) Anesthesia of swine under field conditions. *Journal of the American Veterinary Medical Association*, **174**, 594–596.

124. Thurmon, J. and Tranquilli, W. (1986) Anesthesia for cardiovascular research, in *Swine in Cardiovascular Research* (eds H. Stanton and H. Mersmann), CRC Press, Boca Raton, pp. 39–59.
125. Lacoste, L., Bouquet, S., Ingrand, P. *et al.* (2000) Intranasal midazolam in piglets: Pharmacodynamics (0.2 vs 0.4 mg/kg) and pharmacokinetics (0.4 mg/kg) with bioavailability determination. *Laboratory Animal Science*, **34**, 29–35.
126. Smith, A., Zellner, J., Spinale, F. and Swindle, M. (1991) Sedative and cardiovascular effects of midazolam in swine. *Laboratory Animal Science*, **41**, 157–161.
127. Svendsen, P. and Carter, A. (1997) Blood gas tension, acid-base status and cardiovascular function in miniature swine anesthetized with halothane and methoxyflurane or intravenous metomiolate hydrochloride. *Pharmacology & Toxicology*, **64**, 88–93.
128. Jennings, S. (1971) General anesthesia of ruminants and swine, in *Textbook of Veterinary Anesthesia* (ed L. Soma), Williams & Wilkins, Baltimore, pp. 344–358.
129. Bemis, C., Guard, W. and Covault, C. (1924) Anesthesia, general and local. *Journal of the American Veterinary Medical Association*, **17**, 407–439.
130. Thurmon, J. and Benson, G. (1986) Injectable anesthetic agents and techniques in ruminants and swine. *Veterinary Clinics of North America: Food Animal Practice*, **2**, 567–591.
131. Audisio, S. and Kenia, C. (1979) Use of azaperone combined with chloral hydrate to anesthetize swine. *Gac Vet Buenos Aires*, **41**, 752–753.

Chapter 3

Standing sedation and chemical restraint

HuiChu Lin

Department of Clinical Sciences, College of Veterinary Medicine, Auburn University, USA

Standing sedation and chemical restraint with or without local or regional anesthesia are common techniques used to perform diagnostic and/or surgical procedures in farm animal species. Compared to general anesthesia, ease of drug administration, minimal equipment requirements, low cost, shorter recovery time, and reduced potential for complications are advantages that make these techniques attractive to practitioners, particularly those who often do their work in the field or on the farm. Many minor surgical and diagnostic procedures may only require an animal to remain calm and motionless under the influence of standing sedation or chemical restraint for a short period of time. This is particularly true in the case of large or vigorous animals, where sedation or chemical restraint greatly minimizes the stress caused by forceful restraint. Drugs used for chemical restraint are often similar to the ones used for preanesthetic tranquilization or sedation (refer to Chapter 2). Higher doses of a single tranquilizer/sedative are often needed in order to produce desirable central nervous system (CNS) depression, whereas combinations of different classes of drugs are more likely to achieve the degree of sedation and restraint required for the procedure but with lower doses of each drug and thus reduction of the side effects of each drug.

Cattle

Xylazine produces varying degrees of CNS depression depending on the dose administered. Xylazine is frequently used alone or in combination with other drugs to produce standing sedation and chemical restraint. Intravenous (IV) administration of xylazine at 0.02–0.03 mg/kg induces standing sedation, while recumbency occurs at 0.1–0.18 mg/kg [1]. In adult cattle, intramuscular (IM) or IV administration of xylazine at 0.015–0.025 mg/kg produces standing sedation without recumbency; increasing the dose to 0.1–0.2 mg/kg

Farm Animal Anesthesia: Cattle, Small Ruminants, Camelids, and Pigs, First Edition.
Edited by HuiChu Lin and Paul Walz.

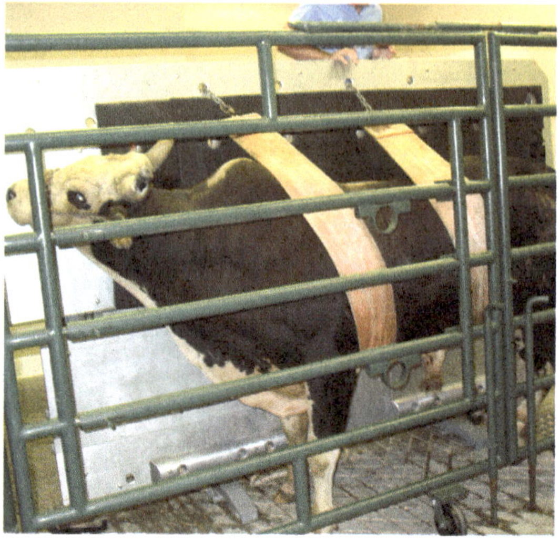

Figure 3.1 Acepromazine-induced calming effect in a rodeo bull prior to induction of anesthesia.

causes recumbency and light anesthesia to occur [2]. However, at standing sedation doses, the analgesic effect of xylazine appears to be minimal. Doses up to 0.025–0.05 mg/kg IV are required to produce standing sedation in extremely anxious or unruly cattle [3]. Similarly, detomidine alone has been administered to produce dose-dependent standing sedation and recumbency. Sedation produced with doses from 0.002 to 0.075 mg/kg IV is adequate to calm tractable and anxious cattle, while doses from 0.01 to 0.015 mg/kg IV are required for unruly cattle [3]. Acepromazine (0.03 mg/kg IV) with or without xylazine (0.03 mg/kg IV) has been administered to facilitate penile extension for examination of preputial injury in bulls (Figure 3.1) [1]. In Norwegian cattle, a higher dose of xylazine (0.55 mg/kg IM) was capable to induce complete immobilization [4].

Butorphanol is an opioid agonist/antagonist. It has agonistic effects on κ receptors but antagonist effects on μ receptors. The analgesic potency of butorphanol is approximately three to five times that of morphine. Butorphanol has a unique "ceiling effect" – that is, after the effective action has been attained, further increases in the dose do not increase or enhance the degree of desired pharmacologic effect [5]. Butorphanol is the most frequently used opioid in ruminants, and recommended doses are 0.02–0.05 mg/kg IV or SC every 4–6 hours [6]. Butorphanol alone has been administered at 0.05–0.07 mg/kg IV to produce adequate standing sedation and analgesia for laparotomy [7]. However, butorphanol alone may cause slight CNS stimulation, especially when used in animals that are not in pain. Twitching of the facial muscles, lips, and head and nystagmus may be observed [8]. One study reported the effectiveness of xylazine (0.02 mg/kg IV) or detomidine (0.01 mg/kg IV) with or without butorphanol (0.05 mg/kg IV) for standing sedation in adult cattle. The result of the study showed that detomidine alone produced more profound sedation for 40–55 minutes than xylazine and xylazine–butorphanol. While butorphanol may enhance the analgesic effect of detomidine, its CNS-stimulating effect at 0.05 mg/kg, as evidenced by nystagmus, seemed to offset the sedative effect of detomidine in three cows [9]. Ataxia and dysphoria have also been reported in sheep when butorphanol was administered intravenously at 0.1–0.2 mg/kg [8].

A combination of low doses of xylazine and ketamine can be used for chemical restraint. IV xylazine (0.05 mg/kg) and ketamine (0.2–0.4 mg/kg) or IM xylazine (0.025–0.05 mg/kg) and ketamine (2 mg/kg) produce chemical restraint with recumbency in combative or unruly ruminants. Opioid analgesics like morphine (0.05 mg/kg) or butorphanol (0.025 mg/kg) have been used with xylazine (0.025–0.05 mg/kg) and ketamine (0.05 mg/kg) administered either intravenously or intramuscularly for standing procedures. A brief period of slight ataxia may occur following IV injection of this combination during standing sedation. Cattle receiving morphine appear to be more alert than those receiving butorphanol [3]. Ketamine can be given 10 minutes after bolus of xylazine and morphine or xylazine and butorphanol to avoid significant ataxia. Longer duration of sedation is produced when ketamine is administered intramuscularly immediately after IV xylazine and morphine or xylazine and butorphanol [10]. This combination is sometimes referred to as **Ketamine Stun**. The low-dose combination of butorphanol, xylazine, and ketamine at 0.02–0.1 mg/kg, 0.02–0.0275 mg/kg, and 0.05–0.1 mg/kg, respectively, administered intramuscularly produces standing sedation. But increasing the doses of butorphanol, xylazine, and ketamine to 0.05–0.1 mg/kg, 0.025–0.05 mg/kg, and 0.3–0.5 mg/kg, respectively, induces chemical restraint with recumbency for 15 minutes [1, 10]. Standing sedation produced by this low-dose combination has been used for laparotomy in range cattle and endoscopy and head examination in rodeo bulls. Chemical restraint with recumbency produced by the high-dose combination along with casting rope and local or regional anesthetic techniques allows the performance of fracture stabilization, unilateral castration, and preputial resection/amputation in bulls [1]. Animals under the sedation of this combination normally appear to be alert but are not bothered by the surroundings and remain quiet for the duration of the procedures [3]. Similar combination of butorphanol, xylazine, and ketamine using a 5–10–20 ratio (5 mg of butorphanol, 10 mg of xylazine, and 20 mg of ketamine) has been administered intramuscularly or subcutaneously to produce effective standing sedation in tame cows and Brahman cows for cesarean section. If repeat dosing is required, ½ of the initial ketamine and ¼ of the initial xylazine doses can be given 30–40 minutes after the initial administration. Adequate sedation with a cooperative animal lasts 60 minutes with this 5–10–20 combination. In adult bulls, 10 mg of butorphanol, 20 mg of xylazine, and 40 mg of ketamine (10–20–40) IM or SC combined with local anesthetic nerve blocks have been used successfully to perform standing preputial surgeries [1, 3].

Standing sedation can be achieved with 0.005 mg/kg IV medetomidine alone in domestic ruminants [11]. Increasing the dose to 0.03 mg/kg and using an IM route of infection, lateral recumbency was induced for 60–75 minutes in domestic calves [12]. When delivered via tranquilizing gun at a higher dose (0.04 mg/kg), medetomidine has been used successfully to produce complete immobilization in capturing free-ranging cattle [4, 13].

A combination of xylazine (0.3–0.5 mg/kg IM), ketamine (0.7–1.0 mg/kg IM), and Telazol (0.7–1 mg/kg IM) has been used to produce dose-dependent chemical restraint and immobilization in free-ranging cattle, for example, Limousin, Scottish highland cattle, and American bison, for nonpainful procedures [14]. Caulkett *et al.* (2000) [15]

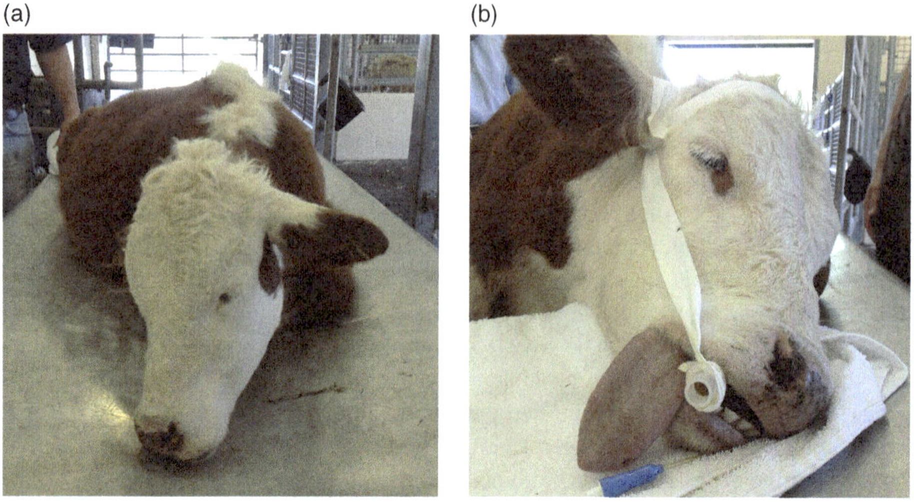

Figure 3.2 (a) Chemical restraint in a calf with xylazine (0.1 mg/kg IV) and diazepam (0.2 mg/kg IV). (b) Chemical restraint in a calf with xylazine (0.1 mg/kg IV) and diazepam (0.2 mg/kg IV) followed by endotracheal intubation.

reported that medetomidine (0.06 mg/kg IM) and Telazol (1.2 mg/kg IM) combination produced immobilization and analgesia adequate for minor procedures for a period of 60 minutes. Atipamezole (0.18 mg/kg) was administered to shorten the recovery time.

Xylazine (0.2 mg/kg IV) and diazepam (0.1 mg/kg IV) have been combined to produce short-term chemical restraint with recumbency in a cow to place wires to stabilize a mandibular fracture. The duration of chemical restraint was 30 minutes and the cow stood approximately 60 minutes following drug administration. Additional analgesia with an opioid or a local anesthetic was not required for this procedure [16]. For procedures that do not require intense analgesia, xylazine at 0.1 mg/kg and diazepam at 0.2 mg/kg can be administered intravenously for a similar duration of recumbency. Tracheal intubation was performed in a calf receiving 0.1 mg/kg of xylazine and 0.2 mg/kg of diazepam (Figure 3.2). Table 3.1 summarizes the doses of drugs and drug combinations used for sedation and chemical restraint in cattle.

Small ruminants and camelids

Goats are more sensitive to xylazine than sheep and camelids; lower doses of xylazine (0.05–0.1 mg/kg IV) are required to produce a similar degree of sedation to that of sheep (0.1–0.4 mg/kg IV) [17]. Compared to sheep and goats, camelids are less sensitive to xylazine and thus require higher doses (0.1–0.2 mg/kg IV) to produce standing sedation [18]. In sheep, approximately 1 hour of standing sedation was produced by 0.3 mg/kg IM, but recumbency of 1.5 hours occurred when 0.6 mg/kg IM was administered [19]. It is recommended that the dose of xylazine should not exceed 0.15 mg/kg IV due to the concern of significant cardiopulmonary depression [20]. Subanesthetic doses of xylazine

Table 3.1 Doses of drugs and drug combinations used for sedation and chemical restraint in cattle.

Drugs	Doses (mg/kg)	Comments
Acepromazine	0.02, IV	Less ↓ in uterine blood flow Less ↑ in uterine vascular resistance
Acepromazine Acepromazine Acepromazine	0.01–0.02, IV 0.033–0.055, IV or IM 0.03–0.1, IM	Chemical restraint – –
Acepromazine	0.03, IV	Facilitate penile extension for exam with or without xylazine 0.03 mg/kg IV for sedation
Acepromazine Morphine Ketamine	0.055–0.088, IV, or 25–40 mg/450 kg 0.1–0.2, IV, or 45–90 mg/45 kg CRI: 0.06 mg/kg/h	Standing chemical restraint
Butorphanol Butorphanol	0.033–0.05, IV 0.22, IM	Analgesia, standing restraint –
Butorphanol	20–30 mg/cow IV with or without xylazine 10 mg/cow	Standing analgesia
Butorphanol	0.022–0.05, IV	Sedation
Acepromazine Butorphanol	0.03, IV 0.01, IV	Sedation
Acepromazine Butorphanol	0.022, IV 0.044, IV	Standing restraint
Chloral hydrate Chloral hydrate	44–66, IV 30–60 gm in 1–2-L water	Standing sedation Sedation with recumbency
Detomidine Detomidine Detomidine	0.002–0.005, IV; 0.006–0.01, IM 0.005–0.0075, IV; 0.01–0.015, IM 0.01–0.015, IV; 0.015–0.02, IM	Standing sedation for tractable cattle Standing sedation for anxious cattle Standing sedation for unruly cattle
Detomidine Detomidine Detomidine Detomidine Detomidine	0.0025–0.01, IV 0.01–0.02, IV 0.03–0.06, IV 0.02–0.04, IM 0.02–0.05, IM	Standing sedation 30–60 min Sedation 60 min Standing sedation Analgesia 20–120 min –
Detomidine	0.04, IV	Profound sedation, recumbency
Detomidine	0.1, IM by dart	Immobilization in free-ranging cattle
Detomidine Butorphanol	0.01, IV 0.05, IV	Enhanced sedation ↓ response to external stimuli Potential significant ptosis, occasional nasopharyngeal edema, and slow nystagmus
Detomidine Butorphanol	15 mg (0.035), IM 15 mg (0.035), IM For 400–450 kg (880–990 lb)	Detomidine less likely to cause recumbency than xylazine or medetomidine

(*Continued*)

Table 3.1 (*Continued*)

Drugs	Doses (mg/kg)	Comments
Detomidine Butorphanol	0.07, IM 0.04, IM	Immobilization in free-ranging cattle
Detomidine Butorphanol Ketamine	0.011–0.022, IV, or 5–10 mg/450 kg 0.011–0.016, IV, or 5–7 mg/450 kg CRI: 0.6 mg/kg/h	Standing chemical restraint
Detomidine	Loading dose: 5–10 mg/450 kg (990 lb), IV CRI: 0.022 mg/kg/h	Standing chemical restraint
Morphine	Loading dose: 45–60 mg/450 kg (990 lb), IV CRI: 0.025–0.05 mg/kg/h	K loading dose may not be required
Ketamine	Loading dose: 100 mg/450 kg (990), IV CRI: 0.6 mg/kg/h	Adjustment CRI to desirable effect
Diazepam Diazepam Diazepam Diazepam	0.25, IM 0.4, IM 0.5, IM 0.4, IV	Inadequate sedation – – 5–10-minute sedation with recumbency
Diazepam Diazepam	0.2–0.5, IV 0.5–1, IM	– –
Medetomidine Medetomidine Medetomidine	0.005, IV 0.01, IV 0.03, IM	Brief standing sedation without analgesia Recumbency Recumbency 60–75 min
Morphine	0.1–0.5, IV	Analgesia
Pentobarbital	2, IV, slow	Moderate standing sedation 30 min, mild sedation for additional 60 min
Romifidine Romifidine	0.02–0.03, IV 0.05, IV	Standing sedation Recumbency
Xylazine Xylazine Xylazine Xylazine	0.0075–0.01, IV; 0.015–0.02, IM 0.01–0.02, IV; 0.02–0.04, IM 0.02–0.03, IV; 0.04–0.06, IM 0.025–0.05, IV; 0.05–0.1, IM	Standing sedation, quiet dairy cattle Standing sedation, tractable cattle Standing sedation, anxious cattle Standing sedation, unruly cattle
Xylazine Xylazine Xylazine Xylazine	0.015–0.025, IV or IM 0.02, IV 0.1, IV, or 0.2, IM 0.055–0.11, IV, or 0.11–0.22, IM	Standing sedation Standing sedation Recumbency 60 min Chemical restraint to light anesthesia
Xylazine Xylazine	0.02–0.03, IV 0.1–0.18, IV	Standing sedation Recumbency
Xylazine	0.66–0.88, IM 2nd dose: 0.52–0.53, IM	Capture wild cattle Recumbency in 3–7 min Fleeing possible Reversal available

Table 3.1 (*Continued*)

Drugs	Doses (mg/kg)	Comments
Xylazine Butorphanol	0.01–0.02, IV 0.01–0.02, IV	Standing sedation Neuroleptanalgesia 60 min
Xylazine Butorphanol	0.05–0.1, IV 0.01–0.02, IV	Deep sedation
Xylazine Butorphanol	0.03, IV 0.033–0.05, IV	Standing restraint
Xylazine Butorphanol	0.055–0.11, IV; 0.11–0.22, IM 0.05–0.07, IV	Standing sedation
Xylazine Diazepam	0.12, IV 0.1, IV	Chemical restraint, analgesia Recumbency 30 min Standing in 45–60 min
Xylazine Diazepam	0.1, IV 0.2, IV	Chemical restraint Standing sedation for tractable cattle
Xylazine Diazepam	0.2, IV 0.1, IV	Chemical restraint, analgesia Standing sedation for tractable cattle
Xylazine Ketamine	0.05, IV 0.2–0.4, IV	Chemical restraint Recumbency Animals appear awake but cooperative ½ original ketamine to extend duration
Xylazine Ketamine	0.025–0.05, IM, or 0.05–0.1, IM 2–4.4, IM	Chemical restraint for **combative** animal Recumbency, extremely unruly animal may remain standing
Ketamine Stun Xylazine Butorphanol Ketamine	 0.02–0.0275, IV 0.02–0.1, IV 0.05–0.1, IV	 Standing sedation Improve patient cooperation Allow exam for penile injury
Ketamine Stun Butorphanol Xylazine Ketamine	(**5–10–20** technique for 450 kg (990 lb)) 5 mg (0.01), IM, SC 10 mg (0.02), IM, SC 20 mg (0.04), IM, SC	Standing sedation, tame Brahman cattle Limit analgesia Combine with local anesthesia for surgery Supplemental dose may cause recumbency
Ketamine Stun Butorphanol Xylazine Ketamine	(**10–20–40** technique for 450 kg (990 lb)) 10 mg (0.02), IM, SC 20 mg (0.04), IM, SC 40 mg (0.08), IM, SC	Standing sedation Combine with local anesthesia Can be used in preputial surgery for adult bulls
Ketamine Stun Xylazine Butorphanol Ketamine	 0.025–0.05, IV 0.05–0.1, IV 0.3–0.5, IV	Recumbency Good analgesia Random head or limb movement Duration 15 minutes

(*Continued*)

Table 3.1 *(Continued)*

Drugs	Doses (mg/kg)	Comments
Ketamine Stun Xylazine Butorphanol Ketamine	 0.05, IM, SC 0.025, IM, SC 0.1, IM, SC	Recumbency, chemical restraint Tolerate endotracheal intubation Ambulatory 30–45 min Combine with local anesthesia, allow umbilical hernia repair; laparotomy in range cattle; endoscopy, head exam for rodeo bulls
Xylazine Butorphanol Ketamine	0.02, IV, IM 0.025, IV, IM 0.05, IV, IM	Standing restraint Longer duration if ketamine is administered 10 minutes after XB ½ original ketamine to extend duration
Xylazine Butorphanol Ketamine	0.05, IV, IM 0.025, IV, IM 0.2–0.4, IV, IM	Recumbency Able to stand and walk upon completion
Xylazine Morphine Ketamine	0.02, IV, IM 0.05, IV, IM 0.05, IV, IM	Standing restraint Longer duration if ketamine is administered 10 minutes following XM ½ original ketamine to extend duration
TKX-Ru Ketamine 2.5 ml (250 mg) Xylazine 1 ml (100 mg) Telazol (500 mg) Final volume 4 ml	 Smaller animals: 1.25–1.5 ml/125 kg (275 lb), IM Larger animals: 1 ml/125 kg (275 lb), IM	Chemical restraint for wild ruminants, large exotic hoofstock Recumbency in 5–10 min Recovery to standing in 40–60 min Leftover TKX-Ru can be frozen for up to 6 months
Xylazine Telazol	0.1–0.2, IM 4, IM	Capture of wild cattle Recumbency
Antagonists		
Doxapram	1, IV	Nonspecific reversal of CNS depression induced by anesthetics to shorten recovery Respiratory stimulant
Atipamezole Atipamezole	0.02–0.05, IV 0.02–0.06, IV	Reversal of α_2 agonists
Idazoxan	0.05, IV	Reversal of α_2 agonists
Tolazoline Tolazoline	0.2–2, IV, IM, or SC 0.5–2, IV	Reversal of α_2 agonists Hyperesthesia at 2 mg/kg IV
Yohimbine Yohimbine Nalorphine	0.12, IV 0.125–0.2, IV 0.0088, IV	Reversal of α_2 agonists Variable efficacy Partially reverse hypoxemia of xylazine t½: 53–76 min Reversal of opioid agonist

(0.025–0.03 mg/kg IV or 1.7–2.2 mg/kg IM) and ketamine (1.1 mg/kg IV or 1.7–2.2 mg/kg IM) have been used to produce chemical restraint with recumbency of 10–25 minutes in camelids. This combination produced better analgesia than that of xylazine alone. Though minor surgical procedures may be performed with subanesthetic doses of xylazine and ketamine combinations, butorphanol (0.05–0.1 mg/kg IV or IM), morphine (0.05–0.1 mg/kg IV or IM), or local or regional anesthetic techniques should be added for more painful procedures [21].

Similar to xylazine, detomidine produces dose-dependent CNS depression. In goats, 0.01–0.02 mg/kg IV of detomidine produces sedation for 30–60 minutes, while severe ataxia and sternal recumbency occur at 0.04 mg/kg administered either intravenously or intramuscularly [22]. Butorphanol (0.05–0.1 mg/kg IV) or morphine (0.01–0.1 mg/kg IV or IM) can be combined with xylazine or detomidine to improve patient cooperation during sedation [3]. Standing sedation occurs when detomidine (0.01 mg/kg IV) is administered concurrently with butorphanol (0.1 mg/kg IV) [23].

Mohammad *et al.* (1993) [24] reported that medetomidine (0.04 mg/kg IM) induced deep sedation with recumbency for a period of 58 minutes in sheep. Good analgesia and muscle relaxation of 30–45 minutes were observed during recumbency. In llamas, medetomidine (0.01 mg/kg IM) induced a brief period of standing sedation with minimal analgesia [25]. Only deep sedation was observed when 0.05 mg/kg of IM medetomidine was combined with 1 mg/kg of IM ketamine to llamas [26].

In sheep and goats, slow injection of diazepam (0.25–0.5 mg/kg IV) produces standing sedation with little analgesia [20, 27]. Transdermal tracheal wash has been performed under the mild sedation produced by 0.2 mg/kg IV of diazepam [28]. A period of 10–20 minutes of recumbency occurred when midazolam (0.3 mg/kg IV, 0.4–0.6 mg/kg IM) was administered to sheep and goats. Increasing the dose of midazolam to 1.2 mg/kg IV prolonged the duration of recumbency up to 30 minutes [29–31].

Butorphanol (0.05 mg/kg IV) can be given alone to sheep and goats to produce light sedation [8, 27, 32]. When xylazine (0.01–0.02 mg/kg IV) and butorphanol (0.01–0.02 mg/kg IV) were administered simultaneously to sheep and goats, deep sedation and recumbency were produced for up to 60 minutes. However, 0.2 mg/kg IV of each drug is required to produce similar sedation in camelids [18]. Barrington *et al.* (1993) [33] described using butorphanol (0.1 mg/kg IM) along with intratesticular injection of 2% lidocaine (2–5 ml) successfully to facilitate standing castration in more than 100 llamas. Diazepam (0.1 mg/kg IV) and butorphanol (0.1 mg/kg IV) are effective in producing short-duration sedation with recumbency in camelids [21].

Johnson (2010) [34] recommended adding 1 ml of butorphanol (10 mg) and 1 ml of xylazine (100 mg) to 10 ml of ketamine (1000 mg) (**Llama Lullaby**) and administering 1 ml/45 kg (99 lb) to camelids for standing sedation. Camelids tend to assume sternal recumbency even under moderate sedation. Therefore, careful selection of the doses of the drugs used is required in order to achieve a desirable effect. Different dose combinations of butorphanol, ketamine, and xylazine have been used in small ruminants and camelids and renamed as **Ketamine Stun** by Abrahamsen [3, 21]. Administered intravenously, 0.08–0.11 mg/kg of butorphanol, 0.22–0.33 mg/kg of ketamine, and 0.22–0.33 mg/kg of xylazine produced reliable recumbency and analgesia for 15–20 minutes. When administered intramuscularly, 0.055–0.11 mg/kg of butorphanol, 0.22 mg/kg of ketamine, and

0.22–0.55 mg/kg of xylazine extended the duration of recumbency to 45 minutes. Less analgesic effect was observed when lower doses were administered. Animals appear to be stunned but alert, oblivious to surroundings and procedures performed. Extension of the duration of restraint can be achieved by administering ½ of the original dose of ketamine IV for additional 5 minutes. If further restraint is desired, then ½ of original xylazine and ketamine IV can be administered to extend recumbency for another 7–10 minutes. Procedures such as castration, biopsies, septic joint flushing, casting of fractured limbs, and flank laparotomy for correction of uterine torsion and cesarean section have been performed under IV **Ketamine Stun** [21].

A mixture of Telazol (500 mg), ketamine (250 mg, 2.5 ml), and xylazine (250 mg, 2.5 ml) is developed to produce chemical restraint and anesthesia in pigs (**TKX-P**). The use of this three-drug combination has also been evaluated in camelids by adding 2.5 ml of ketamine (250 mg) and 1 ml of xylazine (100 mg) into 500 mg of Telazol powder with final solution of 4 ml. This mixture is referred to as **TKX-Ru**. Doses to produce recumbency and chemical restraint for 40–60 minutes in camelids are 1–1.5 ml/110–115 kg (220–253 lb). Sedation occurs within 5–10 minutes following IM injection of **TKX-Ru**, and animals will be awake and assume sternal recumbency by 40–60 minutes and remain in sternal recumbency for another 20–40 minutes [21]. Table 3.2 summarizes the doses of drugs and drug combinations used for sedation and chemical restraint in small ruminants and camelids.

Swine

Pigs do not tolerate restraint, which often poses as stress to these animals. IV injection of pigs is difficult not only because they are resistant to restraint but also because they have very few superficial veins. Therefore, IM injection of drugs is considered less stressful and is often preferred in these animals. Acepromazine (0.05–0.5 mg/kg IM, maximum 10 mg), diazepam (0.5–1 mg/kg), midazolam (0.2–0.4 mg/kg IM), azaperone (2–4 mg/kg IM), or ketamine (20–30 mg/kg IM) can be given alone to produce short duration of sedation (20–30 minutes) [35, 36]. Acepromazine and diazepam are not effective tranquilizers in pigs. Midazolam is another benzodiazepine tranquilizer similar to diazepam but is twice as potent. Unlike diazepam, midazolam is water soluble, and it is easily absorbed from the injection site following IM administration. Sedation with midazolam can be achieved with intranasal administration at doses of 0.2–0.4 mg/kg. IM diazepam and midazolam alone tend to be cost prohibitive due to large volumes of the drugs required to produce effective sedation [37].

Azaperone is the only tranquilizer approved by the Food and Drug Administration (FDA) for use in swine. It can be used to control aggression when mixing commercial pigs. Azaperone should only be given by IM administration, as excitement has been reported when the drug was administered intravenously. In large boars, the dose of azaperone is not recommended to exceed 1 mg/kg to prevent the adverse effect of priapism [37]. For potbellied pigs, azaperone has been used to produce effective tranquilization (2–4 mg/kg IM) and immobilization (8 mg/kg IM) for approximately 20 minutes in order to perform radiography and tusk trimming [38].

Table 3.2 Doses of drugs and drug combinations used for sedation and chemical restraint in sheep, goats, and camelids.

Drugs	Doses for sheep and goats (mg/kg)	Doses for camelids mg/kg)	Comments
Acepromazine Acepromazine	0.03–0.05, IV	0.15, IV, IM, SC	Moderate sedation
	0.05–0.1, IM		May ↑ risk for regurgitation
Acepromazine	<50 kg (110 lb): 0.1–0.2, IV >50 kg (110 lb): 0.05–0.1, IV, IM	–	–
Buprenorphine	0.006, IV	–	Sedation, analgesia
Butorphanol	0.05–0.5, IM	0.05–0.1, IV, IM	Sedation and/or ataxia
Butorphanol	0.4, IV	0.02–0.05, IV, IM for larger camels	Enhance sedation and analgesia of xylazine
Butorphanol	–	5 mg/alpaca (0.07), IM 10 mg/llama (0.07), IM	Analgesia, some sedation Tolerant for procedures like hoot trimming, shearing
Butorphanol	0.05–0.5, IM	0.15, IM	Standing castration
Butorphanol	–	0.1–0.2, IM	Add 1–1.5-ml 2% lidocaine to median raphe of scrotum and 2–3 ml to each spermatic cord Give B 10 minutes prior to local anesthetic
Chloral hydrate	33–55, IV	–	Sedation
Detomidine	0.005–0.02, IV 0.01–0.04, IM	0.01, IM	Sedation for 45–60 min
Detomidine	–	0.03–0.06, IM	Immobilization
Detomidine	0.01–0.02, IV	–	Standing sedation for 30–60 min
	0.02–0.05, IM		Recumbency
Detomidine	0.03, IV	0.04, IV	Mild sedation, no restraint
Detomidine Butorphanol	0.01, IV 0.1, IV	–	Sedation
Diazepam	0.25–0.5, IV, slow	0.1–0.5, IV	Sedation for 30 min
Diazepam	0.44–0.66, IV, IM	–	Sedation
Diazepam	0.2–0.5, IV 0.5–1, IM		Sedation
Diazepam	1–2, IM	–	Light to moderate sedation
	1, IV		
Diazepam	5 mg IV per goat	–	Calming effect Quieting vocalization, movement Lack analgesia

(*Continued*)

Table 3.2 (*Continued*)

Drugs	Doses for sheep and goats (mg/kg)	Doses for camelids mg/kg)	Comments
Diazepam	–	0.1, IV	Short duration of recumbency
Butorphanol		0.1, IV	Less analgesia versus xylazine–butorphanol
Diazepam Xylazine Butorphanol	–	0.2, IM 0.1, IM 0.05, IM	Chemical restraint
Dexmedetomidine	0.002–0.005, IV	–	Deep sedation
Medetomidine	0.001–0.007, IV	–	IV sedation
Medetomidine	Goats 0.01–0.04, IM	–	IM recumbency for 58 min
Medetomidine	Sheep 0.005–0.01, IM	–	
Medetomidine	0.015, IM	–	Recumbency 45 min
Medetomidine	0.025, IM	0.01, IM	Standing sedation
Medetomidine	–	0.02–0.03, IM	Recumbency 60–120 min Analgesia 60 min
Medetomidine Butorphanol	0.01–0.02, IM 0.04, IM	–	Sedation and analgesia
Medetomidine Butorphanol	0.01, IM 0.1, IM	–	Dehorning Block horn buds 0.1–0.2 ml of 1% lidocaine
Meperidine	10, IM	–	–
Midazolam	0.3, IV 0.4–0.6, IM	–	Sedation with recumbency 10–20 min
Midazolam	0.5, IV	–	Moderate sedation
Midazolam	Goats		
	0.6, IV	–	Profound sedation with recumbency
	1, IM		
Midazolam	1.2, IV	–	Recumbency 30 min
Morphine	2, IV	0.05–0.1, IV, IM	↓ Isoflurane MAC 29%
Romifidine	0.05, IV	–	Recumbency
Xylazine	Goats 0.05, IV	0.4, IM 0.1–0.2, IV	Standing castration, add 1–1.5-ml 2% lidocaine infiltration to median raphe of scrotum and 2–3 ml to each spermatic cord
	0.1, IM, IV		Light to moderate sedation
	Sheep 0.1–0.2, IV 0.2–0.3, IM	–	
Xylazine	–	0.3–0.4, IV 0.5, IV	Recumbency 20–30 min Allow tracheal intubation

CHAPTER 3

Table 3.2 (*Continued*)

Drugs	Doses for sheep and goats (mg/kg)	Doses for camelids mg/kg)	Comments
Xylazine	Goats 0.05–0.1, IV Sheep 0.1–0.4, IV	Alpacas 0.3, IV Llamas 0.2, IV	Sedation Combine with local infiltration for dehorning
Xylazine	Loading dose: 0.1 mg/kg IM CRI: 0.04 mg/kg/h	–	–
Xylazine	0.3, IM	–	Standing sedation 60 min
Xylazine	0.6, IM	–	Recumbency 90 min
Xylazine	1.1, IM	–	Analgesia 20–35 min Sedation 60–90 min
Xylazine	0.01–0.02, IV	Alpacas: 0.1–0.15, IV; 0.2–0.3, IM, SQ	Standing sedation
Xylazine	0.1–0.2, IV; 0.2–0.3, IM	Llamas: 0.075–0.1, IV; 0.15–0.2, IM, SQ	
Xylazine	–	Alpacas: 0.33–0.44, IV; 0.66–0.88, IM, SQ Llamas: 0.22–0.33, IV; 0.44–0.66, IM, SQ	Recumbent sedation
Xylazine	–	1, IM	Immobilization
Xylazine	0.1–0.2, IV	–	Enhance patient cooperation and systemic analgesia
Butorphanol	0.01–0.02, IV		Deep sedation to recumbency 60 min
Xylazine Butorphanol	0.1, IM 0.1, IM	0.05–0.1, IM 0.1, IM	Dehorning Block horn buds 0.1–0.2 ml of 1% lidocaine
Xylazine Butorphanol	–	0.2, IV 0.02, IV	Profound sedation Recumbency 20 min
Xylazine Butorphanol	–	0.4, IV 0.1, IV	Recumbency Castration with intratesticular local anesthetic
Xylazine Butorphanol	–	0.2, IM 0.1, IM	Standing castration
Xylazine Butorphanol	–	0.1, IM 0.051, IM	Standing castration
Xylazine Butorphanol	–	Alpacas 0.3, IV 0.05, IV; 0.1 IM, SC Llamas 0.1–0.2, IV 0.05, IV; 0.07–0.1, IM, SC	Standing sedation, analgesia

(*Continued*)

Table 3.2 (*Continued*)

Drugs	Doses for sheep and goats (mg/kg)	Doses for camelids mg/kg)	Comments
Xylazine Butorphanol	–	0.3–0.4, IV 0.1, IV	Castration Recumbency 20–30 min
Xylazine Butorphanol	0.01–0.02, IV 0.01–0.02, IV	0.2, IV 0.2, IV	Neuroleptanalgesia 60 min
Ketamine	20, IM	–	Moderate to deep sedation Immobilization
Xylazine Ketamine	–	0.05, IV 0.5, IV	Sedation
Xylazine	–	0.025–0.03, IV, given 1st	Recumbent chemical restraint 10–15 min
Ketamine		1.1, IV, given when xylazine sedation evident	Better analgesia versus xylazine
Xylazine	–	1.7–2.2, IM	Supplemental dose: ½ of original xylazine and ketamine
Ketamine		1.7–2.2, IM	Recumbency 15–25 min
Ketamine Stun Xylazine	–	0.22–0.33, IV 0.22–0.55, IM	Recumbency 15–20 minute (IV), 45 minute (IM) Animals stunned but alert
Ketamine		0.22–0.33, IV 0.22–0.55, IM	Supplemental dose, ½ of the original K IV extend restraint for 5 min; second supplemental dose, ½ of original X and K IV extend restraint for 7–10 min
Butorphanol		0.08–0.11, IV 0.08–0.11, IM	
TKX-Ru Telazol (500 mg) Ketamine (2.5 ml, 250 mg) Xylazine (1 ml, 100 mg)	–	4-ml mixture 1.25–1.5 ml/110–115 kg (220–253 lb), IM for small patients 1 ml/110–115 kg (220–253 lb), IM for larger patients	Animals awake and sternal in 40–60 min
Antagonists			
Atipamezole	0–0.05, IV	0.125–0.2, slow IV	Reversal for α_2 *agonists*
Atipamezole	0.125–0.2, slow IV	0.3–0.5, slow IV	
Tolazoline	1–2, slow IV	1–2, slow IV	Reversal for α_2 *agonists* Can be given ½ IV, ½ IM Some prefer IM
Yohimbine	0.125–0.22, slow IV	0.125–0.22, slow IV	Reversal for α_2 *agonists*
Doxapram	0.4, IV	0.1, IV	Nonspecific reversal
Flumazenil	–	0.1, IV	Reversal for benzodiazepines
Naloxone	–	0.03, IV	Reversal for opioid *agonists*

Compared to other domestic species, pigs are the least sensitive to xylazine; deep sedation from xylazine alone is rarely observed in pigs even with high doses. Nonetheless, when mild sedation is adequate, the recommended IM doses of xylazine are 0.5–3 mg/kg. One should keep in mind that xylazine can cause vomiting in pigs, particularly in those animals that fasting is not an option [39]. Diazepam (0.5–1 mg/kg IM) or xylazine (4 mg/kg IM) has been combined with ketamine (10–30 mg/kg IM) to produce enhanced degree of sedation and analgesia [35]. In Yucatan minipigs, IM medetomidine (0.2 mg/kg) and ketamine (10 mg/kg) combination induced deep sedation characterized by significant but reversible increase in mean arterial pressures and systemic vascular resistance and a significant decrease in heart rate for 2 hours [40]. However, another report commented that recovery from this combination was rough and prolonged [41], which is conflicting to the observation reported by Nishimura *et al.* [42]. Linkenhoker *et al.* (2010) [41] compared the sedative effects and variable cardiovascular variables of different combinations of ketamine with acepromazine, diazepam, midazolam, or medetomidine. They concluded that midazolam (0.5–0.6 mg/kg SC) with ketamine (25–27 mg/kg SC) produced good sedation for catheterization with little effect on cardiovascular variables. The level of sedation with medetomidine and ketamine combination did not allow for endotracheal intubation; additional mask induction with isoflurane was required to complete endotracheal intubation [41]. In another study, at least 30 minutes of deep sedation was induced with medetomidine (0.2 mg/kg IV) and ketamine (10 mg/kg IV) which was accompanied by hypertension and bradycardia in Yucatan minipigs [40]. This author has used xylazine (4 mg/kg IM) and ketamine (5 mg/kg IM) to produce deep sedation in a potbellied pig for radiograph of the pelvis. The pig assumed sternal recumbency and was immobilized within 10 minutes after drug administration. Though the pig appeared to be deeply sedated, it vocalized when manipulated in order to change position for radiograph (Figure 3.3).

CHAPTER 3

(a) (b)

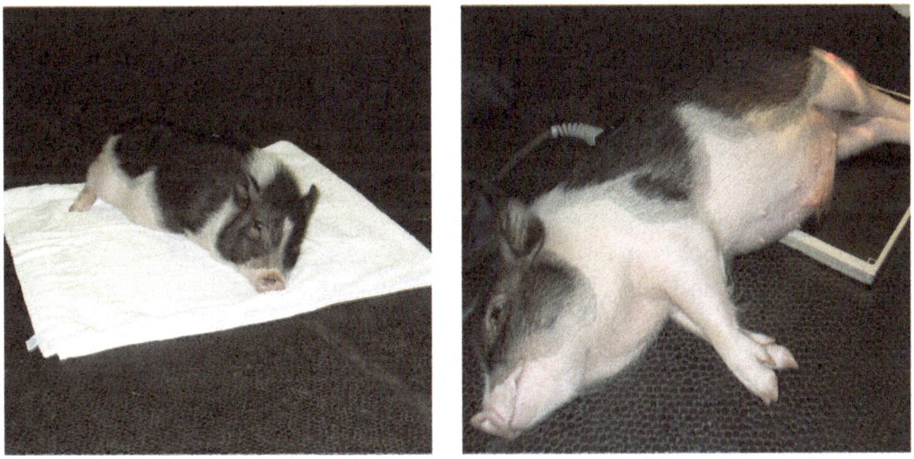

Figure 3.3 (a,b) Chemical restraint in a potbellied pig with diazepam (4 mg/kg IM) and ketamine (5 mg/kg IM) for radiography.

Table 3.3 Doses of drugs and drug combinations used for sedation and chemical restraint in pigs.

Drugs	Doses (mg/kg)	Comments
Acepromazine	0.2, IM	Moderate sedation
Acepromazine	0.05–0.5, IM, IV; maximum 15 mg	Sedation
Acepromazine	0.2–0.5, IM	Onset in 20–30 min
Acepromazine	0.2–01.1, IM	Duration 30–60 min
		–
		–
Acepromazine Ketamine	1, IM 20–27, IM	Light sedation
Acepromazine Ketamine	1, IM 22, IM	Immobilization
Azaperone	0.5–4, IM, IV	Onset in 5–15 min
Azaperone	1–2, IM	Duration 60–120 min
Azaperone	5, IM	–
Azaperone	8, IM	Moderate to deep sedation
		–
Azaperone	0.25–0.5, IM	Mild sedation, no ataxia
Azaperone	0.5–2, IM	Deep sedation, greatly reduced aggression, ataxia
Azaperone	2–4, IM	Recumbency
Azaperone	1–4, IM	–
Azaperone Ketamine	2–8, IM 10–20, IM	Profound sedation
Chloral hydrate	44–66, IV	–
Diazepam	0.1–0.5, PO	Calming effect
Diazepam	0.1–0.2, IV	Sedation 20–30 min
Diazepam	0.5–1.0, IM	Sedation and muscle relaxation
Diazepam	CRI: 0.44–2 mg/kg/h	Long-duration sedation
Diazepam	1–2, IM	Light to moderate sedation
Diazepam	5.5, IM	Tranquilization, posterior ataxia
Diazepam	8.5, IM	Recumbency
		Good sedation prior to general anesthesia
Diazepam Ketamine	0.5–2, IM 10–15, IM	Sedation 20–40 min
Diazepam Ketamine	1–2, IM 10–18, IM	Sedation 20–40 min
Diazepam Ketamine	3.5, SC 27, SC	Adequate sedation for catheterization Time to recovery 70 min
Diazepam Ketamine	0.05–1, IM 10–30, IM	Sedation 20–30 min
Ketamine	10–15, IM	Sedation, immobilization
Ketamine	5–20, IM	Chemical restraint Immobilization Rough recovery
Medetomidine	0.02–0.04, IV 0.04–0.08, IM	Sedation
Medetomidine Ketamine	0.08, IM 10, IM	Sedation 15–30 min
Medetomidine	0.2, IM	Deep sedation

Table 3.3 (*Continued*)

Drugs	Doses (mg/kg)	Comments
Ketamine	10, IM	↑↑ Mean arterial pressure and systemic vascular resistance, ↓↓ heart rate for 120 min
Medetomidine Ketamine	0.1–0.2, SC 5, SC	Rough, prolonged recovery Seizure activity in one pig with 0.1 M Bradycardia in one pig with 0.2 M Time to recovery 210–225 min
Midazolam Midazolam	0.1–0.5, IM 0.2–5, IM	Sedation 40–60 min Sedation and muscle relaxation
Midazolam Midazolam	0.2–0.4, IM 0.2–0.4, intranasal	Sedation 20–30 min Sedation
Midazolam	CRI: 0.6–1.5 mg/kg/h	Long-duration sedation
Midazolam	0.1–0.3, IM	Sedation
Ketamine	3–5, IM	
Midazolam Ketamine	0.5–0.6, SC 25–27, SC	Deep sedation but not allowed for intubation Smooth recovery Time to recovery 165–330 min
Midazolam Ketamine	0.2–0.4, IM 10–30, IM	Sedation 20–30 min
Midazolam Ketamine	0.1–0.5, IM 10–20, IM	Sedation 20–40 min
Butorphanol Atropine Medetomidine Midazolam	0.18 ± 0.04, IM 0.025 ± 0.025, IM 0.01 ± 0.006, IM 0.2 ± 0.07, IM	Deep sedation to immobilization
Xylazine	1, IM	Sedation
Xylazine	0.5–3, IM	Sedation
Butorphanol Atropine Midazolam Xylazine	0.18 ± 0.04, IM 0.025 ± 0.025, IM 0.2 ± 0.07, IM 0.6 ± 0.7, IM	Deep sedation
Xylazine Ketamine	0.44, IM 2.2, IM	Deep sedation 20–40 min
Xylazine Ketamine	4, IM 4–5, IM	Chemical restraint Recumbency
Xylazine Ketamine	4, IM 5–10, IM	Sedation 20–30 min
Telazol	2–4, IM	Moderate to deep sedation
Telazol	3–5, IM	Sedation 20–30 min
Butorphanol Telazol	0.18 ± 0.04, IM 3.7 ± 0.9, IM	Deep sedation to immobilization
Ketamine Telazol	2.2, IM 4.4, IM	Deep sedation 30–35 min Inadequate for tracheal intubation
Xylazine Telazol	5 ml SA X (100 mg) in 500 mg T 1 ml/27.3 kg (60 lb), IM	Short-term sedation
Xylazine Telazol	0.5–2.2, IM 3–6, IM	Deep sedation Adequate for tracheal intubation Analgesia Potential apnea

(*Continued*)

Table 3.3 (*Continued*)

Drugs	Doses (mg/kg)	Comments
Xylazine/ ketamine/Telazol	2.5 ml LA × (250 mg), 2.5 ml K (250 mg) in 500 mg T	Reconstitute Telazol powder with xylazine and ketamine
Ketamine	0.006–0.012 ml/kg, IM	
Telazol	1 ml/75 kg (165 lb)	Low-dose sedation High-dose immobilization
Antagonists		
Flumazenil	1 mg/10–15-mg midazolam IM 0.01 mg/kg, IV	Reversal for benzodiazepines
Atipamezole	0.2, IM	Reversal for α_2 agonists
Tolazoline	1–2, IV, IM	Reversal for α_2 agonists
Yohimbine	0.1–0.2, IV, IM	Reversal for α_2 agonists
Naloxone	0.5–2, IV, IM 4 mg IV, total	Reversal for opioid agonists

Telazol alone (3–5 mg/kg IM) has also been used to produce sedation in potbellied pigs. Though transition into deep sedation and immobilization is usually smooth, recovery to consciousness tends to be rough with Telazol alone [35, 38]. Similar to **TKX-Ru**, Telazol, ketamine, and xylazine mixture has also been used in pigs in that 2.5 ml of ketamine and 2.5 ml of 10% xylazine were used to reconstitute Telazol powder (**TKX-P**). The resulting solution contains 50 mg each of tiletamine, ketamine, zolazepam, and xylazine per milliliter, and the final dissociative concentration (i.e., ketamine and tiletamine) is 100 mg/ml, providing a 2:1 ratio of dissociative anesthetics to either zolazepam or xylazine. The response induced by this combination is dose dependent. For commercial pigs, the dose range from sedation to anesthesia is 1 ml/35–75 kg (77–165 lb) IM. In potbellied pigs, the doses required to induce sedation and immobilization for a duration of 35–40 minutes are 0.007–0.013 ml/kg IM and 0.012–0.018 ml/kg IM, respectively [43, 44]. When administering multiple drugs to achieve desirable effect in pigs, it is better to combine these drugs and give the mixture as a single IM bolus injection. This technique minimizes the stress caused by restraint during injection and the hyperkinetic reaction to the injection, thus ensuring better and more complete drug absorption and more reliable CNS depression. Table 3.3 summarizes the doses of drugs and drug combinations used for sedation and chemical restraint in pigs.

In general, standing sedation in farm animal species presents more of a challenge than other domestic species for the veterinarians. Ruminants and camelids have a tendency to assume sternal recumbency when they are sedated. Therefore, there is a fine line between the doses of a tranquilizer/sedative for standing sedation or chemical restraint, and carefully adjusting the dose should be practiced in order to meet the preference, either standing sedation or chemical restraint, for the individual procedure. Furthermore, pigs are more resistant to the CNS-depressing effects of these anesthetics; standing deep sedation is more difficult to achieve and often requires large doses of the drugs. In either cases, unintended sternal recumbency may complicate the surgical procedure, and adjustment should be made to accommodate this unexpected situation (e.g., recumbency occurs during standing surgical procedure).

References

1. Miesner, M. (2009) Updates in bovine surgery: beef cattle and surgical challenges. *North American Veterinary Community Conference*, pp. 41–43.
2. Ivany, J. and Muir, W. (2004) Farm animal anesthesia in: Fubini S, Ducharme N, eds. *Farm Animal Surgery*. St. Louis: Saunders, An Imprint of Elsevier, pp. 97–112.
3. Abrahamsen, E. (2008) Chemical restraint in ruminants. *Veterinary Clinics of North America: Food Animal Practice*, **24**, 227–243.
4. Arnemo, J. and Søli, N. (1995) Immobilization of free-ranging cattle with medetomidine and its reversal by atipamezole. *Veterinary Research Communications*, **19**, 59–62.
5. Murphy, M. and Hugg, C. (1981) "Ceiling effect" of butorphanol (Stadol) as an anesthetic supplement. *Anesthesiology*, **55**, 261.
6. Jones, M. (2008) Clinical application in pain management. *Can West Veterinary Conference*.
7. Power, J. (1985) Butorphanol tartrate analgesia in a bovine animal. *Proceedings of the Annual Convention – American Association of Bovine Practitioners*, **18,** 158–159.
8. Waterman, A., Linvingston, A. and Amin, A. (1991) Analgesic activity and respiratory effects of butorphanol in sheep. *Research in Veterinary Science*, **51**, 19–23.
9. Lin, H. and Riddell, M. (2003) Preliminary study of the effects of xylazine or detomidine with or without butorphanol for standing sedation in dairy cattle. *Veterinary Therapy*, **4**, 285–291.
10. Anderson, D. (2011) New methods for chemical restraint and field anesthesia in cattle. *North American Veterinary Community Conference,* pp. 6–11.
11. Greene, S. (2003) Protocols for anesthesia of cattle. *Veterinary Clinics of North America: Food Animal Practice*, **19**, 679–693.
12. Sharma, S., Nigam, J., Kumar, A. *et al.* (1994) Preliminary studies on the use of medetomidine in calves and its reversal by atipamezole. *International Congress of Veterinary Anesthesia*, pp. 121.
13. Arnemo, J. and Søli, N. (1993) Chemical capture of free-ranging cattle: immobilization with xylazine or medetomidine, and reversal with atipamezole. *Veterinary Research Communications*, **17**, 469–477.
14. Hofkes, L., Hoyer, M., Dijk, P. and Overgaauw, P. (2005) Immobilization of cattle and bison with a combination of xylazine, zolazepam-tiletamine and ketamine. *Tijdschrift voor Diergeneeskunde*, **130**, 268–272.
15. Caulkett, N., Cattet, M., Cantwell, S. *et al.* (2000) Anesthesia of wood bison with medetomidine-zolazepam/tiletamine and xylazine-zolazepam/tiletamine combinations. *The Canadian Veterinary Journal*, **41**, 49–53.
16. Lin, H. (2012) Large ruminant anesthesia: review and update. *Western Veterinary Conference,* FA#1.
17. Hendrickson, D. (2007) Anesthesia and fluid therapy, in *Techniques in Large Animal Surgery*, 3rd edn (ed D. Hendrickson), Blackwell Publishing, Ames, pp. 7–32.
18. Riebold, T. (2007) Ruminants, in: *Lumb and Jones' Veterinary Anesthesia and Analgesia*, 4th edn (eds W. Tranquilli, J. Thurmon and K. Grimm), Blackwell Publishing, Ames, pp. 731–746.
19. Ali, M., Saleh, A., El-Sebaie, A. and Youssef, H. (1988) Acid-base balance and blood gases alterations under the effect of Rompun in sheep. *Assiut Veterinary Medical Journal*, **19**, 150–155.
20. Gray, P. and McDonell, W. (1986) Anesthesia in goats and sheep, Part II: general anesthesia. *Compendium Continuing Education*, **8**, S127–S135.
21. Abrahamsen, E. (2009) Chemical restraint, anesthesia, and analgesia for camelids. *Veterinary Clinics of North America: Food Animal Practice*, **25**, 455–494.

22. Singh, A., Peshin, P., Singh, J. *et al.* (1991) Evaluation of detomidine as a sedative in goats. *Acta veterinaria Hungarica*, **39**, 109–114.
23. Carroll, G. and Hartsfield, S. (1996) General anesthetic techniques in ruminants. *Veterinary Clinics of North America: Food Animal Practice*, **12**, 627–661.
24. Mohammad, F., Zangana, I. and Abdul-Latif, A. (1993) Medetomidine sedation in sheep. *Zentralbl Veterinarmed A*, **40**, 328–331.
25. Waldridge, B., Lin, H., DeGraves, F. and Pugh, D. (1997) Sedative effects of medetomidine and its reversal by atipamezole in llamas. *Journal of the American Veterinary Medical Association*, **211**, 1562–1565.
26. Jalanka, H. and Roeken, B. (1990) The use of medetomidine, medetomidine-ketamine combinations, and atipamezole in nondomestic mammals: a review. *Journal of Zoo and Wildlife Medicine*, **21**, 259–282.
27. Taylor, P. (1991) Anesthesia in sheep and goats. *In Practice*, **13**, 31–36.
28. Hall, L., Clarke, K. and Trim, C. (2001) Anaesthesia of sheep, goats, and other herbivores, in *Veterinary Anaesthesia*, 10th edn (eds L. Hall, K. Clarke and C. Trim), WB Saunders, London, pp. 341–366.
29. Stegmann, G. and Bester, L. (2001) Sedative-hypnotic effects of midazolam in goats after intravenous and intramuscular administration. *Veterinary Anaesthesia and Analgesia*, **28**, 49–55.
30. Kyles, A., Waterman, A. and Livingston, A. (1995) Antinociceptive activity of midazolam in sheep. *Journal of Veterinary Pharmacology and Therapeutics*, **18**, 54–60.
31. Stegmann, G. (1998) Observations on the use of midazolam in combination for sedation, and induction of anaesthesia with midazolam in combination with ketamine in the goats. *Journal of the South African Veterinary Association*, **69**, 89–92.
32. O'Hair, K., Dodd, K., Phillips, Y. and Beattie, R. (1988) Cardiopulmonary effects of nalbuphine hydrochloride and butorphanol tartrate in sheep. *Laboratory Animal Science*, **38**, 58–61.
33. Barrington, G., Meyer, T. and Parish, S. (1993) Standing castration of the llama using butorphanol tartrate and local anesthesia. *Equine Pract*, **15**, 35–39.
34. Johnson, L. (2010) Keeping small ruminant field anesthesia simple. *North American Veterinary Community Conference*, p. 345.
35. Williams, L. (1992) The Vietnamese pot bellied pig: anesthetic friend or foe? *Symposium of the American College of Veterinary Surgery*, 222–224.
36. Anderson, D. and St Jean, G. (2012) Anesthesia and surgical procedures in swine, in *Diseases of Swine*, 10th edn (eds J. Zimmerman, L. Karriker, A. Ramirez *et al.*), Ames, Wiley-Blackwell, pp. 119–140.
37. Moon, P. and Smith, L. (1996) General anesthetic techniques in swine. *Veterinary Clinics of North America: Food Animal Practice*, **12**, 663–691.
38. Boldrick, L. and Blackburn, A. (1993) Anesthesia. *Veterinary Care of Pot-bellied Pigs*. Orange: All Publishing Co, pp. 104–110.
39. Braun, W. (1993) Anesthetic and surgical techniques useful in the potbellied pig. *Veterinary Medicine*, **88**, 441–447.
40. Vainio, O., Bloor, B. and Kim, C. (1992) Cardiovascular effects of a ketamine-medetomidine combination that produces deep sedation in Yucatan mini swine. *Laboratory Animal Science*, **42**, 582–588.
41. Linkenhoker, J., Burkholder, T., Linton, C. *et al.* (2010) Effective and safe anesthesia for Yorkshire and Yucatan swine and without cardiovascular injury and intervention. *Journal of the American Association for Laboratory Animal Science*, **49**, 344–351.

42. Nishimura, R., Kim, H., Matsunaga, S. *et al.* (1993) Comparative of sedative and analgesic-anesthetic effects induced by medetomidine, acepromazine, azaperone, droperidol and midazolam in laboratory pigs. *The Journal of Veterinary Medical Science*, **55**, 687–690.
43. Thurmon, J. and Benson, G. (1993) Anesthesia in ruminants and swine, in *Current Veterinary Therapy: Food Animal Practice*, 3rd edn (ed J. Howard), WB Saunders, Philadelphia, pp. 58–76.
44. Ko, J., Thurmon, J., Benson, G. and Olson, W. (1993) A new drug combination for use in porcine cesarean sections. *Veterinary Medicine*, **88**, 466–472.

Chapter 4

Injectable anesthetics and field anesthesia

HuiChu Lin

Department of Clinical Sciences, College of Veterinary Medicine, Auburn University, USA

Injectable anesthetics can be used to produce short-term anesthesia for minor diagnostic and surgical procedures, or they can be used for induction of general anesthesia followed by maintenance of inhalation anesthesia for longer procedures. Short-term injectable anesthesia is often preferred for field procedures. Compared to inhalation anesthesia, injectable anesthesia offers the advantages of ease of administration, rapid transition from awake to unconsciousness, and minimal apparatus required for its use. However, it is often difficult to maintain a consistent level of anesthesia with an injectable anesthetic, particularly when it is administered by intermittent repeated dosing. When an injectable anesthetic is used repeatedly to prolong anesthesia, accumulation of the anesthetics may cause prolonged recovery. The goal of balanced anesthesia is to provide narcosis (unconsciousness), analgesia, and muscle relaxation, which ideally can be produced by administration of a single drug. But in reality, the large dose of an injectable anesthetic which is often required to achieve balanced anesthesia and maintain anesthesia for lengthy procedures is often associated with severe adverse effects. The combinations of different classes of anesthetics are frequently used to achieve desirable anesthetic effects with as few side effects as possible. The choice of the anesthetics used for field anesthesia should be based on the intrinsic pharmacological effects of each anesthetic, types of surgery or diagnostic procedures performed, and the duration of the procedure. This chapter describes the pharmacology of commonly used injectable anesthetics and their uses for field anesthesia in farm animal species.

Farm Animal Anesthesia: Cattle, Small Ruminants, Camelids, and Pigs, First Edition.
Edited by HuiChu Lin and Paul Walz.

Injectable anesthetics

Ketamine

Ketamine is a dissociative anesthetic. Presently, ketamine is the most commonly used injectable anesthetic in large animal practice. It has a rapid onset of action following intravenous (IV) administration with the maximal effect occurring within 1 minute as a result of its small molecular weight, high lipid solubility, and a dissociation constant (pK_a, 7.5) value near the physiologic pH allowing rapid diffusion of the anesthetic across the blood–brain barrier into the central nervous system (CNS). Ketamine produces dose-dependent unconsciousness and analgesia. Termination of the anesthetic effect after a single dose of ketamine depends on rapid redistribution of the drug from the CNS to peripheral muscle and fat tissues [1]. The primary CNS site of action appears to be mediated through the thalamoneocortical projection system. Ketamine selectively depresses neuronal function of the neocorticothalamic axis and the central nucleus of the thalamus, and at the same time, it stimulates parts of the limbic system, including the hippocampus [2, 3]. Therefore, ketamine anesthesia is characterized by unconsciousness while maintaining eye reflexes (palpebral and corneal reflexes) and pharyngeal–laryngeal reflexes (e.g., swallowing reflex). Evidence indicates that antagonism of ketamine on the *N*-methyl-D-aspartate (NMDA) receptors is responsible for most of the anesthetic, analgesic, psychotomimetic, and neuroprotective effects of the drug [4]. On the cellular level, ketamine-induced anesthesia is believed to be mediated through (1) non-competitive antagonism on the NMDA glutamate receptors, (2) action on the voltage-dependent sodium and potassium channels and calcium channels, (3) depression of the acetylcholine receptors, (4) enhancement and prolongation of the γ-amino-butyric acid (GABA) receptors that link to chloride channels ($GABA_A$) [5], and (5) depression of nociceptive cells in the medial medullary reticular formation and activity of the laminae I and V of the dorsal horn [6, 7].

Ketamine does not depress cardiovascular function; instead, it causes direct stimulation of the CNS leading to increased sympathetic outflow, resulting in increased heart rate and arterial blood pressures during anesthesia [8]. Several contributing factors for the ketamine-induced increased sympathetic outflow have been identified including (1) sympathomimetic effects mediated within the CNS [9], (2) inhibition of the neuronal uptake of catecholamines by sympathetic nerve endings [10], (3) direct vasodilation of the vascular smooth muscle [11], and (4) an inotropic effect on the myocardium [12]. Plasma concentrations of epinephrine and norepinephrine increase within 2 minutes after IV administration of ketamine and return to control concentrations 15 minutes later; this increase is a reflection of increased sympathetic outflow due to sympathomimetic effect induced by ketamine [13]. As a result, heart rate and arterial blood pressure increase transiently following IV administration of the drug. However, the cardiovascular-stimulating effects of ketamine can be blunted or prevented by prior administration of a benzodiazepine [14, 15], droperidol [16], acepromazine, and α_2 agonists or by concomitant administration of inhalation anesthetics, including nitrous oxide [17, 18]. In the CNS, ketamine induces significant increases in cerebral blood flow (CBF), intracranial pressure (ICP), and cerebrospinal fluid (CSF) pressure as a result of cerebral vasodilation and elevated systemic arterial blood pressure [19–25]. Direct smooth muscle relaxation of bovine middle cerebral arteries via inhibition of calcium uptake has been reported, supporting the finding that ketamine causes cerebral vasodilation [26]. However, the mechanism of ketamine-induced elevated ICP remains controversial. In awake goats, ketamine increases CBF and ICP when $PaCO_2$ is allowed to rise, but CBF and ICP remain unchanged when $PaCO_2$ is maintained at a preketamine concentration [27, 28]. In piglets with increased ICP, a further increase in ICP paralleling a rise in $PaCO_2$ was observed during ketamine anesthesia. When ventilation was controlled, no increase in ICP was observed in piglets with normal or elevated ICP [28]. Increased skeletal, thoracic, and abdominal muscle tone can impede venous return from the head to cause an increase in intracranial blood volume and pressure [28, 29].

Ketamine does not depress ventilatory responses to hypoxia at clinically recommended doses [30]. Hypoxic pulmonary vasoconstriction is preserved during ketamine anesthesia but potentiated during propofol anesthesia in dogs [31]. Nonetheless, arterial oxygenation and functional residual capacity are usually well maintained during ketamine anesthesia [32–35]. Ketamine is a potent bronchodilator capable of preventing and reversing wheezing in human patients with asthma requiring anesthesia and intubation [36, 37]. At clinically useful doses, this bronchoprotective effect is mediated primarily via depression of neurally (vagally) induced vasoconstriction [38]. In sheep, ketamine induces a transient decrease in PaO_2 in the presence of decreased or increased respiratory rate [39–41]. The transient apnea induced by ketamine appears to be dose dependent. At higher doses, respiration is characterized by an apneustic, shallow, and irregular pattern [42–44]. Severe respiratory depression or arrest due to overdosage has been reported in human patients, cats, and ponies [44–46].

Ketamine often causes increased salivation and secretion of mucus in the respiratory tract, which can be reduced by administration of an anticholinergic drug. Laryngeal and pharyngeal reflexes usually are well maintained during ketamine anesthesia. Swallowing reflexes may be present but somewhat obtunded because most animals can be intubated when anesthetized with ketamine [47]. Ruminants normally salivate profusely during ketamine anesthesia. Total amounts of salivary secretion in conscious adult cattle and sheep have been reported to be 50L and 6–16L per 24 hours, respectively [48, 49]. If the trachea is left unprotected during anesthesia, aspiration of large amount of saliva can cause pneumonia.

Ketamine alone does not provide muscle relaxation. Muscle jerking and sometimes rigidity are present following the induction of anesthesia. Acepromazine, diazepam, xylazine, and medetomidine can be used in combination with ketamine to enhance the degree of analgesia and muscle relaxation during anesthesia. Ketamine has been shown to produce intense analgesia even at subanesthetic doses [50]. Proposed mechanisms responsible for the analgesic actions of ketamine include blockade of spinoreticular tracts [51, 52], depression of nuclei of the medial medullary reticular formation [6], suppression of lamina in the dorsal horn of the spinal cord [7, 53, 54], interaction with CNS and spinal cord opiate receptors [55–58], and antagonism of NMDA receptor [4]. Studies also indicate that ketamine induces visceral analgesia as evidenced by inhibition of nociceptive responses to graded test in rats [59–61]. Furthermore, NMDA receptors appear to be more involved in hyperalgesic responses after peripheral tissue injury and inflammation rather than nonnoxious somatic inputs [60, 62]. Ketamine has been used in combination with opioids or nonsteroidal anti-inflammatory drugs (NSAIDs) administered at 0.25–0.5 mg/kg intramuscularly every 6–8 hours to provide pain relief in goats suffering severe pain due to burn injury, polyarthritis, or osteomyelitis [63].

Cattle

An IV bolus injection of ketamine (2 mg/kg) followed by continuous infusion of 0.2% (2 mg/ml) ketamine in physiologic saline at a rate of 10 ml/min induces dissociative anesthesia for both minor and major surgeries (toe amputation, laparotomy, etc.) in cows [64]. Intramuscular (IM) administration of ketamine alone or in various combinations with other drugs in calves has been used to induce chemical restraint or anesthesia, but this technique is impractical for adult cattle due to the large volume of drug required for the size of the animal. Presently, IV ketamine (2.2 mg/kg) is commonly administered concomitantly with or after IV administration of xylazine (0.1–0.2 mg/kg) for short-term anesthesia in both large and small ruminants. Tracheal intubation is easily achieved in cattle anesthetized with this combination. Anesthesia may be safely prolonged by intermittent IV injection of 1–2 mg/kg of ketamine given slowly to effect. Alternatively, a continuous infusion of 2 mg/ml of ketamine in 0.9% NaCl solution, 5% dextrose solution, or 5% guaifenesin in 5% dextrose solution is administered at a rate of 10 ml/min to prolong anesthesia [65].

Small ruminants and camelids

In sheep, ketamine alone (22 mg/kg IV) may cause side effects such as tachycardia, muscle rigidity, and mild salivation during anesthesia and marked ataxia during recovery [66]. However, at a low IV bolus dose of 2 mg/kg followed by 4 ml/min of continuous infusion of 0.2% ketamine in 5% glucose solution (2 mg/ml) for up to 2 hours, ketamine produced safe anesthesia in pregnant ewes [67]. In goats, IM ketamine (10 mg/kg, 84 minutes) [68] produced longer duration of anesthesia than in goats that were administered with IV ketamine (6 mg/kg, 15–30 minutes) [69]. Levinson *et al.* (1973) [70] reported that ketamine caused an increase in uterine blood flow but did not produce detrimental effects on fetal cardiovascular or acid–base status. When administered intramuscularly or intravenously to pregnant goats, ketamine rapidly traversed the placental membrane, resulting in an increase in fetal heart rate and blood pressure. Fetal pHa and PaO_2 decreased while $PaCO_2$ increased during anesthesia. The detrimental effects of ketamine on the fetus appeared to be greater with IV administration than with IM administration [71]. When administered to induce general anesthesia, ketamine reportedly increased basal uterine tone as well as the intensity of the contractions in both pregnant and nonpregnant women. Nonetheless, the study showed that human fetal mortality is less with ketamine than with other anesthetics [72].

Similar to cattle and small ruminants, ketamine (1 mg/ml) is often combined with 5% guaifenesin and given to effect (1.5–2.2 ml/kg IV) to induce and maintain general anesthesia for 15–20 minutes in camelids. When using xylazine and ketamine combination to induce satisfactory anesthesia and to facilitate tracheal intubation, camelids appear to require a higher dose of ketamine (3–5 mg/kg) [73] as opposed to the lower dose of 2.2 mg/kg normally used for cattle and small ruminants [74].

Swine

Ketamine administered intramuscularly alone (11 mg/kg) to pigs provides anesthesia that may more appropriately be considered chemical restraint [42]. Although immobilization occurred within 3–5 minutes, muscle relaxation was considered poor with only a brief period of analgesia. IV administration of an additional 2–4 mg/kg of ketamine prolonged immobilization [42]. Violent reactions in pigs to initial IM injection of ketamine with subsequent muscle tremor, extensor rigidity, panting respiration, and erythema have been reported [75]. Other side effects including tachycardia, hypertension, and poor muscle relaxation, as seen in other species, are also observed in pigs. Concurrent administration of diazepam (1 mg/kg IM) or xylazine (2 mg/kg IM) with ketamine provided deep sedation and good muscle relaxation and minimized adverse reactions, but unforutunately pigs still responded to surgical stimulus, for example, incision of the abdominal wall [75, 76].

Telazol

Telazol, a proprietary combination of tiletamine (dissociative derivative) and zolazepam (benzodiazepine derivative), produces anesthesia similar to the commonly used anesthetic combination, diazepam and ketamine. Tiletamine and zolazepam are combined in a 1:1 ratio by weight of base and marketed as Telazol. The combination of the drugs is supplied in a sterile vial as a lyophilized powder containing 250 mg of tiletamine and 250 mg of zolazepam. It is recommended that the drug be reconstituted immediately before use with 5 ml of sterile water, resulting in a combination of 50 mg of tiletamine and 50 mg of zolazepam per ml of the solution. Telazol has a wide margin of safety and has been used to produce safe anesthesia in a wide variety of animal species including wildlife. The pH of the injectable solution of Telazol is between 2 and 3.5; though acidic, it does not cause tissue irritation and the animal's reactions to IM injection of the drug are minimal. Induction of anesthesia is rapid and smooth, as is recovery in most species. Compared with ketamine, Telazol anesthesia produces better muscle relaxation, more profound analgesia, and longer-lasting effects. The swallowing and eructation/vomiting reflexes are retained. Muscle relaxation and general lack of response to external stimuli add to Telazol's usefulness. Telazol induces analgesia from interruption of sensory input into the brain, which usually persists after the anesthetic effect has subsided. The animal's eyes remain open, even during surgical anesthesia. Protective reflexes, such as coughing, swallowing, and corneal and pedal reflexes, are maintained. Increased salivation is a common occurrence in most animals administered with Telazol. An anticholinergic drug (e.g., atropine and glycopyrrolate) can be administered with Telazol to reduce salivation [77].

In llamas, Telazol causes no significant changes in heart rate [78]. In calves, Telazol (4 mg/kg IV) induces a transient decrease followed by an increase in heart rate. The mechanism of the transient decrease in heart rate is believed to be caused by tiletamine's negative inotropic and chronotropic effects [79]. The direct depressant effect of tiletamine was clearly demonstrated in denervated myocardium [80]. A decreased amplitude of myocardial contraction was observed when tiletamine (0.5–5 mg) was administered into the coronary circulation of an isolated rabbit heart preparation [81]. The subsequent increase in heart rate is attributed to direct CNS stimulation leading to increased sympathetic tone and perhaps decreased vagal tone [82]. Changes in arterial blood pressure and systemic vascular resistance induced by Telazol are characterized by a decrease followed by an increase after IV injection to calves. Tiletamine may play a major role in the unique biphasic hemodynamic changes occurring after Telazol administration [79]. In calves, the biphasic response in arterial blood pressure induced by Telazol (4 mg/kg IV) is reversed when Telazol is combined with xylazine (0.1 mg/kg IV). The hemodynamic effects of Telazol are offset by the initial vasoconstrictive effect and delayed sympatholytic and parasympathomimetic effects of IV xylazine [83]. In sheep, butorphanol (0.5 mg/kg IV) administered preanesthetically does not influence the decrease in mean systemic and pulmonary arterial pressures induced by Telazol (12 mg/kg IV). Heart rate does not change significantly when butorphanol is administered with or prior to Telazol, although increased systemic vascular resistance is observed [84]. In calves, left ventricular stroke work index and rate pressure product follow a similar biphasic response as seen with blood pressure and systemic vascular resistance after Telazol injection [79]. Cardiac output remains unchanged in calves and llamas [78, 79]. Decreased cardiac output is observed in sheep given butorphanol/Telazol [84]. In calves receiving xylazine and Telazol, cardiac output decreased transiently and was associated with an increase in afterload and a decrease in heart rate [83].

Respiratory rate usually increases in most species following Telazol injection. In calves, low doses of Telazol (4–8 mg/kg IV or IM) increase respiratory rate for 30–60 minutes. Apnea may occur when larger doses (10 mg/kg IM) of Telazol are administered, but spontaneous breathing usually soon resumes without respiratory support. In sheep, although respiratory rate remains unchanged, apneustic breathing and decreased inspired minute ventilation and tidal volume are observed after Telazol administration (12 or 24 mg/kg IV) [74]. In llamas, mild respiratory depression accompanied by hypoxemia is also evident [78]. Hypothermia may occur after Telazol injection as a result of profound muscle relaxation. Body temperature should be monitored, as supplemental heat may be required during Telazol anesthesia, particularly in small patients.

Cattle

In ruminants, Telazol produces smooth induction of anesthesia rapidly with gradual and prolonged recovery [85]. The pharmacologic effect of Telazol is predominated by tiletamine since zolazepam has very minimal cardiovascular effect, but it is capable of enhancing the anesthetic effect and muscle relaxation of tiletamine. As a result, Telazol causes cardiovascular stimulation rather than depression [85, 86]. In calves, Telazol alone (4 mg/kg IV) induced 45–60 minutes of satisfactory anesthesia with minimal cardiovascular depression [79]. Telazol comes as 500-mg powder, and it is usually reconstituted with 5 ml of sterile water into 100 mg/ml solution. The drug is very water soluble; thus, it can be reconstituted with a smaller volume of sterile water into an injectable solution with higher concentration. For example, adding 2.5 ml of sterile water into 500-mg Telazol powder results in an injectable solution with final concentration of 250 mg/ml. Because of this, Telazol has been recommended for use to capture free-ranging cattle when smaller volume are necessary to fill darts of a tranquilizing gun [65]. Xylazine or detomidine can be used to substitute sterile water to reconstitute Telazol powder to ensure effective chemical restraint of free-ranging cattle. A combination of Telazol, ketamine, and xylazine (**TKX-Ru**) has been used successfully to capture wild ruminants.

Small ruminants and camelids

Telazol (8–20 mg/kg IV) has been used successfully to anesthetize sheep undergoing surgical procedures. Induction is rapid and exceptionally smooth, and duration of surgical anesthesia ranges from 40 minutes to 3.7 hours. Excessive salivation can be controlled by administration of 0.066 mg/kg of atropine sulfate [87]. IV doses of 12 or 24 mg/kg of Telazol cause a significant decrease in minute ventilation and respiratory airflow that is characterized by an apneustic breathing pattern [88]. IM administration of 12 mg/kg of Telazol appears to be the optimal dose, with surgical anesthesia lasting approximately 30 minutes. The analgesic effect was found to be most profound around the head, the neck, and the trunk, whereas poor analgesia was found in the distal portion of the limb and perineal area [89]. Hypoventilation and hypothermia have been observed in sheep anesthetized with Telazol alone or with xylazine. Assisted or controlled ventilation with O_2 supplementation may be required in the presence of severe hypoventilation and hypoxemia [90].

In llamas, Telazol (4.4 mg/kg IM) provides good chemical restraint and immobilization for 2 hours, but the degree of muscle relaxation and the quality of analgesia are not sufficient for major surgery [78]. In free-ranging adult guanacos, Telazol (4–6 mg/kg) produced immobilization for an average duration of 7 minutes (1.5–53 minutes) [91].

Swine

Telazol alone in pigs (doses range from 4.4 to 22 mg/kg) induces rapid immobilization but does not produce adequate muscle relaxation and analgesia sufficient for surgery. A hyperresponsive reflex characterized by exaggerated limb withdrawal is common and often persists throughout the course of immobilization. Similar responses have been described in swine receiving ketamine alone [42]. Ganter and Ruppert [92] reported that 10 mg/kg of Telazol given intramuscularly induced rapid immobilization with an average duration of 33.7 ± 15 minutes. Although muscle relaxation was described as good, analgesia was poor. During recovery, the pigs were excited and salivated excessively. It appears that zolazepam in pigs does not induce the same degree of muscle relaxation or suppress hyperresponsiveness as effectively as it does in other species [93–96].

Propofol

Propofol (PropoFlo™) is a unique short-acting anesthetic. Structurally, propofol does not relate to any of the injectable anesthetics currently available in veterinary practice. Propofol is only slightly water soluble and comes as a white, oil-in-water emulsion containing 10 mg of propofol, 100 mg of soybean oil, 22.5 mg of glycerol, and 12 mg of egg lecithin per ml in sterile glass ampules. Because this emulsion contains no preservative, after the ampule is opened, the contents should be used or discarded within 8 hours. Rapid recovery from propofol is believed to be the result of a combination of rapid redistribution of the drug to peripheral muscle and fat tissues as well as rapid hepatic and extrahepatic metabolism [97, 98]. Complete recovery without residual sedation and ataxia makes propofol a popular choice for outpatient procedures. A single dose of propofol (2 mg/kg IV) produces approximately 10 minutes of anesthesia with complete recovery occurring in 20–30 minutes [99, 100]. Propofol is best used for induction before inhalation anesthesia; it also can be used as a continuous infusion to maintain short-term anesthesia [101–103]. Supplemental analgesic drug should be administered to provide pain relief following surgery since propofol at subanesthetic dose does not provide analgesia [104]. A comparative study was performed to evaluate propofol (3 mg/kg IV), thiopental (8 mg/kg IV), or ketamine (10 mg/kg IV) as induction agents in goats. The result of this study indicated that propofol was superior to thiopental or ketamine as an induction agent because of the rapid and uneventful recovery it produced [105]. A new formulation of propofol, PropoFlo™ 28, recently has become available. The injectable solution is also white, water-in-oil emulsion. Twenty mg/ml instead of 1 mg/ml of benzyl alcohol is added to the original propofol to extend its shelf life up to 28 days. Due to its extremely short duration of action and high cost, clinical use of propofol and PropoFlo™ 28 is somewhat limited in farm animal species, especially in adult cattle.

Small ruminants and camelids

A single dose of propofol (2–6 mg/kg) induces approximately 10 minutes of anesthesia with complete recovery in 20–30 minutes in sheep [100, 101, 106, 107]. Propofol is best used for induction before inhalation anesthesia; it also can be used as a continuous infusion to maintain short-term anesthesia [101–103]. Propofol alone does not provide good analgesia. Concurrent administration of an analgesic such as opioids or NSAIDs is beneficial to provide pain relief during painful procedures.

In camelids, 2 mg/kg of propofol does not induce muscle relaxation adequate for tracheal intubation. However, a light plane of anesthesia can be achieved with additional infusion of 24 mg/kg/hour. Llamas were able to maintain a sternal recumbency position 10–15 minutes after the discontinuation of the propofol infusion [108]. For cesarean section, pregnant camelids can be sedated with xylazine (0.1–0.2 mg/kg IM) and butorphanol (0.06–0.12 mg/kg IM) and general anesthesia induced with propofol (3.5 mg/kg IV) with diazepam (0.5 mg/kg IV) or guaifenesin. Though anesthesia can be maintained with propofol infusion for cesarean section, fetal ventilatory function may be better maintained when isoflurane in O_2 is used [109].

Swine

In pigs, 2 mg/kg of propofol was administered intravenously as loading dose, and anesthesia maintained with a continuous infusion of 9–13 mg/kg/hour. Decreased heart rate and cardiac index and dose-dependent ventilatory depression were observed with a high dose of propofol. Depending on the total dose of propofol administered, pigs recovered and assumed sternal recumbency within 30 minutes after being administered a low dose, while

60 minutes was required for pigs that received a high dose [110]. Endotracheal intubation and positive pressure ventilation may be required immediately following induction as transient apnea occurred frequently with propofol. The cardiovascular effects of propofol administered at 7.5, 15, and 30 mg/kg/hour in newborn piglets were studied. Only mean arterial blood pressure decreased 25% from baseline values; heart rate and left ventricular pressure remained unchanged for all doses [111].

Guaifenesin

Guaifenesin is a central muscle relaxant frequently used in large animal practice. The drug acts by interrupting impulse transmission in the internuncial neurons of the spinal cord, brain stem, and subcortical areas of the brain. Unlike neuromuscular blocking drugs, guaifenesin produces muscle relaxation, not muscle paralysis. In cattle, IV guaifenesin when administered at 50 mg/kg induced ataxia and muscle relaxation. Recumbency occurred at a dose of 100 mg/kg [112]. Only minimal changes on respiratory muscle activity and respiratory and cardiovascular functions were observed when guaifenesin was administered at the therapeutic dose [113]. However, a significant decrease in arterial blood pressure and acute respiratory acidosis occurred following the administration of guaifenesin (165 mg/kg) to buffalo calves [114]. Guaifenesin doses three to four times higher than the dose required to induce recumbency can result in respiratory paralysis [115]. Guaifenesin is not an anesthetic, and it does not produce anesthesia or analgesia. Therefore, guaifenesin should always be used in combination with other anesthetic(s), for example, ketamine, thiopental, or propofol, to provide good muscle relaxation during anesthesia [65]. Nevertheless, guaifenesin alone at 15–25 mg/kg IV induces mild standing sedation in large ruminants and camelids; but the amount of the drug administered should be carefully titrated to avoid excessive muscle relaxation and recumbency [116]. Guaifenesin comes as a powder and can be reconstituted with 5% dextrose to make up 5% (50 mg/ml) or 10% (100 mg/ml) injectable solution by a compounding pharmacist. Thrombophlebitis has occurred following the administration of 5% guaifenesin solution [117]. However, hemolysis, hemoglobinuria, and venous thrombosis are more likely to occur with solution of 10% or greater [118]. Guaifenesin, xylazine, and ketamine combination, referred to as **Triple Drip**, is a popular injectable anesthetic combination for short-term anesthesia in large and small ruminants, camelids, and pigs. Because of the breed and species variation in sensitivity to xylazine and individual difference for the anesthetic dose requirement, adjustment of the concentration of each drug in the **Triple Drip** and the rate of infusion of the mixture is very important to ensure safe anesthesia.

Field anesthesia

Cattle

Acepromazine, diazepam, xylazine, and medetomidine can be used in combination with ketamine to enhance analgesia and muscle relaxation during anesthesia. IV administration of xylazine (0.1–0.2 mg/kg) prior to or concomitantly with ketamine (2–3 mg/kg) is the

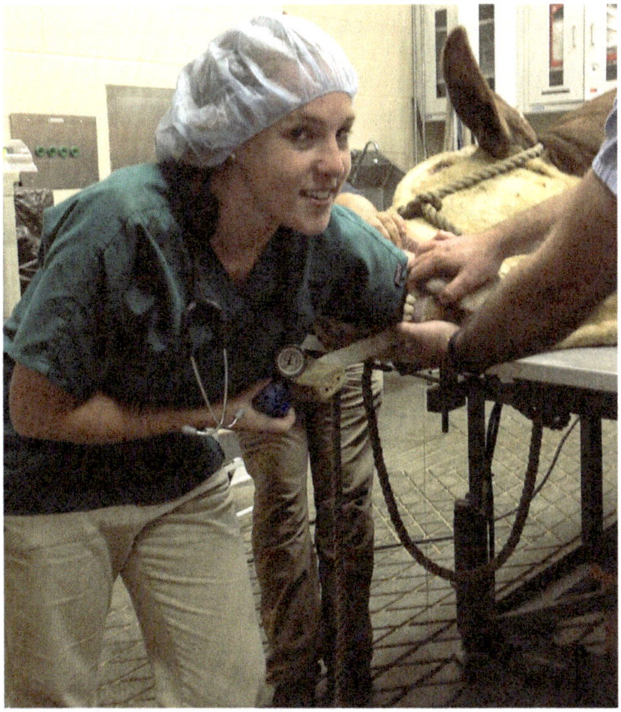

Figure 4.1 Endotracheal intubation using digital palpation technique in a bull anesthetized with xylazine (0.1 mg/kg IV) and ketamine (2.2 mg/kg IV).

most commonly used combination to induce short-term anesthesia in cattle of all ages. Lowering the dose of xylazine in cattle weighing more than 600 kg (1320 lb) may be appropriate [119]. While IM xylazine (0.1–0.2 mg/kg) and ketamine (10–15 mg/kg) can be used in young calves, this is impractical for adult cattle because of the large amount of ketamine required [99]. Tracheal intubation is easily achieved in cattle anesthetized with this combination (Figure 4.1). Duration of anesthesia with IV xylazine and ketamine is approximately 20–30 minutes in most cases. Anesthesia may be safely prolonged by IV administration of ⅓ to ½ of the original dose of each drug or 1–2 mg/kg of ketamine given slowly to effect for additional 15 minutes [65]. In calves anesthetized with xylazine and ketamine, the decrease in heart rate induced by xylazine is offset by the subsequent administration of ketamine. When xylazine and ketamine are administered simultaneously, no significant changes in heart rate, cardiac output, and arterial blood pressure are observed [120, 121]. Thus, it appears that administration of xylazine prior to or simultaneously with ketamine offers the advantage of minimizing the decrease in heart rate and arterial blood pressure induced by xylazine alone [122]. Respiratory rate often increases after xylazine and ketamine administration, but it is usually accompanied by a decrease in PaO_2 and an increase in $PaCO_2$ [123, 124]. Arterial pH decreases slightly as a result of accumulation of $PaCO_2$. Only minor changes in base excess and bicarbonate are observed during xylazine and ketamine anesthesia, indicating hypoventilation is minor without need for metabolic compensation [123]. Alternatively, anesthesia can be maintained with a continuous infusion of ketamine (2 mg/ml) in 0.9% NaCl solution or 5% dextrose solution at a rate of 10 ml/min [65]. A bolus injection of ketamine (2 mg/kg IV) followed by continuous IV infusion of 0.2% (2 mg/ml) ketamine in 0.9% NaCl solution at a rate of 10 ml/min in cows produces anesthesia appropriate for minor and major surgeries (e.g., toe amputation, laparotomy, etc.) [64]. Low doses of xylazine (0.05 mg/kg IV, 0.05–0.1 mg/kg IM) and ketamine (2 mg/kg IV, 4 mg/kg IM) combined have been used to produce anesthesia with less intensity of analgesia and shorter duration of recumbency [116]. As mentioned in Chapter 3 (Standing Sedation and Chemical Sedation), IV xylazine (0.1–0.2 mg/kg) and diazepam (0.1–0.2 mg/kg) induce approximately 30 minutes of immobilization with analgesia in adult cattle [125]. Depending on the desired level of analgesia, high dose of xylazine with low dose of diazepam is suitable for procedures requiring a greater degree of analgesia, whereas low dose of xylazine with high dose of diazepam is preferred for animals with high anesthetic risk.

Ketamine (1 mg/ml) can be mixed with 5% guaifenesin (50 mg/ml) solution to maintain short duration of anesthesia in ruminants [86]. A combination of guaifenesin (50 mg/ml), ketamine (1–2 mg/ml), and xylazine (0.1 mg/ml), often referred to as **Bovine Triple Drip** or **GKX**, can be used for procedures that require longer duration of anesthesia [126]. Anesthesia using **Bovine Triple Drip** can be induced with 0.55–1.1 ml/kg initially and maintained with 2.2 ml/kg/hour in adult cattle and 1.65 ml/kg/hour in calves. Onset of anesthesia is gradual but smooth; muscle relaxation is excellent and tracheal intubation is easy. Supplementation with O_2 (5–10 l/min) during prolonged procedures may help prevent hypoxemia. Mild hypoventilation is observed when this anesthetic mixture is used. Recovery to standing with **Bovine Triple Trip** usually occurs within 40–45 minutes after discontinuation of the infusion. Surgical procedures that can be performed in cattle anesthetized with **Bovine Triple Trip** include femoral fracture plating and pinning, penile surgery, umbilical hernia repair, cesarean section, and celiotomy [74]. The concentration of xylazine and/or ketamine should be reduced to 0.05 and 1 mg/ml, respectively, for procedures lasting longer than 2 hours to prevent accumulation of the drugs and prolonged recovery. Because cattle anesthetized with **Bovine Triple Drip** may regurgitate due to profound muscle relaxation, tracheal intubation is recommended immediately following induction [99].

Higher doses of ketamine, xylazine, and butorphanol combination (**Ketamine Stun**) than those used for standing sedation and chemical restraint can be used to produce a short duration of recumbency and anesthesia. Onset of recumbency occurs within 1 minute following IV bolus injection of ketamine (0.3–0.5 mg/kg), xylazine (0.025–0.05 mg/kg), and butorphanol (0.05–0.1 mg/kg). Animals may appear to be "awake" but are not responsive to external stimulations. Many minor surgical procedures can be performed under this level of light anesthesia. Mild involuntary head or limb movements can occur which may not be a response to surgical stimulation. Only purposeful movement or vocalization indicates inadequate depth of anesthesia, and half of the initial doses of xylazine and ketamine should be administered to produce appropriate depth of anesthesia. Surgical anesthesia is produced with this combination; however, local anesthetic solution can be administered to the surgical field to enhance analgesia. A short period of anesthesia (15–20 minutes) is achieved with this combination. IM or subcutaneous (SC) administration of the same combination–ketamine (0.1 mg/kg), xylazine (0.05 mg/kg), and butorphanol

(0.025 mg/kg)–produces recumbency but with less analgesia as compared to that produced when the combination is administered by IV injection. Recumbency occurs within 3–10 minutes and lasts for 45 minutes following SC injection. Endotracheal intubation can be accomplished with this technique [116]. Initially, the combination of butorphanol (0.0375 mg/kg), ketamine (3.75 mg/kg), and xylazine (0.375 mg/kg) was described by Dr. Larue Johnson at Colorado State University. The combination was made by adding 1 ml of xylazine (100 mg) and 1 ml of butorphanol (10 mg) to 10 ml (1,000 mg) of ketamine and administering the combination at a dose of 1 ml/20 kg (44 lb) IM. Recumbency occurs within 3–5 minutes with 20–30 minutes of anesthesia. Half of the original dose of each drug can be administered to extend the duration of anesthesia. This dose combination is recommended only for normal, healthy animals as the combination contains a higher dose of xylazine [127] than that described by Abrahamsen [116]. Recovery to standing time is expected to be longer with this dose combination. In clinical practice, IV butorphanol (0.025–0.05 mg/kg), xylazine (0.1–0.15 mg/kg), and ketamine (0.5–1 mg/kg) have been used to produce 30 minutes of surgical anesthesia for complicated umbilical surgery. Xylazine and butorphanol are administered to produce profound sedation and followed by ketamine to induce anesthesia. Miesner [128] indicated that endotracheal intubation during these surgical procedures greatly improved the quality and duration of the anesthesia. If surgery requires an hour or longer, IV infusion of **Bovine Triple Drip** can be used to extend the duration of anesthesia.

IV administration of medetomidine (20 μg/kg) and ketamine (2.2 mg/kg) induced lateral recumbency for 94 ± 25 minutes in Holstein calves [129]. Muscle relaxation was adequate for endotracheal intubation in all calves. During anesthesia, heart rate remained unchanged, but arterial blood pressure increased significantly. Respiratory rate increased significantly immediately following drug administration, but mean values for PaO_2, $PaCO_2$, and pHa remained within normal ranges. Atipamezole and tolazoline were each effective in reversing medetomidine and ketamine anesthesia with recovery to standing occurring in 4 ± 3 and 16 ± 9 minutes, respectively, after injection. Yohimbine is the least effective of the three α_2 antagonists in shortening the duration of medetomidine and ketamine anesthesia; calves did not stand for 48 ± 20 minutes after the injection [129]. Medetomidine (0.02 mg/kg IV) combined with lower dose of ketamine (0.5 mg/kg IV) was reported to produce anesthesia of 32 minutes for calves undergoing umbilical hernia surgery. The intensity of analgesia produced by the lower dose of ketamine in this combination was not sufficient to prevent signs of pain during surgery, and administration of a local anesthetic solution at the incision site was required. Similar to xylazine and ketamine combination, anesthesia can be prolonged with administration of ½ of the initial dose of each drug if needed [130]. In cattle, diazepam (0.1 mg/kg IV) administered prior to ketamine (4.5 mg/kg IV) produces 10–15 minutes of surgical anesthesia. Endotracheal intubation can be achieved with this combination, but swallowing reflex may still be present. Animals usually stand 30 minutes after this combination of drugs is administered [99, 119].

In calves, Telazol (4 mg/kg IV) induces 45–60 minutes of satisfactory anesthesia with minimal cardiovascular depression [79]. In calves, Telazol induces rapid immobilization when administered in doses of 4–12 mg/kg intramuscularly. When Telazol is administered at a dose of 10 mg/kg or greater, apnea occurs. Muscle relaxation is profound, but analgesia is minimal. The overall response is characteristic of general anesthesia. Xylazine can be administered at a dose of 0.1–0.2 mg/kg IM in combination with Telazol (4 mg/kg IV) to increase the duration of anesthesia for an additional 15 and 25 minutes for 0.1 and 0.2 mg/kg, respectively. However, higher doses of xylazine tend to increase the incidence of apnea [131]. By administering a combination of xylazine (0.1 mg/kg IV) with Telazol (4 mg/kg IV), a longer duration of profound muscle relaxation and analgesia was observed when compared to Telazol (4 mg/kg IV) administered alone [83, 131].

A combination of Telazol, ketamine, and xylazine (**TKX-Ru**) has been used successfully to capture wild ruminants. When 500 mg of Telazol is reconstituted with 2.5 ml of ketamine (100 mg/ml) and 1 ml of xylazine (100 mg/ml) with a final volume of 4 ml, the concentration of each drug is 125 mg/ml of Telazol, 62.5 mg/ml of ketamine, and 25 mg/ml of xylazine, respectively. The recommended IM dose of the mixture is 1.25–1.5 ml/125 kg (275 lb) for small cattle and 1 ml/125 kg (275 lb) for larger, adult cattle. Recumbency usually occurs within 5–10 minutes following IM administration of **TKX-Ru**. Twenty minutes is required for the initial administration to reach peak anesthetic effect before repeat dosing is considered. Recovery to standing with this combination usually occurs within 40–60 minutes following **TKX-Ru** administration. Ketamine and guaifenesin mixture or **Bovine Triple Drip** described previously can be administered following **TKX-Ru** to maintain longer duration of anesthesia [132]. Table 4.1 summarizes the doses of injectable anesthetic and anesthetic combinations used in cattle.

Small ruminants and camelids

Ketamine (1 mg/ml) and guaifenesin mixture can be used to induce and maintain anesthesia in small ruminants and camelids. **Bovine Triple Drip** is a commonly used anesthetic combination for induction and maintenance of anesthesia in these animals [126]. Xylazine and ketamine are another effective and widely used anesthetic combination for these two species. In general, doses of xylazine (0.1–0.2 mg/kg IV) and ketamine (2–3 mg/kg IV) used in cattle produce similar short-term anesthesia in sheep and goats. This combination can be administered either intravenously or intramuscularly. IM xylazine (0.1–0.2 mg/kg) and ketamine (6.6–11 mg/kg) are a more convenient way to induce anesthesia in less cooperative animals [133]. Camelids are less sensitive to xylazine than are sheep and goats; thus, the dose of xylazine required in the xylazine and ketamine combination is higher when used in camelids. Short duration of anesthesia can be achieved with 0.15–0.25 mg/kg IV or 0.25–0.35 mg/kg IM of xylazine combined with 3–5 mg/kg IV or 5–8 mg/kg IM of ketamine. Longer duration of anesthesia (30–45 minutes) is produced when higher IM doses of xylazine (0.5–0.7 mg/kg) and ketamine (5–7 mg/kg) are administered. Castration can be performed successfully with 0.6 mg/kg of xylazine and 6 mg/kg of ketamine for llamas and 0.7 mg/kg of xylazine and 7 mg/kg of ketamine for alpacas [134]. Alpacas tend to be temperamental as compared to llamas; thus, high-dose ranges of xylazine and ketamine are needed to produce desirable anesthesia (Figure 4.2). **Llama Lullaby** or **BKX**, a combination of ketamine, butorphanol, and xylazine, has been used effectively to produce short-term anesthesia in alpacas and llamas [127]. The injectable solution of the combination is made up by adding 1 ml of xylazine (100 mg) and 1 ml of butorphanol (10 mg) into 10 ml of ketamine (1000 mg) with the concentration of each drug being 0.83, 83.3, and 8.3 mg/ml for butorphanol, ketamine,

Table 4.1 Doses of injectable anesthetic and anesthetic combinations used in cattle.

Drugs	Doses (mg/kg)	Comments
Ketamine	Loading dose: 2, IV CRI: 600 ml/hour of 2 mg/ml K in saline	–
Diazepam Xylazine	0.1, IV 0.2, IV	Immobilization with good analgesia
Diazepam Ketamine	0.1, IV, followed immediately 4.5, IV	Adequate muscle relaxation for tracheal intubation Anesthesia 10–15 minutes Total recumbency 30 minutes
Medetomidine Ketamine	0.02, IV 0.5, IV	Used in calves Incomplete analgesia, requires local anesthetic at the incision site
Medetomidine Ketamine	0.02, IV 2.2, IV	Anesthesia 70–120 minutes in calves
Xylazine Ketamine	0.1–0.2, IM 10–15, IM	Used in calves Anesthesia for 45 minutes Supplemental dose: K 3–5, IM, or 1–2, IV
Xylazine Ketamine	0.05–0.1, IM 4, IM	Anesthesia 30–40 minutes ½ of each IM for additional 15–20 minutes
Xylazine Ketamine	0.05, IV, wait for sedation or recumbency or mix with K 2, IV	Surgical analgesia 15–20 minutes ½ dose ketamine to extend duration for 10 minutes
Xylazine Ketamine	0.03–0.05, IV 3–5, IV	Anesthesia 15–20 minutes
Xylazine Ketamine	0.1–0.2, IV; 0.1 for>600 kg (1,320 lb) 2, IV	Preferred combination for adult large ruminants Can be given together as a bolus injection or separately with K following X Anesthesia 30 min Additional K 0.75–1.25 mg/kg for another 15 minutes
Xylazine Butorphanol Ketamine	0.1–0.15, IV 0.025–0.05, IV 0.5–1, IV, after sign of sedation with XB	Anesthesia 30 minutes Surgery for umbilical hernia repair
BKX Butorphanol Ketamine Xylazine	 0.0375, IM 3.75, IM 0.375, IM	 Anesthesia 20–30 minutes Mixture: add 1 ml LA x (100 mg) and 1 ml B (10 mg) into 10 ml K (1,000 mg); give 1 ml/20 kg (44 lb) IM Additional ½ BKX for total duration of 25–35 minutes

(Continued)

Table 4.1 (*Continued*)

Drugs	Doses (mg/kg)	Comments
Double drip Ketamine Guaifenesin	 1 mg/ml K in 5% guaifenesin 1.5–2.2 ml/kg, IV	 Morphine 0.05–0.3 mg/kg IM or butorphanol 0.05–0.2 mg/kg IM for analgesia
Bovine Triple Drip (GKX) Xylazine (1 mg/ml) Ketamine (1–2 mg/ml) in guaifenesin (5%)	 Induction: 0.67–1.1 ml/kg Maintenance: 2.2 ml/kg/hour	Adjustable dose for induction Stable plane of anesthesia Maintenance CRI to effect (1.5 ml/kg/hour for calves; 2 ml/kg/hour for adult cattle) Smooth recovery
Telazol	4, IV	Minimal cardiovascular depression in healthy calves Anesthesia 45–60 minutes Zolazepam lasts longer than tiletamine, smooth but gradual recovery
Xylazine Telazol	0.1, IM 4, IM	Anesthesia 60 min Standing in 130 minutes
Xylazine Telazol	0.05, IV 1, IV	Shorter duration than IM
Propofol	4–6, IV	Anesthesia 5–10 min Transient apnea may occur CRI 0.4 mg/kg/minutes for maintenance of light anesthesia

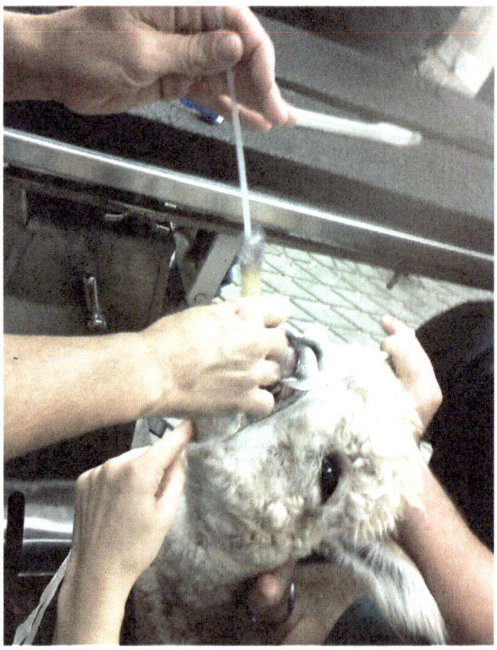

Figure 4.2 Endotracheal intubation in an alpaca anesthetized with xylazine (0.35 mg/kg IM) and ketamine (8 mg/kg IM).

and xylazine, respectively. The dose to produce 20–30 minutes of anesthesia for llamas is 1 ml/23 kg (50.6 lb) IM and for alpacas is 1 ml/18 kg (39.6 lb) IM. The resulting individual dose of each drug in this mixture for llamas is 0.036, 3.6, and 0.36 mg/kg for butorphanol, ketamine, and xylazine, respectively, and 0.046, 4.6, and 0.46 mg/kg, respectively, for alpacas [127, 135]. The same **Llama Lullaby** or **BKX** combination has also been administered at 1 ml/91 kg (200.2 lb) IM to goats to produce anesthesia. More rapid and complete anesthetic response occurs when the IM injection is made in the triceps muscles [127, 136]. Lateral recumbency generally occurs within 4–7 minutes after **BKX** administration with anesthetic effect sufficient for minor surgical procedures. However, endotracheal intubation may be difficult to accomplish with this combination at this dose. Addition of infiltration of local anesthetic to the incision site may be required for more painful surgery, for example, castration. The times to return to sternal recumbency and standing in llamas and alpacas anesthetized with **BKX** were 43 ± 14.6 minutes and 62.9 ± 12.6 minutes, respectively, for llamas and 18.4 ± 7.7 minutes and 21.9 ± 10.4 minutes, respectively, for alpacas [136]. This shows that at this dosage range, the duration of anesthesia is shorter in alpacas and repeat dosing to prolong anesthesia is more likely to be needed for alpacas. A **modified BKX** has been described, using 8 mg of xylazine, 8 mg of butorphanol, and 400 mg of ketamine mixture with the final concentration of each drug being 1.6, 8, and 1.6 mg/ml for butorphanol, ketamine, and xylazine, respectively. Safe anesthesia is produced in sheep when the combination is given at 0.022 ml/kg IV (xylazine 0.03 mg/kg, ketamine 1.6 mg/kg, butorphanol 0.03 mg/kg) [127]. Anderson [137] reported that a combination of xylazine (0.2 mg/kg IV, 0.4 mg/kg IM), butorphanol (0.1 mg/kg IV or IM), and ketamine (2 mg/kg IV, 4 mg/kg IM) provided 20 minutes of surgical anesthesia for minor surgical procedures, such as castration, in camelids. However, careful titration of the IV dose of ketamine is required as respiratory depression, or even arrest has been observed after bolus IV injection of 2 mg/kg of ketamine.

Other α_2 agonists such as detomidine and medetomidine have also been used in combination with ketamine to produce short-term anesthesia. A combination of detomidine (0.02–0.04 mg/kg IM) and ketamine (2–4 mg/kg IM) has been used in New World camelids with subsequent administration of atipamezole to shorten the recovery time [91]. Only deep sedation was observed when 0.05 mg/kg of medetomidine was combined with 1 mg/kg of ketamine and administered intramuscularly to llamas. Surgical anesthesia was produced when a higher dose of ketamine (2 mg/kg IV) was administered with medetomidine (0.02 mg/kg IV) in sheep and goats. For more vigorous small ruminants, diazepam (0.44 mg/kg) and ketamine (6.6 mg/kg) combination can be administered intravenously as a bolus injection to induce short-term anesthesia [138]. α_2 agonists such as xylazine, detomidine, and medetomidine are associated with a significant increase in urine output and may be contraindicated in animals with urethral obstruction. Hyperkalemia with characteristic bradycardia, arrhythmias, and occasional cardiac arrest has been observed in goats with urethral obstruction (personal observation). Therefore, the minimal cardiovascular depression produced by diazepam makes this drug a good substitution for α_2 agonists to combine with ketamine for use in severely compromised animals. Diazepam (5 mg/ml) can be mixed with ketamine (100 mg/ml) at equal volumes and administered at 1 ml/18–22 kg (39.6–48.4 lb) to sheep and goats for short-term anesthesia of 15–20 minutes. Administration of an analgesic such as butorphanol (0.05–0.1 mg/kg IV or IM) or morphine (0.05–0.1 mg/kg IV or IM) may be needed for painful procedures [116].

Telazol (2.2–6.6 mg/kg IM) can be administered to small ruminants to induce general anesthesia lasting 60–100 minutes. When given intravenously, higher doses of Telazol (8–20 mg/kg) produce surgical anesthesia. The induction is reported to be exceptionally smooth with surgical anesthesia ranging from 40 minutes to 3.7 hours. Significant decrease in minute ventilation and respiratory airflow that is characterized by apneustic breathing pattern occurred with Telazol when administered at an IV dose of 12 or 24 mg/kg [139]. Twelve mg/kg of Telazol administered intramuscularly appears to be the optimal dose to produce surgical anesthesia lasting approximately 30 minutes. Administering butorphanol (0.5 mg/kg IV) along with Telazol (12 mg/kg IV) anesthesia simultaneously or prior to administration of Telazol provides good analgesia for 25–50 minutes [84]. In goats, Telazol (5 mg/kg IV) with or without butorphanol (0.1 mg/kg IV) has been used for laparotomy and embryo collecting procedures. Supplemental doses of Telazol (0.5–1 mg/kg IV) were administered to extend anesthesia. At the completion of the surgery, the average total dose of Telazol was 10.46 ± 1.64 mg/kg when administered alone and 10.53 ± 2.0 mg/kg when administered with butorphanol. Interestingly, Carroll *et al.* (1997) [140] reported that adding butorphanol to Telazol anesthesia did not improve visceral analgesia or prolong the duration of Telazol-induced anesthesia. Compared to Telazol alone, xylazine (0.11 mg/kg IV) combined with Telazol (13.2 mg/kg IV) produces a longer duration of analgesia in sheep, 41.6 and 101.7 minutes, respectively. Apnea may occur after administering this combination, and sheep may require assisted ventilation immediately after IV injection of the combination. Nonetheless, apnea is short-lived with spontaneous breathing returning within 2 minutes [90]. In llamas, Telazol (4.4 mg/kg IM) provides good chemical restraint, but muscle relaxation and analgesia are not sufficient for surgery [78].

Propofol is best used for induction before inhalation anesthesia, and it is also used as a continuous infusion to maintain longer duration of anesthesia in small ruminants [101–103]. A single dose of propofol (2 mg/kg) produces approximately 10 minutes of anesthesia with complete recovery occurring within 20–30 minutes [99, 100]. Duke *et al.* (1997) [108] evaluated the cardiopulmonary effects of propofol infusion in llamas. Anesthesia was induced with 2 mg/kg IV and maintained using two different infusion rates, 12 and 24 mg/kg/hour, for 1 hour. Only the higher infusion rate induced adequate anesthesia. Increased heart rate and mean carotid arterial pressure were observed during anesthesia. Three llamas became dyspneic and required nasotracheal intubation to maintain a patent airway even though $PaCO_2$ in these llamas remained within normal range. All llamas recovered and stood at 13–20 minutes after discontinuation of infusion with little to no ataxia [108]. In goats, a combination of detomidine, butorphanol, and propofol has been used for induction followed by continuous IV infusion for maintenance to provide surgical anesthesia for castration or ovariectomy [141]. Comparing propofol (3 mg/kg IV), thiopental (8 mg/kg IV), or ketamine (10 mg/kg IV) as induction agents in goats, propofol was reported to be superior to thiopental or ketamine because recovery was rapid and uneventful [105]. Total intravenous anesthesia (TIVA) with ketamine and propofol infusion has been used successfully to maintain immobilization and anesthesia in goats undergoing magnetic resonance imaging procedure. These goats were sedated with midazolam (0.4 mg/kg IV), and anesthesia was induced with propofol (1 mg/kg IV) and ketamine (3 mg/kg IV) and maintained with constant infusion rates of propofol (18 mg/kg/hour) and ketamine (1.8 mg/kg/hour) with or without sevoflurane [142]. Table 4.2 summarizes the doses of injectable anesthetic and anesthetic combinations used in sheep, goats, and camelids.

Table 4.2 Doses of injectable anesthetic and anesthetic combinations for sheep, goats, and camelids.

Drugs	Dosage in sheep and goats (mg/kg)	Dosage in camelids (mg/kg)	Comments
Ketamine (1 mg/ml) in 5% guaifenesin	Induction: 2 ml/kg, 50–75% of calculated dose first Maintenance: 2.2 ml/kg/hour or to effect	Induction: 2 ml/kg, 65–75% of calculated dose first Maintenance: 2.2 ml/kg/hour or to effect	–
Acepromazine Ketamine	0.55, IV 2.2, IV	N/A	–
Detomidine Ketamine Butorphanol	0.022, IV 2.2, IV 0.4, IV	0.02, IV 2.2, IV 0.4, IV	–
Diazepam Ketamine	Mix 1 ml D (5 mg) and 1 ml K (100 mg); give 1 ml/18–22 kg (40–48 lb), IV	–	Anesthesia 15–20 minutes Additional analgesia: butorphanol 0.05–0.1 mg/kg IV, IM, or morphine 0.05–0.1 mg/kg, IV, IM
Diazepam Ketamine	1–2, IM 10–15, IM	0.2–0.3, IM 5–8, IM	Light to medium anesthesia 20–30 minutes
Diazepam Ketamine	0.5–1, IV 4, IV	–	Anesthesia 15–20 minutes Recumbency 30 minutes
Diazepam Ketamine	0.25–0.5, IV 4–7.5, IV	–	Anesthesia 15–20 minutes Recumbency 30 minutes
Diazepam Ketamine	–	0.1, IV 2.2–4.4, IV	Anesthesia 5–10 minutes
Diazepam Ketamine	–	0.05–0.2, IV 4, IV	Anesthesia 10–20 minutes
Diazepam Ketamine	0.11, IV 4.4, IV	0.2–0.3, IM 5–8, IM	Anesthesia 10–20 minutes
Diazepam Ketamine	–	0.1, IV 2.2, IV	Anesthesia 5–10 minutes
Diazepam Ketamine	0.25–0.5, IV 4–7.5, IV	0.05–0.2, IV 4, IV	Anesthesia 5–10 minutes
Ketamine Guaifenesin (5%)	–	1.6, IV 80, IV	Anesthesia 15–20 minutes

(*Continued*)

Table 4.2 (*Continued*)

Drugs	Dosage in sheep and goats (mg/kg)	Dosage in camelids (mg/kg)	Comments
Medetomidine Ketamine	0.015, IM 5, IM	–	Anesthesia 45 minutes
Medetomidine Ketamine	0.02, IV 2, IV	0.05, IM 1, IM	Deep sedation in camelids
Medetomidine Ketamine	0.025, IV 1, IV	0.025–0.035, IM 1–1.5, IM	Light anesthesia 30–60 minutes
Midazolam Ketamine	0.4, IM 4, IV	–	Anesthesia 15 minutes
Xylazine Ketamine	0.1, IV 2.2, IV	0.22–0.44 IV 2.2–2.5, IV	Anesthesia 30–60 minutes
 Xylazine Ketamine Ketamine Xylazine	Goats 0.1, IM 3–5, IM Sheep 0.2, IM 3–5, IM	 0.03–0.05, IV 3–5, IV 0.5, IM 2.2, IV	High range for alpacas Anesthesia 15–20 minutes –
Xylazine Ketamine	–	0.44, IV 4.4, IV	Anesthesia 15–25 minutes
Xylazine Ketamine	–	0.25–0.35, IM 6–10, IM	Recumbency 30–60 minutes
Xylazine Ketamine Xylazine Ketamine Xylazine Ketamine	0.11–0.22, IM, wait for 10 min 10–15, IM – – 	0.35, IM 5–8, IM 0.8, IM 8, IM 1.2, IM 12, IM	Induction of anesthesia& intubation Analgesia 15–45 min Anesthesia 30 min Analgesia 50–70 min
Xylazine Ketamine	0.2, IM 15, IM	0.22, IM, wait for 10 minutes 10–15, IM	High-dose range for alpacas
Xylazine Ketamine	–	Add 1 ml X (100 mg/ml) to 10 ml (100 mg/ml) K, 1 ml/23 kg (51 lb) IV, IM	Anesthesia 15–25 minutes
Xylazine Ketamine	–	0.5–0.7, IM 5–7, IM	Low dose range for llamas High-dose range for alpacas Anesthesia 30–45 minutes

CHAPTER 4

Table 4.2 (*Continued*)

Drugs	Dosage in sheep and goats (mg/kg)	Dosage in camelids (mg/kg)	Comments
BKX **(Llama Lullaby)*** Butorphanol Ketamine Xylazine Butorphanol Ketamine Xylazine	 **1 ml/91 kg (200 lb), IM** 0.009, IM 0.92, IM 0.09, IM **1 ml/23 kg (51 lb), IM; 1 ml/45 kg (99 lb), IV** 0.037, IM 0.018, IV 3.7, IM 1.8, IV 0.37, IM 0.18, IV	 **Llamas 1 ml/23 kg (51 lb), IM** 0.037, IM 3.7, IM 0.37, IM **Alpacas 1 ml/18 kg (40 lb), IM** 0.046, IM 4.6, IM 0.46, IM	*Add 1 ml of X (100 mg/ml), 1 ml of B (10 mg/ml) to 10 ml of K (100 mg/ml) Concentration of mixture: 8.3 mg/ml X, 83.3 mg/ml K, and 0.83 mg/ml B Recumbency 18–43 minutes
Modified BKX[£] Xylazine Ketamine Butorphanol	0.02 ml/kg, IV 0.03, IV 1.6, IV 0.03, IV	–	[£]Add 8 mg of xylazine, 8 mg of butorphanol to 400 mg (4 ml) of ketamine; total volume 5 ml; concentration of mixture: 1.6 mg/ml X, 80 mg/ml K, and 1.6 mg/ml B Reduce xylazine dose
Xylazine Ketamine Butorphanol	–	0.22–0.33, IV 0.077–0.11, IV 0.22–0.33, IV	Recumbency 15–20 minutes Analgesia
Xylazine Ketamine Butorphanol	–	0.22–0.55, IM 0.22–0.55, IM 0.055–0.11, IM	Recumbency 45 minutes
Butorphanol Ketamine Xylazine	–	0.1 1.5 0.2	Anesthesia 20 minutes Castration
Bovine Triple Drip (GKX) Xylazine (1 mg/ml) Ketamine (1–2 mg/ml) in 5% guaifenesin	Induction: 0.67–1.1 ml/kg Maintenance: 2.2 ml/kg/hour	Induction: 0.67–1.1 ml/kg Maintenance: 2.2 ml/kg/hour	Adjustable dose for induction Stable plane of anesthesia Maintenance CRI to effect Smooth recovery
Propofol	4–6, IV	–	Light anesthesia 5–10 minutes
Propofol	Induction: 3–4, IV, or Induction: 4–8, IV Maintenance: 18–40 mg/kg/hour IV infusion or to effect	Induction: 2–3.5, IV Maintenance: 24 mg/kg/hour	Rapid induction Rapid recovery

(*Continued*)

CHAPTER 4

Table 4.2 (Continued)

Drugs	Dosage in sheep and goats (mg/kg)	Dosage in camelids (mg/kg)	Comments
Xylazine Butorphanol Diazepam Propofol	–	0.1–0.2, SC, IM 0.06–0.12, IM 0.5, IV 3.5, IV	For cesarean section Anesthesia maintained with isoflurane Minimal fetal effect
Telazol	–	2, IV	Anesthesia 15–20 minutes Recumbency 25–35 minutes Poor muscle relaxation
Telazol	2–4, IV, or 5.5, IV	4.4, IM	Anesthesia 100 minutes Butorphanol 0.1, IV, can be added
Telazol Butorphanol	2–5, IV 0.1, IV	2–5, IV 0.1, IV	Anesthesia
Atropine Xylazine Telazol	–	0.04, IV 0.25, IV 1, IV	Anesthesia for laparotomy

Swine

Pigs do not tolerate restraint well, and they often protest strongly with loud noises and vigorous struggling. Gentle handling with little restraint should be practiced to avoid stress and overheating, particularly during hot and humid weather as pigs are known to be more susceptible to malignant hyperthermia than other domestic species. Thus, IM administration of anesthetic drugs is preferred over more stressful IV injection. Adverse effects such as muscle tremor and extensor rigidity observed with IM ketamine alone can be minimized by combining ketamine (10–20 mg/kg IM) with drugs that produce central muscle relaxation such as diazepam (1 mg/kg IM) or xylazine (2–3 mg/kg IM). Addition of diazepam or xylazine to ketamine also reduces the potential for excitement to occur during recovery. IM diazepam (1 mg/kg) or xylazine (2 mg/kg) can be combined with ketamine (11–17.6 mg/kg) for minor procedures of short duration. Though deep sedation and good muscle relaxation occur with these combinations, pigs may still respond to noxious stimuli such as incision of the abdominal wall [75, 76, 138]. Supplemental dosing with ½ of the original dose of xylazine and ketamine may be required for tracheal intubation [76]. This author (Lin) prefers simultaneous administration of xylazine (2.2 mg/kg IV) and ketamine (2.2 mg/kg IV) to induce a short period of satisfactory anesthesia when IV injection is possible. Alternatively, a combination of oxymorphone (0.075 mg/kg), xylazine (2 mg/kg), and ketamine (2 mg/kg) mixed in the same syringe and given intravenously induces surgical anesthesia with good analgesia and muscle relaxation. When given intramuscularly, satisfactory response can be achieved by doubling the dose of each drug [65, 143]. Short-term anesthesia in pigs can also be achieved by administering either of these two-drug combinations: butorphanol (0.2 mg/kg IM), xylazine (2 mg/kg IM), and ketamine (10 mg/kg IM) or butorphanol (0.2 mg/kg IM), medetomidine (0.08 mg/kg IM), and ketamine (10 mg/kg IM). Rapid induction of anesthesia occurs with either combination. The combination of butorphanol, medetomidine, and ketamine induces more adequate anesthesia for 98.8 ± 22.5 minutes, which is characterized by good muscle relaxation appropriate for endotracheal intubation. Atipamezole (0.24 mg/kg IV or IM) can be administered to shorten the duration of anesthesia from either combination [144]. Another report shows that medetomidine and ketamine combination induces longer duration of muscle relaxation (43.6 ± 12.7 minutes vs. 21.0 ± 14 minutes) and anesthesia (49.4 ± 13.5 minutes vs. 34.6 ± 17.2 minutes) than xylazine and ketamine combination in pigs. Slight cardiovascular stimulation with minimal respiratory effect is observed during medetomidine and ketamine anesthesia [145]. Intratesticular injection of xylazine (1–2 mg/kg) and ketamine (3–5 mg/kg) has been used to induce immobilization and anesthesia for castration of mature boars. Half the calculated dose of the combination is injected into each testicle. Surgical removal of the testicle removes the drugs not yet absorbed from the testicle, which, as a result, shortens the duration of immobilization and hastens the recovery from anesthesia [65].

As in horses and ruminants, the combination of guaifenesin (50 mg/ml), xylazine (1 mg/ml), and ketamine (1 mg/ml) (**Swine Triple Drip**) is a very useful anesthetic regimen for pigs of all ages. It should be recognized that the concentration of xylazine in this mixture is twice that used in horses and ten times that used in ruminants. With this combination, anesthesia can be induced rapidly when administered at 0.55–1 ml/kg via a catheterized auricular vein. For prolonged procedures, anesthesia can be maintained by continuous infusion at 2.2–4.4 ml/kg/hour. Mean arterial pressure and systemic vascular resistance increase in pigs anesthetized with **Swine Triple Drip**. During anesthesia, heart rate decreases but the rate remains within an acceptable range. The $PaCO_2$ decreases, while PaO_2 remains unaffected. In general, continuous infusion of **Swine Triple Drip** induces minimal cardiopulmonary changes similar to those observed in pigs anesthetized with inhalation anesthetics. This mixture has been used to induce satisfactory anesthesia in healthy swine for up to 2 hours [146].

In miniature swine, acepromazine (0.39 mg/kg IM) and ketamine (15 mg/kg IM) combination produces anesthesia for 65–80 minutes [147]. When used with **Innovar-Vet** (proprietary combination of droperidol and fentanyl, 1 ml/15 kg IM), ketamine (12–16 mg/kg IM) induces surgical anesthesia of 30–40 minutes. Prolongation of anesthesia can be achieved with supplemental ketamine (2.2 mg/kg IV or 6.6 mg/kg IM) [148].

Xylazine (2 mg/kg IM), ketamine (5 mg/kg IM), and butorphanol (0.1 mg/kg IM) have been used successfully to produce light anesthesia in Vietnamese potbellied pigs for electroejaculation and artificial insemination [149]. Ketamine has also been combined with diazepam (0.5–1 mg/kg IM) or midazolam (0.2–0.4 mg/kg IM) to produce short-term anesthesia [138, 150, 151]. In miniature pigs, the anesthetic effect produced by xylazine (2 mg/kg IM), ketamine (5 mg/kg IM), and butorphanol (0.22 mg/kg IM) is reported to be better, more potent, and longer lasting (62 ± 13 minutes vs. 28 ± 19 minutes) than that of xylazine (2 mg/kg IM) and ketamine (15 mg/kg IM). The quality of recovery is also believed to be better and smoother when the xylazine, ketamine, and butorphanol combination is administered [152].

Telazol alone (2–4 mg/kg) can be administered intramuscularly to induce immobilization and anesthesia adequate for minor diagnostic procedures in pigs, but muscle relaxation and analgesia are deemed insufficient for surgery. Butorphanol (0.2 mg/kg) can be given concomitantly for more painful procedures. Combining xylazine (1.1 or 2.2 mg/kg IM) with Telazol (6 mg/kg IM) induces effective and safe anesthesia with good muscle relaxation for approximately 1 hour. Pigs become recumbent within 1–2 minutes following xylazine and Telazol injection. Heart rate increases but decreases gradually below baseline values at 45 minutes. Respiratory rate also increases but returns to baseline 15 minutes later. Duration of analgesia is prolonged when higher doses of xylazine are administered (68 minutes vs. 47 minutes) [153]. IV administration of xylazine (2.2 mg/kg) and Telazol (2.2 mg/kg) combination has been recommended for short-term anesthesia or for induction where anesthesia is to be maintained with an inhalation anesthetic. Repeat dosing of Telazol to extend the duration of anesthesia is not recommended since prolonged recovery may occur, especially in older pigs. Xylazine and ketamine combination may be a better option to extend the duration of xylazine and Telazol anesthesia if needed. In feral swine (*Sus scrofa*) and wild collard peccaries (*Tayassu tajacu*), IM xylazine and Telazol combination has been a very effective immobilizing drug combination. The combination is given at 4–5 mg/kg of each drug or by mixing 1 ml of Telazol (100 mg/ml) with 1 ml of xylazine (100 mg/ml) and administering 0.04–0.05 ml/kg of the mixture. Immobilization occurs within 5 minutes with the pigs recovering to standing in 54–78 minutes after administration of the drugs [154]. Female babirusa (*Babyrousa babyrussa*: deer hog of Indonesia) was shown to require higher doses of xylazine and Telazol (xylazine 1.88 ± 0.37 mg/kg IM, Telazol 2.2 mg/kg IM) than males (xylazine 1.22 ± 0.16 mg/kg IM, Telazol 1.7 mg/kg IM). Rapid immobilization with good analgesia and muscle relaxation are the characteristic anesthetic effects of this combination. In this report, yohimbine (0.15 mg/kg IM) and flumazenil (1 mg/20 mg of zolazepam IM) are administered to antagonize the pharmacological effects of xylazine and zolazepam, respectively. Compared to yohimbine, atipamezole (0.2–0.3 mg/kg IM) appears to be more effective in reversing xylazine's effects [155].

Prolonged recovery associated with Telazol anesthesia in swine is believed to be due to zolazepam. When using Telazol alone, it is impossible to increase the concentration of tiletamine without increasing the concentration of zolazepam since the drug is a proprietary combination. In an effort to reduce the dose of zolazepam used for Telazol anesthesia and to shorten recovery, 2.5 ml of ketamine and 2.5 ml of 10% xylazine were used to reconstitute Telazol powder (**TKX-P**). The resulting solution contains 50 mg each of tiletamine, ketamine, zolazepam, and xylazine per ml, and the final dissociative concentration (i.e., ketamine and tiletamine) is 100 mg/ml, providing a 2:1 ratio of dissociative anesthetics to either zolazepam or xylazine. The addition of xylazine and ketamine in this combination increases the anesthetic action and dissociative anesthetic concentrations relative to the concentration of zolazepam. The dose volume necessary to produce anesthesia is decreased, as is the dose component of zolazepam. Consequently, prolonged recovery often observed when Telazol alone is administered is shortened with **TKX-P** [65, 151, 156, 157]. The anesthetic effect induced by this combination

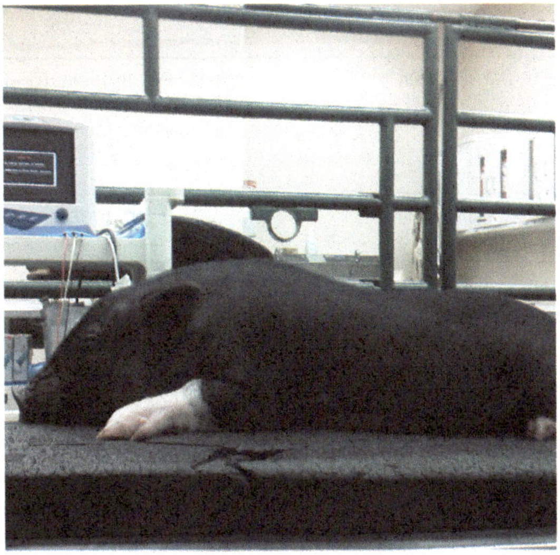

Figure 4.3 A potbellied pig anesthetized with Telazol, ketamine, and xylazine (**TKX-P**) combination.

is dose dependent. For commercial pigs, the dose recommended for sedation to anesthesia is 1 ml/35–75 kg (77–165 lb) IM. In potbellied pigs, the dose required to induce sedation and immobilization for a duration of 35–40 minutes is 0.007–0.013 ml/kg IM. Doses of 0.02–0.026 ml/kg IM induce muscle relaxation adequate for tracheal intubation and surgical anesthesia for 25–35 minutes (Figure 4.3). Anesthesia can be safely extended by a supplemental IV dose of 0.006 ml/kg of **TKX-P** given slowly over 60 seconds. When this combination is used to induce anesthesia, the inhalation anesthetic requirement for maintenance is decreased by approximately 40–50%. The anesthetic effects of IM **TKX-P** (Telazol 4.4 mg/kg, ketamine 2.2 mg/kg, and xylazine 2.2 mg/kg), xylazine (4 mg/kg) and ketamine (8 mg/kg) combination, and xylazine (2.2–4.4 mg/kg) and Telazol (4.4 mg/kg) combination were studied [158]. The results showed that all four combinations produced safe and satisfactory anesthesia. However, **TKX-P** and xylazine and Telazol (xylazine 4.4 mg/kg, Telazol 4.4 mg/kg) were preferred drug combinations for injectable anesthesia. Many practitioners commented that **TKX-P** produced reliable anesthesia with good analgesia and muscle relaxation. In addition, only one single IM injection of **TKX-P** was needed to induce anesthesia as compared to the need of IV catheter for administration of **Swine Triple Drip** [65, 156, 159].

In pigs weighing 30–60 kg, medetomidine (0.02–0.04 mg/kg) and propofol (2–4 mg/kg) combination induces a light plane of anesthesia. Though medetomidine may provide some degree of analgesia, adding a potent analgesic may be necessary for painful procedures [160]. Martin-Cancho *et al.* (2004) [161] reported that combining propofol (11 mg/kg IV) with an opioid analgesic, fentanyl (2.5 mg/kg IV, every 30 minutes), produced surgical anesthesia for abdominal surgery [161]. The need for IV administration of propofol limits its use in pigs. Table 4.3 summarizes the doses of injectable anesthetic and anesthetic combinations used in pigs.

Table 4.3 Doses of injectable anesthetic and anesthetic combinations used in pigs.

Drugs	Doses (mg/kg)	Comments
Ketamine	10–20, IM	–
Acepromazine Ketamine	0.1–0.4, IM 10–20, IM	Anesthesia 15–30 minutes
Acepromazine Ketamine	0.5, IM 15, IM	Recumbency 18 minutes
Acepromazine Ketamine	1.1, IM 10, IM	Light anesthesia 20–30 minutes
Azaperone Ketamine Propofol	2, IM 10, IM 1.87 ± 0.6, IV	Maintenance of anesthesia: isoflurane
Azaperone Xylazine Ketamine	2, IM 0.2, IM 2, IM	40–60 minutes
Azaperone Meperidine Morphine Ketamine	2.2, IM 2.2, IM 1.7, IM 22, IM	Ketamine–morphine 20 minutes after azaperone–meperidine Surgical anesthesia for 60–120 minutes
Detomidine Butorphanol Midazolam	0.125, IM 0.3, IM 0.3, IM	Anesthesia
Detomidine Butorphanol Ketamine	0.1, IM 0.1–0.2, IM 5, IM	–
Diazepam Ketamine	1–2, IM 12–20, IM	Duration 20–40 minutes
Diazepam Ketamine	2, IM 15, IM	–
Diazepam Ketamine	1.1, IM 11–17.6, IM	Short-term anesthesia
Diazepam Ketamine	1:2 ratio of D:K 1 ml/10 kg (22 lb), IV	–
Medetomidine Ketamine	0.1, IM 1, IM	–
Medetomidine Ketamine	0.08, IM 10, IM	Light anesthesia for 40–90 minutes
Medetomidine Butorphanol Ketamine	0.03–0.08, IM 0.1–0.2, IM 5, IM	Anesthesia for 60–120 minutes
Medetomidine Butorphanol Ketamine	0.08, IM 0.2, IM 2, IM	Anesthesia for 60–120 minutes
Medetomidine Butorphanol Ketamine	0.08, IM 0.2, IM 10, IM	Anesthesia for 75–100 minutes
Medetomidine Midazolam Butorphanol	0.04–0.07, IM 0.08–0.3, IM 0.15–0.3, IM	–
Medetomidine Midazolam Butorphanol	0.06, IM 0.3, IM 0.3, IM	Good anesthesia Analgesia

Table 4.3 (*Continued*)

Drugs	Doses (mg/kg)	Comments
Midazolam Ketamine	0.1–0.5, IM 10–15, IM	Duration 20–40 minutes
Midazolam Ketamine	0.5–2, IM 10–15, IM	Light anesthesia for 20–30 minutes
Midazolam Ketamine	0.5, SC 25, SC	Effective anesthesia for instrumentation for cardiovascular catheterization
Midazolam Ketamine	0.5, IM 33, IM	–
Propofol	2.5–3.5, IV	Surgical anesthesia for 5–10 minutes
Propofol	2–5, IV	Duration 2–5 minutes
Propofol	6.6–8.8, IV	–
Propofol	9–11, IV	–
Fentanyl Propofol	2.5, IV CRI: 11 mg/kg/hour	Fentanyl every 30 minutes
Medetomidine Propofol	0.02–0.04, IM, IV 2–4, IV	Light anesthesia
Xylazine Propofol	1–2, IM, IV 2–4, IV	Light anesthesia
Romifidine Butorphanol Ketamine	0.12, IM 0.1, IM 5–8, IM	–
Xylazine Ketamine	0.2, IM 11, IM	Recumbency 25 minutes
Xylazine Ketamine	0.5, IM 5, IM	Anesthesia 5–15 minutes
Xylazine Ketamine	2, intratesticularly 6, intratesticularly	Castration
Xylazine Ketamine	2, IM 20, IM	Duration 20–40 minutes ½ of each drug needed for tracheal intubation
Xylazine Ketamine	2.2, IM 12–20, IM	Anesthesia extended with 2–4 mg/kg K IV
Xylazine Ketamine	1.1, IM 11–17.6, IM	Short-term anesthesia
Azaperone Xylazine Ketamine	2, IM 0.2, IM 2, IM	Duration 40–60 minutes
Xylazine Butorphanol Ketamine	2, IM 0.22, IM 10–11, IM	Short-term anesthesia for abdominal surgery Duration 60–120 minutes
Xylazine Medetomidine Ketamine	0.2, IM 0.08, IM 2, IM	Duration 60–120 min
Xylazine Midazolam Ketamine	2, IM 0.25, IM 20, IM	Anesthesia 70–100 minutes

(*Continued*)

Table 4.3 *(Continued)*

Drugs	Doses (mg/kg)	Comments
Swine Triple Drip (GKX) Guaifenesin (5%) Xylazine Ketamine	Add 1 mg/ml X, 1–2 mg/ml K in 5% guaifenesin Induction: 0.67–1.1 ml/kg, IV CRI maintenance: 2.2 ml/kg/hour, IV	–
Xylazine Ketamine Oxymorphone	4, IM 4, IM 0.15, IM	Anesthesia 40–60 minutes
Xylazine Ketamine Oxymorphone	2.2, IV 2, IV 0.075, IV	Anesthesia 20–30 minutes
Xylazine Ketamine Tramadol	2.5, IM 25, IM 5, IM	Anesthesia 30–60 minutes
Telazol	2.2, IV	–
Telazol Telazol Telazol	2–4, IM 1–5, IM 6.6, IM	Short-term anesthesia for 20–30 minutes Diagnostic procedures Smooth induction, poor muscle relaxation and recovery
Telazol	6–8, IM	Light anesthesia for 20–30 minutes
Butorphanol Telazol	0.2, IM 2–4, IM	Painful procedures
Xylazine Telazol	0.2–1, IM 2–7, IM	Light to medium anesthesia for 30–40 minutes
Xylazine Telazol	0.5–2.2, IM 3–6, IM	Anesthesia for 30–50 minutes
Xylazine Telazol	0.22–2.2, IM 6.6, IM	X improves muscle relaxation and ease of recovery
Xylazine Telazol	1–4, IM 4–6, IM	Anesthesia for 30–60 minutes
Xylazine Telazol	5 ml LA × (500 mg) in 500 mg T 1 ml/45 kg (99 lb)	Anesthesia
Xylazine Telazol Tramadol	1.2, IM 3, IM 1.6, IM	Anesthesia for 78 minutes Excellent muscle relaxation and analgesia
Acepromazine Ketamine Telazol	0.03–0.1, IM 2.2, IM 4.4, IM	Anesthesia 40–50 minutes
Xylazine Ketamine Telazol	2.5 ml LA × (250 mg) and 2.5 ml K (250 mg) in 500 mg T 0.012–0.018 ml/kg, IM; 1 ml/83–56 kg (183–123 lb), IM 0.018–0.024 ml/kg, IM; 1 ml/56–42 kg (123–92 lb), IM 1 ml/35 kg (77 lb), IM	Smooth induction Immobilization Good muscle relaxation for tracheal intubation Duration 20–35 minutes Duration 45–60 minutes
Xylazine Ketamine Telazol	2.2, IM 2.2, IM 4.4, IM	Anesthesia for 47–60 minutes
Xylazine Ketamine Telazol	4.4, IM 2.2, IM 4.4, IM	Anesthesia for 60–75 minutes

Field anesthesia with injectable anesthetics provides a convenient method allowing many minor procedures to be completed in the field. Knowledge of the pharmacologic effects of the anesthetic used alone and in combination, type of procedure to be performed, and the duration required to complete the procedure are important for selecting an appropriate anesthetic or anesthetic combination to ensure safe anesthesia and uneventful recovery of the patient.

References

1. Cohen, M., Chan, S., Way, W. and Trevor, A. (1973) Distribution in the brain and metabolism of ketamine in the rat after intravenous administration. *Anesthesiology*, 39, 370–376.
2. Miyasaka, M. and Domino, E. (1968) Neuronal mechanisms of ketamine-induced anesthesia. *International Journal of Neuropharmacology*, 7, 557–573.
3. Massopust, L., Wolin, L. and Albin, M. (1973) The effect of a new phencyclidine derivative and diazepinone derivative on the electroencephalographic and behavioral responses in the cat. *Tower International Technomedical – Journal of Life Sciences*, 3, 1–10.
4. Kohrs, R. and Durieux, M. (1998) Ketamine: teaching an old drug new tricks. *Anesthesia and Analgesia*, 87, 1186–1193.
5. Brockmeyer, D. and Kendig, J. (1995) Selective effects of ketamine on amino acid-mediated pathways in neonatal rat spinal cord. *British Journal of Anaesthesia*, 74, 79–84.
6. Ohtani, M., Kikuchi, H., Kitahata, L. *et al.* (1979) Effects of ketamine on nociceptive cells in the medial medullary reticular formation of the cat. *Anesthesiology*, 51, 414–417.
7. Kitahata, L., Taub, A. and Kosaka, Y. (1973) Lamina-specific suppression of dorsal-horn unit activity by ketamine hydrochloride. *Anesthesiology*, 38, 4–11.
8. Wong, D. and Jenkins, L. (1974) An experimental study of the mechanism of action of ketamine on the central nervous system. *Canadian Anaesthetists' Society journal*, 21, 57–67.
9. Ivankovitch, A., Miletich, D., Reinmann, C. *et al.* (1974) Cardiovascular effects of centrally administered ketamine in goats. *Anesthesia and Analgesia*, 53, 924–933.
10. Salt, P., Barnes, P. and Beswick, F. (1979) Inhibition of neuronal and extraneuronal uptake of noradrenaline by ketamine in the isolated perfused rat heart. *British Journal of Anaesthesia*, 51, 835–838.
11. Altura, B., Altura, B. and Carella, A. (1980) Effects of ketamine on vascular smooth muscle function. *British Journal of Pharmacology*, 70, 257–267.
12. Tweed, W., Minuck, M. and Mymin, D. (1972) Circulatory responses to ketamine anesthesia. *Anesthesiology*, 37, 613–619.
13. Baraka, A., Harrison, T. and Kachachi, T. (1973) Catecholamine levels after ketamine anesthesia in man. *Anesthesia and Analgesia*, 52, 198–200.
14. Zsigmond, E., Kothary, S., Kumar, S. *et al.* (1980) Counteraction of circulatory side effect of ketamine by pretreatment with diazepam. *Clinical Therapeutics*, 3, 28–32.
15. Jackson, A., Dhadphale, P., Callaghan, M. and Alseri, S. (1978) Haemodynamic studies during induction of anaesthesia for open-heart surgery using diazepam and ketamine. *British Journal of Anaesthesia*, 50, 375–378.
16. Bålfors, E., Haggmark, S., Nyhman, H. *et al.* (1983) Droperidol inhibits the effects intravenous ketamine on central hemodynamics and myocardial oxygen consumption in patients with generalized atherosclerotic disease. *Anesthesia and Analgesia*, 62, 193–197.
17. Bidwai, A., Stanley, H., Graves, C. *et al.* (1975) The effects of ketamine on cardiovascular dynamics during halothane and enflurane anesthesia. *Anesthesia and Analgesia*, 54, 588–592.

18. Reich, D. and Silvay, G. (1989) Ketamine: an update on the first twenty five years of clinical experience. *Canadian Journal of Anesthesia*, 36, 186–197.
19. Evans, J., Rosen, M., Weeks, R. and Wise, C. (1971) Ketamine in neurosurgical procedures. *Lancet*, 1, 40–41.
20. Gardner, A., Olson, B. and Lichtiger, M. (1971) Cerebrospinal-fluid pressure during dissociative anesthesia with ketamine. *Anesthesiology*, 35, 226–228.
21. Shapiro, H., Wyte, S. and Harris, A. (1972) Ketamine anesthesia in patients with intracranial pathology. *British Journal of Anaesthesia*, 44, 1200–1204.
22. Takeshita, H., Okuda, Y. and Sari, A. (1972) The effects of ketamine on cerebral circulation and metabolism in man. *Anesthesiology*, 36, 69–75.
23. List, W., Crumrine, R., Cascorbi, H. and Weiss, M. (1972) Increased cerebrospinal fluid pressure after ketamine. *Anesthesiology*, 36, 98–99.
24. Wyte, S., Shapiro, H., Turner, P. and Harris, A. (1972) Ketamine-induced intracranial hypertension. *Anesthesiology*, 36, 174–176.
25. Schulte, E., Pfeifer, G., Thiemig, I. and Entzian, W. (1978) The influence of intravenous anaesthetic agents on primarily increased intracranial pressure. *Acta Neurochirurgica*, 45, 15–25.
26. Wendling, W., Daniels, F., Chen, D. *et al.* (1994) Ketamine directly dilates bovine cerebral arteries by acting as a calcium entry blocker. *Journal of Neurosurgical Anesthesiology*, 6, 186–192.
27. Schwedler, M., Miletich, D. and Albrecht, R. (1982) Cerebral blood flow and metabolism following ketamine administration. *Canadian Anaesthetists' Society Journal*, 29, 222–226.
28. Pfenninger, E. and Reith, A. (1990) Ketamine and intracranial pressure, in *Status of Ketamine in Anesthesiology* (ed E. Domino), NPP Books, Ann Arbor, pp. 109–118.
29. Lassen, N. (1986) Cerebral and spinal cord blood flow, in *Anesthesia and Neurosurgery* (eds J. Cottrell and H. Turndoff), CV Mosby, St. Louis, p. 1.
30. Booth, N. (1988) Intravenous and other parenteral anesthetics, in *Veterinary Pharmacology and Therapeutics*, 6th edn (eds N. Booth and L. McDonald), Iowa State University Press, Ames, pp. 212–274.
31. Nakayama, M. and Murray, P. (1999) Ketamine preserves and propofol potentiates hypoxic pulmonary vasoconstriction compared with the conscious state in chronically instrumented dogs. *Anesthesiology*, 91, 760–771.
32. Domino, E., Chodoff, P. and Corssen, G. (1965) Pharmacologic effects of CI 581, a new dissociative anesthetic, in man. *Clinical Pharmacology & Therapeutics*, 6, 279–291.
33. Gooding, J., Dimick, A., Tavakoli, M. and Corssen, G. (1977) A physiologic analysis of cardiopulmonary responses to ketamine anesthesia in noncardiac patients. *Anesthesia and Analgesia*, 56, 813–816.
34. Mankikian, B., Cantineau, J., Sartene, R. *et al.* (1986) Ventilatory pattern and chest wall mechanics during ketamine anesthesia in humans. *Anesthesiology*, 65, 492–499.
35. Shulman, D., Beardsmore, C., Aronson, H. and Godfrey, S. (1985) The effects of ketamine on the functional residual capacity in young children. *Anesthesiology*, 62, 551–556.
36. Corssen, G., Gutierrez, J., Reves, J. and Huber, F. (1972) Ketamine in the anesthetic management of asthmatic patients. *Anesthesia and Analgesia*, 51, 588–596.
37. Huber, F., Gutierrez, J. and Corssen, G. (1972) Ketamine: its effect on airway resistance in man. *Southern Medical Journal*, 65, 1176–1180.
38. Brown, R. and Wagner, E. (1999) Mechanisms of bronchoprotection by anesthetic induction agents: propofol vs ketamine. *Anesthesiology*, 90, 822–828.
39. Short, C. (1987) Dissociative anesthesia, in *Principles and Practice of Veterinary Anesthesia* (ed C. Short), Williams & Wilkins, Baltimore, pp. 158–169.

40. Waterman, A. and Livingston, A. (1978) Some physiological effects of ketamine in sheep. *Research in Veterinary Science*, 25, 225–233.
41. Thurmon, J., Kumar, A. and Link, R. (1973) Evaluation of ketamine hydrochloride as an anesthetic in sheep. *Journal of the American Veterinary Medical Association*, 162, 293–297.
42. Thurmon, J., Nelson, D. and Christie, G. (1972) Ketamine anesthesia in swine. *Journal of the American Veterinary Medical Association*, 160, 1325–1330.
43. Evans, A., Krahwinkel, D. and Sawyer, D. (1972) Dissociative anesthesia in the cat. *Journal of the American Animal Hospital Association*, 8, 371–373.
44. Child, K., Davis, B., Dodds, M. and Twissell, D. (1972) Anaesthetic, cardiovascular and respiratory effects of a new steroidal agent CT 1341: a comparison with other intravenous anaesthetic drugs in the unrestrained cat. *British Journal of Pharmacology*, 46, 189–200.
45. Sears, B. (1971) Complications of ketamine. *Anesthesiology*, 35, 231.
46. Szappanyas, G., Gemperle, M. and Rifat, K. (1971) Selective indications for ketamine anesthesia. Proceeding of the Royal Society of Medicine, 1156–1159.
47. Wright, M. (1982) Pharmacologic effects of ketamine and its use in veterinary medicine. *Journal of the American Veterinary Medical Association*, 180, 1462–1471.
48. Somers, M. (1958) Comparison of the salivary secretion of both parotid glands in a sheep. *Nature*, 182, 400.
49. Kay, R. (1960) The rate of flow and composition of various salivary secretion in sheep and calves. *The Journal of Physiology*, 150, 515–537.
50. Nimmo, W. and Clements, J. (1984) Ketamine, in: *Pharmacokinetics of Anesthesia (eds C. Prys-Roberts and C. Hug), Blackwell Scientific Publications, Boston,* pp. 235.
51. Sparks, D., Corssen, G., Sides, J. *et al.* (1973) Ketamine induced anesthesia: neural mechanisms in the rhesus monkey. *Anesthesia and Analgesia*, 52, 288–297.
52. Sparks, D., Corssen, G., Aizenman, B. and Black, J. (1975) Further studies of the neural mechanisms of ketamine-induced anesthesia in the rhesus monkey. *Anesthesia and Analgesia*, 54, 189–195.
53. Conseiller, C., Benoist, J., Hamann, K. *et al.* (1972) Effects of ketamine (CI 581) on cell responses to cutaneous stimulations in laminae IV and V in the cat's dorsal horn. *European Journal of Pharmacology*, 18, 346–352.
54. Tang, A. and Schroeder, L. (1973) Spinal-cord depressant effects of ketamine and etoxadrol in the cat and the rat. *Anesthesiology*, 39, 37–43.
55. Vincent, J., Cavey, D., Kamenka, J. *et al.* (1978) Interaction of phencyclidines with the muscarinic and opiate receptors in the central nervous system. *Brain Research*, 152, 176–182.
56. Finck, A. and Ngai, S. (1982) Opiate receptor mediation of ketamine analgesia. *Anesthesiology*, 56, 291–297.
57. Smith, D., Pokoe, G., Monroe, P. *et al.* (1990) Ketamine analgesia in rats may be mediated by an interaction with opiate receptors, in *Status of Ketamine in Anesthesiology* (ed E. Domino), NPP Books, Ann Arbor, pp. 199–209.
58. Hanaoka, K., Tagami, M., Nagase, M. *et al.* (1990) Spinal analgesia mechanisms of ketamine: Antagonism by naloxone, in *Status of Ketamine in Anesthesiology* (ed E. Domino), NPP Books, Ann Arbor, pp. 229–246.
59. Olivar, T. and Laird, J. (1999) Differential effects of N-methyl-D-aspartate receptor blockade on nociceptive somatic and visceral reflexes. *Pain*, 79, 67–73.
60. Alam, S., Saito, Y. and Kosaka, Y. (1996) Antinociceptive effects of epidural and intravenous ketamine to somatic and visceral stimuli in rats. *Canadian Journal of Anaesthesia*, 43, 408–413.
61. Iwasaki, H., Collins, J., Namiki, A. *et al.* (1991) Effects of ketamine on behavioral responses to somatic and visceral stimuli in rats. *Masui*, 40, 1691–1694.

62. Castroman, P. and Ness, T. (2002) Ketamine, an N-methyl-D-aspartate receptors antagonist, inhibits the spinal neuronal responses to distension of the rat urinary bladder. *Anesthesiology*, 96, 1410–1419.
63. Wegner, K. (2008) Anesthesia and analgesia, in *Blackwell's Five-Minute Veterinary Consult: Ruminant* (ed S. Hankell), Wiley-Blackwell, Ames, pp. 66–69.
64. Fuentes, V. and Tellez, E. (1974) Ketamine dissociative analgesia in the cow. *The Veterinary Record*, 94, 482.
65. Thurmon, J. and Benson, G. (1993) Anesthesia in ruminants and swine, in *Current Veterinary Therapy: Food Animal Practice*, 3rd edn (ed J. Howard), WB Saunders, Philadelphia, pp. 58–76.
66. Nowrouzian, I., Schels, H., Ghodsian, I. and Karimi, H. (1981) Evaluation of the anesthetic properties of ketamine and a ketamine/xylazine/atropine combination in sheep. *The Veterinary Record*, 108, 354–356.
67. Taylor, P., Hopkins, L., Young, M. and McFadyen, I. (1972) Ketamine anesthesia in the pregnant sheep. *The Veterinary Record*, 90, 35–36.
68. Dehghani, S., Sharifnia, N., Yahyaei M. and Souri A. (1991) Clinical, haematological and biochemical effects of xylazine, ketamine, and their combination in caprine and feline. The 3rd International Congress of Veterinary Anaesthesia, Brisbane, p. 30.
69. Smith, M. and Sherman, D. (2009) Anesthesia, in: *Goat Medicine (eds M. Smith and D. Sherman), Wiley-Blackwell, Philadelphia,* pp. 709–722.
70. Levinson, G., Shnider, S., Gildea, J. and DeLorimier, A. (1973) Maternal and foetal cardiovascular and acid-base changes during ketamine anaesthesia in pregnant ewes. *British Journal of Anaesthesia*, 45, 1111–1115.
71. Kumar, A., Thurmon, J., Nelson, D. and Link, R. (1978) Effects of ketamine hydrochloride on maternal and fetal arterial pressure and acid base status in goats. *Veterinary Anesthesiologist*, 5, 28–33.
72. White, P. (1990) Ketamine update: its clinical uses in anesthesia, in *Status of Ketamine in Anesthesiology* (ed E. Domino), NPP Books, Ann Arbor, pp. 343–366.
73. Riebold, T., Kaneps, A. and Schmotzer, W. (1989) Anesthesia in the llama. *Veterinary Surgeons*, 18, 400–404.
74. Thurmon, J. and Benson, G. (1986) Injectable anesthetic agents and techniques in ruminants and swine. *Veterinary Clinics of North America: Food Animal Practice*, 2, 567–591.
75. Green, C., Knight, J., Precious, S. and Simpkin, S. (1981) Ketamine alone and combined with diazepam or xylazine in laboratory animals: a 10 years experience. *Laboratory Animals*, 15, 163–170.
76. Kyle, O., Novak, S. and Bolooki, H. (1979) General anesthesia in pigs. *Laboratory Animal Science*, 29, 123–124.
77. Lin, H. (2007) Dissociative anesthesia, in *Lumb and Jones' Veterinary Anesthesia and Analgesia*, 4th edn (eds W. Tranquilli, J. Thurmon and K. Grimm), Blackwell Publishing, Ames, pp. 301–353.
78. Klein, L., Tomasic, M. and Olson, K. (1989) Evaluation of Telazol in llamas. Annual Meeting of the American College of Veterinary Anesthesiologists, pp. 23.
79. Lin, H., Thurmon, J., Benson, G. *et al.* (1989) The hemodynamic response of calves to tiletamine-zolazepam anesthesia. *Veterinary Surgeons*, 18, 328–334.
80. Parke-Davis. (1974) Pharmacology of CI 716, in: *Detroit* (ed. P-D. Co).
81. Chen, G., Ensor, C. and Bohner, B. (1969) The pharmacology of 2-(ethylamino)-2-(2-thienyl)-cyclohexamine·HCl (CI 634). *The Journal of Pharmacology and Experimental Therapeutics*, 168, 171–179.
82. McGrath, J., MacKenzie, J. and Miller, R. (1975) Effects of ketamine on central sympathetic discharge and baroreceptor reflex during mechanical ventilation. *British Journal of Anaesthesia*, 47, 1141–1147.

83. Lin, H., Thurmon, J., Benson, G. *et al.* (1991) Hemodynamic responses of calves to tiletamine-zolazepam-xylazine anesthesia. *American Journal of Veterinary Research*, 52, 1606–1610.
84. Howard, B., Lagutchik, M., Januszkiewicz, A. and Martin, D. (1990) The cardiovascular response of sheep to tiletamine zolazepam and butorphanol tartrate anesthesia. *Veterinary Surgeons*, 19, 461–467.
85. Lin, H., Thurmon, J., Benson, G. and Tranquilli, W. (1993) Telazol – a review of its pharmacology and use in veterinary medicine. *Journal of Veterinary Pharmacology and Therapeutics*, 16, 383–418.
86. Lin, H. (1996) Dissociative anesthetics, in *Lumb and Jones' Veterinary Anesthesia*, 3rd edn (eds J. Thurmon, W. Tranquilli and G. Benson), Lea & Febiger, Baltimore, pp. 241–296.
87. Williams, L., Levy, J., Robertson, S. *et al.* (2002) Use of the anesthetic combination of Tiletamine, zolazepam, ketamine, and xylazine for neutering feral cats. *Journal of the American Veterinary Medical Association*, 220, 1491–1495.
88. Short, C. (1989) Talking about Telazol: roundtable. *Veterinary Medicine*, 84, 1–8.
89. Taylor, J., Botha, C., Swan, G. *et al.* (1992) Tiletamine hydrochloride in combination with zolazepam hydrochloride as an anesthetic agent in sheep. *Journal of the South African Veterinary Association*, 63, 63–65.
90. Lin, H., Tyler, J., Wallace, S. *et al.* (1993) Telazol and xylazine anesthesia in sheep. *The Cornell Veterinarian*, 83, 117–124.
91. Fowler, M. (2010) Anesthesia, in *Medicine and Surgery of Camelids*, 3rd edn (ed M. Fowler), Wiley-Blackwell, Ames, pp. 111–127.
92. Ganter, M. and Ruppert, K. (1990) The effect of the anesthetic Tilest in swine. *Deutsche Tierarztliche Wochenschrift*, 97, 360–364.
93. Bree, M. (1972) Dissociative anesthesia in Macaca mulatta: clinical evaluation of CI 744. *Journal of Medical Primatology*, 1, 256–260.
94. Hellyer, P., Muir, W., Hubbell, J. and Sally, J. (1988) Cardiorespiratory effects of the intravenous administration of tiletamine-zolazepam to cats. *Veterinary Surgeons*, 17, 105–110.
95. Schobert, E. (1987) Telazol use in wild and exotic animals. *Veterinary Medicine*, 82, 1080–1088.
96. Ward, G., Johnson, D. and Roberts, C. (1974) The use of CI 744 as an anesthetic for laboratory animals. *Laboratory Animal Science*, 24, 732–742.
97. Zoran, D., Riedesel, D. and Dyer, D. (1993) Pharmacokinetics of propofol in mixed breed dogs and greyhounds. *American Journal of Veterinary Research*, 54, 755–760.
98. Langley, M. and Heel, R. (1988) Propofol: a review of its pharmacodynamics and pharmacokinetic properties and use as an intravenous anesthetic. *Drug*, 35, 334–372.
99. Riebold, T. (1996) Ruminants, in *Lumb & Jones' Veterinary Anesthesia*, 3rd edn (eds J. Thurmon, W. Tranquilli and G. Benson), Lea & Febiger, Baltimore, pp. 610–626.
100. Handel, I., Weaver, B., Staddon, G. and Cruz Madorran, J. (1991) Observation on the pharmacokinetics of Propofol in sheep. International Congress of Veterinary Anesthesia, pp. 143–154.
101. Waterman, A. (1988) Use of propofol in sheep. *The Veterinary Record*, 122, 260.
102. Reid, J., Nolan, A. and Welsh, E. (1993) Propofol as an induction agent in the goats: a pharmacokinetic study. *Journal of Veterinary Pharmacology and Therapeutics*, 16, 488–493.
103. Lin, H., Purohit, R. and Powe, T. (1997) Anesthesia in sheep with propofol or with xylazine-ketamine followed by halothane. *Veterinary Surgeons*, 26, 247–252.
104. Tranquilli, W. and Grimm, K. (1996) Pharmacology of drugs used for anesthesia and sedation. *Veterinary Clinics of North America: Food Animal Practice*, 12, 501–529.
105. Prassinos, N., Galatos, A. and Raptopoulos, D. (2005) A comparison of propofol, thiopental or ketamine as induction agents in goats. *Veterinary Anaesthesia and Analgesia*, 32, 289–296.
106. Taylor, P. (1991) Anesthesia in sheep and goats. *In Practice*, 13, 31–36.

107. Nolan, A., Reid, J. and Welsh, E. (1991) The use of Propofol as an induction agent in goats. *Journal of Veterinary Anaesthesia*, 18, 53–54.
108. Duke, T., Egger, C., Ferguson, J. and Frketic, M. (1997) Cardiopulmonary effects of Propofol infusion in llamas. *American Journal of Veterinary Research*, 58, 153–156
109. Tibary, A. (2009) Reproductive surgery in camelids. *North American Veterinary Community Conference*, pp. 342–345.
110. Mascøas, M., Pera, A., Santos, M. *et al.* (1993) Total intravenous anesthesia with Propofol in pigs. *Journal of Veterinary Anaesthesia*, 20, 53–54.
111. Graham, M., Thiessen, D. and Mutch, W. (1998) Left ventricular systolic and diastolic function is unaltered during propofol infusion in newborn swine. *Anesthesia and Analgesia*, 86, 717–723.
112. Muir, W., Hubbell, J., Bednarski, R. and Skarda, R. (eds) (2007) Anesthetic procedures and techniques in ruminants, in: *Handbook of Veterinary Anesthesia, Mosby/Elsevier,* St. Louis, pp. 402–411.
113. Tavernor, W. (1970) The influence of guaiacol glycerol ether on cardiovascular and respiratory function in the horse. *Research in Veterinary Science*, 11, 91–93.
114. Singh, J., Sobti, V., Kohli, R. *et al.* (1981) Evaluation of glyceryl guaiacolate as a muscle relaxant in buffalo calves. *Zentralbl Veterinarmed A*, 28, 60–69.
115. Funk, K. (1973) Glyceryl guaiacolate: some effects and indications in horses. *Equine Veterinary Journal*, 5, 15–19.
116. Abrahamsen, E. (2009) Ruminant field anesthesia, in *Current Veterinary Therapy: Food Animal Medicine*, 5th edn (eds D. Anderson and D. Rings), Saunders/Elsevier, St. Louis, pp. 552–558.
117. Schatzman, U. (1974) The induction of general anesthesia in the horse with glyceryl guaiacolate. Comparison when used alone and with sodium thiamylal (Surital). *Equine Veterinary Journal*, 6, 164–169.
118. Hall, L., Clarke, K. and Trim, C. (2001) Anaesthesia of sheep, goats, and other herbivores, in *Veterinary Anaesthesia*, 10th edn (eds L. Hall, K. Clarke and C. Trim), WB Saunders, London, pp. 341–366.
119. Riebold, T. (2001) Anesthetic management of cattle, in *Recent Advances in Anesthetic Management of Large Domestic Animals* (ed E. Steffey), International Veterinary Information Service, Ithaca.
120. Waterman, A. (1981) Preliminary observations on the use of a combination of xylazine and ketamine hydrochloride in calves. *The Veterinary Record*, 109, 464–467.
121. Rings, D. and Muir, W. (1982) Cardiopulmonary effects of intramuscular xylazine-ketamine in calves. *Canadian Journal of Comparative Medicine*, 46, 386–389.
122. Campbell, K., Klavano, P., Richardson, P. and Alexander, J. (1979) Hemodynamic effects of xylazine in the calf. *American Journal of Veterinary Research*, 40, 1777–1780.
123. Waterman, A. (1983) Effects of a combination of ketamine and xylazine on respiratory gas tensions and acid base status in calves. *The Veterinary Record*, 113, 517.
124. Blaze, C., Holland, R. and Grant, A. (1988) Gas exchange during xylazine-ketamine anesthesia in neonatal calves. *Veterinary Surgeons*, 17, 155–159
125. Lin, H. (2012) Large ruminant anesthesia: review and update. *Western Veterinary Conference*, FA#1.
126. Lin, H., Tyler, J., Welles, E. *et al.* (1993) Effects of anesthesia induced and maintained by continuous intravenous administration of guaifenesin, ketamine, and xylazine in spontaneously breathing sheep. *American Journal of Veterinary Research*, 54, 1913–1916.
127. Johnson, L. (2010) Keeping small ruminant field anesthesia simple. North American *Veterinary Community Conference*, p. 345.

128. Miesner, M. (2009) Updates in bovine surgery: beef cattle and surgical challenges. *North American Veterinary Community Conference*, pp. 41–43.
129. Lin, H., Riddell, M. and DeGraves, F. (1999) Comparison of three alpha 2-antagonists, Yohimbine, tolazoline, or atipamezole for reversing the anesthetic effects of medetomidine and ketamine in dairy calves. *The Bovine Practitioner*, 33, 21–26.
130. Raekallio, M., Kivalo, M., Jalanka, H. and Vainio, O. (1991) Medetomidine/ketamine sedation in claves and its reversal with atipamezole. *Journal of Veterinary Anaesthesia*, 18, 45–47.
131. Thurmon, J., Lin, H., Benson, G. *et al.* (1989) Combining Telazol and xylazine for anesthesia in calves. *Veterinary Medicine*, 84, 824–830.
132. Anderson, D. (2011) New methods for chemical restraint and field anesthesia in cattle. *North American Veterinary Community Conference*, pp. 6–11.
133. Trim, C. (1987) Special anesthesia considerations in the ruminant, in *Principles and Practice of Veterinary Anesthesia* (ed C. Short), Williams and Wilkins, Baltimore, pp. 285–300.
134. Washburn, K. (2012) Common surgical and nonsurgical procedures of camelids. *Western Veterinary Conference*, pp. FA #44.
135. Abrahamsen, E. (2009) Chemical restraint, anesthesia, and analgesia for camelids. *Veterinary Clinics of North America: Food Animal Practice*, 25, 455–494.
136. Van Metre, D. (2012) Handling, restraint, and practical tips for working with sheep and goats. *North American Veterinary Community Conference*, pp. 676–682.
137. Anderson, D. (2009) Field anesthetic techniques for camelids. Annual Convention of the American Association of Bovine Practitioners, pp. 103–104.
138. Matthews, N. (1992) Anesthesia of small ruminants, llamas and miniature pigs in small animal practice. *North American Veterinary Community Conference*, pp. 17–18.
139. Lagutchik, M., Januszkiewicz, A., Dodd, K. and Martin, D. (1991) Cardiopulmonary effects of tiletamine-zolazepam combination in sheep. *American Journal of Veterinary Research*, 52, 1441–1447.
140. Carroll, G., Hartsfield, S. and Hambleton, R. (1997) Anesthetic effects of Tiletamine-zolazepam, alone or in combination with butorphanol, in goats. *Journal of the American Veterinary Medical Association*, 211, 593–597.
141. Carroll, G., Hooper, R., Slater, M. *et al.* (1998) Detomidine-butorphanol-propofol for carotid artery translocation and castration or ovariectomy in goats. *Veterinary Surgeons*, 27, 75–82.
142. Larenza, M., Bergadano, A., Iff, I. and Schatzmann, U. (2005) Comparison of the cardiopulmonary effects of anesthesia maintained by continuous infusion of ketamine and propofol with anesthesia maintained by inhalation of sevoflurane in goats undergoing magnetic resonance imaging. *American Journal of Veterinary Research*, 66, 2135–2141.
143. Breese, C. and Dodman, N. (1984) Xylazine-ketamine-oxymorphone: an injectable anesthetic combination in swine. *Journal of the American Veterinary Medical Association*, 184, 182–183.
144. Sakaguchi, M., Nishimura, R., Sasaki, N. *et al.* (1996) Anesthesia induced in pigs by use of a combination of medetomidine, butorphanol, and ketamine and its reversal by administration of atipamezole. *American Journal of Veterinary Research*, 57, 529–534.
145. Sakaguchi, M., Nishimura, R., Sasaki, N. *et al.* (1995) Chemical restraint by medetomidine-ketamine and its cardiopulmonary effects in pigs. *Zentralbl Veterinarmed A*, 42, 293–299.
146. Thurmon, J., Tranquilli, W. and Benson, G. (1986) Cardiopulmonary responses of swine to intravenous infusion of guaifenesin, ketamine, and xylazine. *American Journal of Veterinary Research*, 47, 2138–2140.
147. Gray, K., Raulston, G., Flow, B. *et al.* (1978) Repeated immobilization of miniature swine with an acepromazine-ketamine combination. Southwest Veterinary Symposium, 31, 27–30.
148. Benson, G. and Thurmon, J. (1979) Anesthesia of swine under field conditions. *Journal of the American Veterinary Medical Association*, 174, 594–596.

149. Evans, L. and Ko, J. (1990) Electroejaculation and artificial insemination in Vietnamese potbellied miniature pigs. *Journal of the American Veterinary Medical Association*, 197, 1366–1367.
150. Williams, L. (1992) The Vietnamese pot bellied pig: anesthetic friend or foe? American College of Veterinary Surgeons Symposium, 222–224.
151. Braun, W. (1993) Anesthetic and surgical techniques useful in the potbellied pig. *Veterinary Medicine*, 88, 441–447.
152. Nishimura, R., Sakaguchi, M., Mochizuki, M. *et al.* (1992) A balanced anesthesia with a combination of xylazine, ketamine and butorphanol anesthesia and its antagonism by yohimbine in pigs. *The Journal of Veterinary Medical Science*, 54, 615–620.
153. Thurmon, J., Benson, G., Tranquilli, W. *et al.* (1988) The anesthetic and analgesic effects of Telazol and xylazine in pigs: evaluating clinical trials. *Veterinary Medicine*, 83, 841–845.
154. Gabor, T., Hellgren, E. and Silvy, N. (1997) Immobilization of collared peccaries (*Tayassu tajacu*) and feral hogs (*Sus scrofa*) with Telazol and xylazine. *Journal of Wildlife Diseases*, 33, 161–164.
155. James, S., Cook, R., Raphael, B. *et al.* (1999) Immobilization of babirusa (*Babyrousa babyrussa*) with xylazine and tiletamine/zolazepam and reversal with yohimbine and flumazenil. *Journal of Zoo and Wildlife Medicine*, 30, 521–525.
156. Ko, J., Thurmon, J., Benson, G. and Olson, W. (1993) A new drug combination for use in porcine cesarean sections. *Veterinary Medicine*, 88, 466–472.
157. Ko, J., Thurmon, J., Tranquilli, W. *et al.* (1993) Problems encountered when anesthetizing potbellied pigs. *Veterinary Medicine*, 88, 435–440.
158. Ko, J., Williams, B., Smith, V. *et al.* (1993) Comparison of Telazol, Telazol-ketamine, Telazol-xylazine, and Telazol-ketamine-xylazine as chemical restraint and anesthetic induction combination in swine. *Laboratory Animal Science*, 43, 476–480.
159. Ko, J., Williams, B., Rogers, E. *et al.* (1995) Increased xylazine dose-enhanced anesthetic properties of Telazol-xylazine combination in swine. *Laboratory Animal Science*, 45, 290–294.
160. Thurmon, J. and Smith, G. (2007) Swine, in *Lumb & Jones' Veterinary Anesthesia and Analgesia*, 4th edn (eds W. Tranquilli, J. Thurmon and K. Grimm), Blackwell Publishing, Ames, pp. 747–763.
161. Martin-Cancho, M., Carrasco-Jimenez, M., Lima, J. *et al.* (2004) Assessment of the relationship of bispectral index values, homodynamic changes, and recovery times associated with sevoflurane or propofol anesthesia in pigs. *American Journal of Veterinary Research*, 65, 409–416.

Chapter 5

Inhalation anesthesia

HuiChu Lin
Department of Clinical Sciences, College of Veterinary Medicine, Auburn University, USA

When general anesthesia is considered in farm animal species, factors that affect the decision between injectable and inhalation anesthesia include the type of procedure to be performed, anticipated duration of the procedure, inhalation anesthetic equipment availability, familiarity of the veterinarians with the anesthetic technique, and anesthetic costs. Injectable anesthesia has the advantages of easy drug administration and relatively low cost of specific anesthetic equipment or accessories required for delivery and monitoring. Delivery of an inhalation anesthetic requires expensive and specialized equipment and accessories to be able to deliver the anesthetic to the patient. However, accumulation of injectable anesthetics in the patient following repeated dosing, or extended infusion required for completion of a procedure, can result in delayed drug elimination and prolonged recovery. Because of the ease and speed in adjusting the depth of anesthesia with the currently available inhalation anesthetics (e.g., isoflurane, sevoflurane, and desflurane), inhalation anesthesia is often preferred for use in long procedures and also for patients that are considered at higher anesthetic risk as a result of preexisting systemic conditions. Isoflurane was first synthesized in 1965 and subsequently became a popular inhalation anesthetic in human patients in 1981. It is still a very commonly utilized inhalation anesthetic in veterinary practice. Sevoflurane was synthesized in the early 1970s. At that time, it was difficult to synthesize the drug and therefore was expensive to manufacture. It wasn't until the late 1980s that sevoflurane was introduced in Japan and was later marketed in the US in 1995 [1]. Special preanesthetic considerations and preparations with respect to laryngeal and gastrointestinal anatomy and physiology prior to general anesthesia in farm animal species are discussed in detail in Chapter 1.

The goal of delivering surgical anesthesia with an inhalation anesthetic is to maintain a constant and optimal partial pressure of the anesthetic in the alveoli of the lungs and central nervous systems (CNS). Currently available inhalation anesthetics, isoflurane, sevoflurane, and desflurane, have low blood solubility (isoflurane, 1.46; sevoflurane, 0.68; desflurane, 0.42) and minimal hepatic metabolism (isoflurane, 0.2%; sevoflurane, 3–5%; desflurane, 0.02%) [2].

Farm Animal Anesthesia: Cattle, Small Ruminants, Camelids, and Pigs, First Edition.
Edited by HuiChu Lin and Paul Walz.

Blood solubility of an inhalation anesthetic is referred to as blood–gas partition coefficient which is a ratio of the distribution of an inhalation anesthetic between the blood and the gas. Partition coefficient is the concentration ratio of an anesthetic between the solvent and gas phase, for example, blood and gas, or between two tissue solvents, for example, brain and blood. As an example, an inhalation anesthetic with a blood–gas partition coefficient of 10 at equilibrium (i.e., the partial pressure of that anesthetic is identical in the blood and in the gas phase) implies that the concentration of that anesthetic is 10 in the blood and 1 in the gas phase. An anesthetic with a lower blood solubility has a lower blood–gas partition coefficient. In other words, a smaller amount of the anesthetic is dissolved in the blood than in the gas phase when their partial pressures reach equilibrium. Therefore, the speed of achieving surgical plane of anesthesia, the rate of anesthetic depth variation, and the time until consciousness is regained and recovery is achieved are normally faster for an inhalation anesthetic with a lower blood solubility than anesthetics with higher blood solubility. In this case, the time of induction to surgical plane of anesthesia and the time to recovery of full motor function of a patient are faster with desflurane (0.42), intermediate with sevoflurane (0.69), and slower with isoflurane (1.41) [2].

Under ideal conditions, the partial pressure of an anesthetic from the alveoli (P_A) to the pulmonary arterial blood (P_a) and then to the brain (P_{br}) should be close, if not equal, to the inspired anesthetic partial pressure (P_I), that is, $P_I \approx P_A \approx P_a \approx P_{br}$, at equilibrium. Changes in P_I, alveolar ventilation, and characteristics of an anesthetic breathing system will affect the uptake of the anesthetic from the inspired anesthetic gas flow delivered by the anesthesia machine to the alveoli. Variation of the blood–gas partition coefficient of the anesthetics, cardiac output of the patients, and alveoli to venous partial pressure difference affect the transfer of an inhalation anesthetic from the alveolar tissues to pulmonary arterial blood. Factors that determine how quickly the inhalation anesthetic accumulates in the brain include the brain–blood partition coefficient, the cerebral blood flow, and the cerebral arterial to venous partial pressure difference. Because the brain–blood partition coefficient for isoflurane (1.6) and sevoflurane (1.7) is very similar, there should be no significant difference in the speed of the transfer from blood to brain between these two anesthetics [1]. Therefore, increasing P_I and alveolar ventilation and reducing anesthesia breathing system volume decrease the time of the partial pressure of an inhalation anesthetic to equilibrium between alveoli and pulmonary arterial blood, and therefore result in a faster induction of anesthesia for that anesthetic. Vice versa, decreasing P_I and alveolar ventilation and increasing the volume of the anesthesia breathing system prolong the time to equilibrium and result in a slower induction of anesthesia. Furthermore, anesthetics with a low blood–gas partition coefficient, patients with a low cardiac output, and small differences between alveolar and venous partial pressures tend to result in faster induction than an anesthetic with greater blood–gas partition coefficient, patients with an increased cardiac output, and larger differences between alveolar and venous partial pressures. Similarly, an anesthetic with a low brain–blood partition coefficient, patients with increased cerebral blood flow, and small differences between cerebral arterial and venous partial pressures tend to result in a faster induction than those with a greater brain–blood partition coefficient, patients with decreased cerebral blood flow, and larger differences between cerebral arterial and venous partial pressures. These tend to result in a slower induction of anesthesia [1, 3]. Return of consciousness and recovery from inhalation anesthesia is an inverse process of induction which is a result of the elimination of the anesthetic from the CNS. Therefore, factors that affect the speed of induction, for example, alveolar ventilation, cardiac output, and blood and tissue solubility, also affect the speed of recovery. In the presence of normal alveolar ventilation and cardiac output, recovery is generally faster for an anesthetic with lower blood and tissue solubility. Hence, recovery from desflurane (0.42) and sevoflurane (0.69) tends to be faster than isoflurane (1.41).

Isoflurane and sevoflurane are the two most commonly used inhalation anesthetics in current veterinary practice (Figure 5.1 and Figure 5.2). Both anesthetics can be used safely and effectively for general anesthesia in farm animal species. Desflurane is a newer inhalation anesthetic with a chemical structure similar to isoflurane with the exception of the substitution of a fluorine for the chlorine on the alpha-ethyl carbon. Desflurane is unique among the conventional inhaled anesthetics. It has a vapor pressure of 681 mmHg at 20°C, which is very close to the atmospheric pressure (760 mmHg) and a boiling point of 22.8°C. At normal operating room temperature, desflurane can boil with a saturated vapor concentration of 87% (681 mmHg/760 mmHg), which is approximately 10 times the minimum alveolar concentration (MAC) of desflurane for humans (6.6%). Because of these unique characteristics, desflurane requires a specially designed vaporizer that is pressurized and heated to provide precise control of anesthetic output from the vaporizer and prevent overanesthetizing the patient [4]. Because of this special vaporizer requirement, desflurane has not been used as commonly as isoflurane and sevoflurane. Isoflurane and sevoflurane require a standard vaporizer calibrated specifically for each anesthetic. Compared to older inhalation anesthetics, isoflurane and sevoflurane have lower potency with a MAC value of 1.29% and 2.33%, respectively [5]. The MAC value of an inhalation anesthetic is the minimum alveolar anesthetic concentration required to prevent gross purposeful movement in 50% of the patients in response to obnoxious stimuli such as surgical incision. The MAC value is used as an indicator of the potency of the anesthetic.

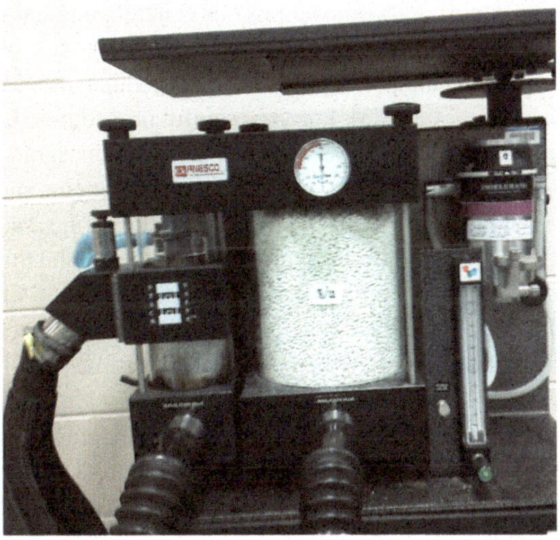

Figure 5.1 Anesthesia machine with isoflurane vaporizer.

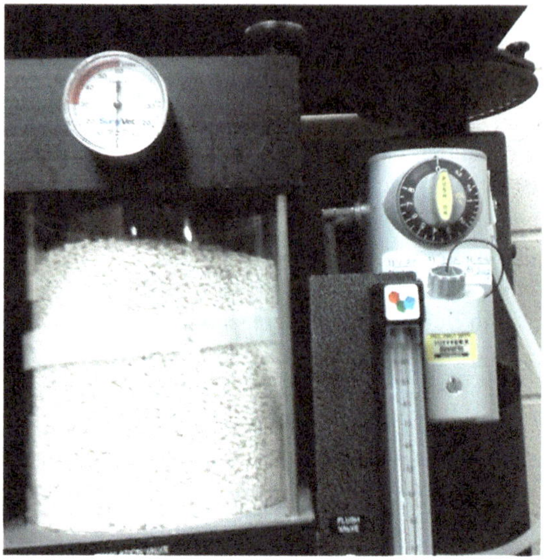

Figure 5.2 Anesthesia machine with sevoflurane vaporizer.

The higher the MAC value, the lower the potency of the anesthetic. From the physicochemical properties of the inhalation anesthetics, MAC values are inversely related to the blood solubility of the anesthetic. Therefore, an inhalation anesthetic with high potency normally has a high blood solubility but a low MAC value. Vice versa, an inhalation anesthetic with low potency generally has a low blood solubility but a high MAC value [1]. Sevoflurane is less potent than isoflurane as reflected in the higher MAC values (2.33% vs. 1.29%) and lower blood solubility (0.69 vs. 1.41). One should always keep in mind that at 1 MAC (1 × MAC), only 50% of the patients will not respond to obnoxious stimulation. In other words, the remainder of the patients may respond to an obnoxious stimulation, resulting in gross purposeful movement. In general, surgical anesthesia requires maintaining anesthetic concentration at 1.3 MAC to prevent 95% of the patients from responding to surgical stimulation. Thus, 1.3 MAC of an inhalation anesthetic is referred to as ED_{95} or surgical anesthesia [1, 3]. For very painful procedures, 1.5 MAC of an inhalation anesthetic concentration may be required to maintain surgical anesthesia. The MAC value is measured and determined in normal healthy patients anesthetized with that inhalation anesthetic alone with no other CNS-depressing drugs such as tranquilizers, sedatives, analgesics, and injectable anesthetics administered at the time of measurement. The MAC values can be influenced by concurrent administration of anesthetic-related drugs, alterations of the physiological conditions of the patient, or concurrent administration of medications for the treatment of other conditions or illness. Factors that may increase the MAC value of an inhalation anesthetic for a particular patient include hyperthermia (fever), hypernatremia, and drug-induced increased CNS catecholamine levels. Increased age, hypothermia, hyponatremia, pregnancy, and concurrent administration of tranquilizers, sedatives, analgesics, injectable anesthetics, local anesthetics, neuromuscular blocking drugs, and drugs that decrease CNS catecholamine levels tend to decrease the MAC value. Duration of anesthesia and magnitude of individual anesthetic metabolism

Table 5.1 Blood–gas solubility, metabolism, and MAC of isoflurane, sevoflurane, and desflurane in farm animal species.

	Isoflurane	Sevoflurane	Desflurane
Blood–gas solubility [7]	1.46	0.68	0.42
Hepatic metabolism [7]	0.2%	3–5%	0.02%
MAC values (%)			
Cattle	Calves: 1.47 [8]	N/A	N/A
Goats	1.13 ± 0.03 [9] 1.29 ± 0.11 [5] 1.63 ± 0.17 [11]	2.3–2.7 [10] 2.33 ± 0.15 [5]	N/A
Sheep	1.01–1.58 [12, 13] 1.51 [16]	3.3 [14]	9.5 [15]
Llamas/alpacas	1.05 ± 0.17 [17]	L: 2.29 ± 0.14 [18] A: 2.33 ± 0.09 [18]	L: 7.99 ± 0.58 [19] A: 7.83 ± 0.51 [19]
Pigs	1.65 ± 0.36–2.04 ± 0.19 [20]	4.1 (3.65–4.5) [21] 3.5 ± 0.1 [22]	8.28 ± 1.34%–10 ± 0.94 [20]

have no effect on the MAC value [6, 7]. Table 5.1 summarizes blood–gas solubility, metabolism, and MAC of isoflurane, sevoflurane, and desflurane in farm animal species. Table 5.1 summarizes the blood–gas partition coefficient, metabolism, and MAC values of isoflurane, sevoflurane, and desflurane in farm animal species.

Eger [23] and Malan *et al.* [24] reported that the circulatory effects produced by desflurane closely resemble those produced by isoflurane. Sevoflurane-induced circulatory effects have the characteristics of both isoflurane and halothane. In humans, isoflurane and sevoflurane produce a dose-dependent decrease in mean arterial pressure primarily due to the decrease in systemic vascular resistance produced by these anesthetics. Heart rate tends to increase up to 1 MAC (1.29%) during isoflurane anesthesia, while heart rate does not increase until the concentration of sevoflurane anesthesia is greater than 1.5 MAC ($1.5 \times 2.3\% = 3.5\%$). An abrupt increase in alveolar concentration of isoflurane from 0.55 to 1.66 MAC produces an increase in sympathetic nervous system and renin–angiotensin activities. As a result, transient increases in heart rate and mean arterial blood pressure occur, which may cause the anesthetist to misinterpret as insufficient anesthetic depth and further increase the anesthetic concentration delivered to the patient [25]. The transient increase in heart rate and mean arterial pressure associated with an abrupt increase in anesthetic concentration has not been observed during sevoflurane anesthesia [26]. It is believed that the neurocirculatory excitatory effect of isoflurane is caused by stimulation of the sympathetic nervous system located in the upper airway and in the lung in response to a sudden increase in alveolar concentration of the anesthetic. This effect is more likely to occur for inhalation anesthetics with low blood solubility and is capable of causing a rapid rise in alveolar concentration by increasing the inspired concentration delivered to the patient [27]. However, prior administration of fentanyl, alfentanil, or clonidine has been shown to blunt the neurocirculatory excitatory effect of desflurane concentration increase [28, 29]. It is believed that a similar suppression response can occur if these drugs are administered prior to isoflurane anesthesia.

In general, isoflurane does not affect cardiac output as much as sevoflurane. Cardiac output decreases significantly at 1 and 1.5 MAC of sevoflurane but returns to near awake values at 2 MAC [30]. It is believed that isoflurane may possess mild β agonist effects and the resultant sympathomimetic effect is reflected as an increased heart rate, decreased systemic vascular resistance, and overall unchanged cardiac output in human patients [30]. However, this theory has not been supported by animal data [31]. Neither isoflurane nor sevoflurane overly sensitizes the myocardium to circulating catecholamines; thus, they are unlikely to cause cardiac dysrhythmias in susceptible patients [30].

Hypoventilation and increased $PaCO_2$ are often observed during inhalation anesthesia as a result of medullary respiratory center depression and reduced chest wall expansion due to anesthetic-induced intercostal muscle relaxation [4]. Furthermore, positioning of ruminant patients in lateral or dorsal recumbency for surgery results in compression of the diaphragm, which collapses the caudal lung lobes by the cranial shifting of the rumen and further debilitates the ventilation function of an anesthetized ruminant patient [32, 33]. Sevoflurane produces a dose-dependent increase in respiratory rate in human volunteers. Isoflurane increases the respiratory rate up to a concentration of 1 MAC. A further increase in isoflurane concentration is not associated with a further increase in the respiratory rate. Awake patients may be able to compensate for a decrease in respiratory rate by increasing the tidal volume in order to maintain normal minute ventilation and preventing the increase in $PaCO_2$. However, dose-dependent depression of the response of the medullary respiratory center to the increased $PaCO_2$ is often observed which prohibits central compensatory mechanism by increasing respiratory rate or tidal volume in an effort to maintain normal $PaCO_2$ during isoflurane or sevoflurane anesthesia [23, 34]. Isoflurane and sevoflurane both produce bronchodilation in patients suffering from chronic obstructive pulmonary disease. Isoflurane vapor has a special pungent odor and has been shown to cause airway irritation, coughing, and breath holding during induction. On the contrary, sevoflurane has been described as "pleasant smelling," and it does not irritate the airway. Therefore, sevoflurane is often preferred for mask inductions [35].

Isoflurane, sevoflurane, and desflurane have little effect in overall hepatic and renal function in healthy patients. Isoflurane has been reported to decrease portal venous blood flow at 1.5 MAC, but total hepatic blood flow and hepatic arterial blood flow are shown to be within normal range. Therefore, hepatic perfusion is well maintained, which when combined with isoflurane-induced vasodilation ensures adequate hepatic O_2 delivery [36]. Of the three most popular inhalation anesthetics, isoflurane is probably the one that better maintains hepatic O_2 supply and is least likely to cause hepatic injury. Nevertheless, sevoflurane and desflurane produce hepatic effects similar to isoflurane [37–39]. The elimination of these inhalation anesthetics depends primarily on ventilation rather than the hepatic metabolism. Sevoflurane has a higher hepatic metabolism (3%) than isoflurane (0.2%) and desflurane (0.02%). Apparently, sevoflurane is 10 times more vulnerable than isoflurane and 100 times more than desflurane to hepatic metabolism and the subsequent production of inorganic and organic fluoride [23]. Fluoride-induced renal toxicity and renal dysfunction with a fluoride concentration of 50 µmol/l or greater have been previously documented with the administration of one of the older-generation inhalation anesthetics, methoxyflurane [40]. Clinical studies in humans showed that plasma fluoride concentrations can be maintained below 80 µmol/l, even though peak plasma fluoride concentration is rarely reached due to methoxyflurane's high blood solubility and slow rise in blood concentration [41]. Further evidence shows that renal dysfunction rarely occurs even with a peak plasma fluoride concentration of greater than 50 µmol/l, but less than 80 µmol/l, in the presence of high sevoflurane concentration and prolonged duration of anesthesia [41–46]. That being said, sevoflurane-induced cardiovascular depression may enhance the renal toxicity effect by detrimental hepatic or renal effects, for example, hepatocellular injury due to reduced hepatic blood flow and decreased O_2 delivery and diminished renal function as a result of the decreased renal blood flow and glomerular filtration rate. Therefore, it is important to maintain normal cardiovascular function and ensure adequate hepatic and renal perfusion in anesthetized patients.

Compound A is a vinyl ether produced as one of the degradation products of sevoflurane presented in the CO_2-absorbent canister as a trace contaminant. Breakdown of sevoflurane to compound A has been associated with administration of high sevoflurane concentrations, presence of the dry alkaline CO_2 absorbent (e.g., soda lime or baralyme), use of the low O_2 flow in the breathing circuit, and the production of high temperature from the chemical interaction of exhaled CO_2 with the CO_2 absorbent [47–56]. In rats, inhalation of high compound A concentrations has been shown to cause fatal renal injuries [56]. However, it is believed that compound A is less toxic in humans due to lower β-lyase enzyme activity as compared to rats [57]. When a fresh O_2 flow rate of 2 l/min was used in rats during sevoflurane anesthesia, which provided much higher O_2 than the minimum metabolic O_2 requirement of the rats, a very low concentration of compound A in the breathing circuit of the anesthetic machine was analyzed, and renal toxicity to the rats was not reported [34]. Increased production of compound A has been associated with higher CO_2 absorbent at temperatures up to 46°C. Also, studies have shown that CO_2 absorbent that contained NaOH and/or KOH often resulted in higher compound A production. No compound A was produced when NaOH- and KOH-free CO_2 absorbent was used [55, 58]. In rats, the concentrations of compound A that are associated with renal toxicity and the median lethal concentration following 1 hour of sevoflurane anesthesia are reported to be 100–300 ppm [59] and 1050–1090 ppm [60], respectively. In humans, peak compound A concentration of less than 40 ppm was reported even after prolonged duration of sevoflurane anesthesia [49, 61]. Similarly, a peak compound A concentration of 61 ppm was reported in dogs anesthetized with sevoflurane using a low-flow (fresh O_2 flow rate: 3 ml/kg/min), closed circuit system for 1 hour [62]. Kandel *et al.* [60] reported that renal injury in rats only occurred in the presence of a compound A concentration of at least 200 ppm with a maximum of 1 hour of exposure time. Fortunately, there is no report of compound A-related renal toxicity under normal clinical conditions in humans or domestic animals.

Cattle

In steers anesthetized for rumenotomy with atropine/guaifenesin/thiamylal for induction and either isoflurane or halothane for maintenance, higher heart rate and lower respiratory rates were observed during isoflurane than those observed during halothane anesthesia. Mean arterial blood pressure was not significantly different between the two anesthetics.

Surprisingly, the end-tidal isoflurane concentration required for rumenotomy surgery (1.7% at 15 minutes and 1.3% at 90 minutes) was lower than that of halothane (2.6% at 15 minutes and 1.7% at 90 minutes) [63]. In most of the other domestic species, isoflurane is reported to be less potent than halothane with 1.5 MAC values being 1.95% (1.5 × 1.3%) and 1.35% (1.5 × 0.9%) vapor concentration for isoflurane and halothane, respectively. The reason for this discrepancy remains unknown [63]. Both anesthetics produced a similar degree of respiratory depression which was reflected in the same level of $PaCO_2$ accumulation during anesthesia. However, it seems that animals anesthetized with isoflurane tend to breath with greater tidal volume so as to compensate for the lower respiratory rate caused by isoflurane. On the contrary, a decreased tidal volume accompanied by an increased respiratory rate in isoflurane-anesthetized calves was not able to prevent hypoventilation as evidenced by a significant increase in $PaCO_2$ throughout the anesthesia period. In normal, awake animals, an increase in $PaCO_2$ (hypoventilation) and a decrease in PaO_2 (hypoxia) are the primary stimulants for the medullary respiratory center and peripheral chemoreceptors to increase respiratory rate or tidal volume in order to maintain normal $PaCO_2$ and PaO_2. When the medullary respiratory center and peripheral chemoreceptors are depressed by isoflurane during anesthesia, hypoxia becomes the primary stimulant responsible to improve ventilation. However, 100% O_2, typically used as the carrier gas for all the inhalation anesthetics, more specifically isoflurane in this case, eliminated the ventilatory drive that normally responds to hypoxia, resulting in an accumulation and subsequent increase in $PaCO_2$ despite an increased respiratory rate [64, 65]. Nonetheless, calves induced with xylazine (0.1 mg/kg IM) and ketamine (2 mg/kg IV) and maintained with isoflurane in O_2 for repair of umbilical hernia had better arterial oxygenation, less degree of pulmonary vascular shunting, and better quality of anesthesia than those induced with xylazine (0.2 mg/kg IM) and ketamine (5 mg/kg IV) and maintained with intermittent IV ketamine (2.5 mg/kg) [66].

In calves, mask induction with desflurane to tracheal intubation only required 151 ± 32.8 seconds. No struggling, breath holding, or coughing was observed during the induction period, indicating lack of upper airway irritation from desflurane. Anesthesia was maintained at mean end-tidal desflurane concentration of 10 ± 0.76% with control ventilation. No surgery was performed in these calves during desflurane anesthesia. The only cardiovascular changes observed were significant decreases in arterial blood pressures and systemic vascular resistance. Heart rate and cardiac output did not change from baseline values, suggesting that the decrease in systemic vascular resistance was responsible for the decrease in arterial blood pressure observed in these calves, similar to that seen with isoflurane and sevoflurane. Desflurane anesthesia was discontinued after 45 minutes of recording of cardiovascular variables, and isoflurane was then used to maintain anesthesia for surgical placement of a duodenal cannula and thymectomy. All calves in this study recovered uneventfully. Compared to isoflurane and sevoflurane, desflurane, due to its low blood solubility, has the advantage of having a very rapid induction and recovery and the ease of adjustment of anesthetic depth [67]. There is no report on the alveolar concentration of desflurane required during surgical anesthesia in calves. In other domestic animals, the MAC value of desflurane ranges from 7.6% in horses [68], 9.5% in sheep [69], and 10% in pigs [20]. The authors of the study in calves suggested that the 10% end-tidal desflurane concentration used resulted in the maintenance of a light plane of anesthesia which was sufficient for the nonpainful instrumentation procedure but higher concentrations would be required for actual surgery [67].

In Holstein cows induced with thiopental and guaifenesin and maintained under sevoflurane anesthesia, heart rate increased above preanesthetic values throughout the anesthesia period. Atropine administered during the preanesthetic period may be responsible for the increased heart rate observed in this study. Arterial blood pressure and respiratory rate remained unchanged during sevoflurane anesthesia. However, a decrease in pHa and an increase in $PaCO_2$ were reported in these cows, indicating the presence of respiratory depression produced by sevoflurane. Cows in this study recovered from anesthesia smoothly and rapidly. All cows had normal aspartate aminotransferase (AST), alanine aminotransferase (ALT), alkaline phosphatase (ALP), blood urea nitrogen (BUN), and creatinine for 7 days, suggesting a normal hepatic and renal function following 75 minutes of sevoflurane anesthesia [70]. A comparison study in Holstein calves anesthetized with either isoflurane or sevoflurane reported no significant difference in cardiopulmonary parameters between the two anesthetics. However, recovery from sevoflurane appeared to be more rapid, and more attempts were required for the calves to stand unassisted than those receiving isoflurane [71].

Small ruminants and camelids

In newborn lambs, isoflurane induced significant decreases in heart rate, stroke volume, cardiac output, and mean arterial blood pressures when compared to baseline values, but only cardiac output and mean arterial blood pressure decreased in a dose-dependent manner [16]. Conflicting results were reported by Hikasa *et al.* [5], in that isoflurane and sevoflurane both induced a dose-dependent decrease in arterial blood pressure and systemic vascular resistance, but the cardiac index (cardiac output/body weight in kg), a reflection of cardiac output, did not decrease further with increasing either isoflurane or sevoflurane concentration in adult goats. Isoflurane induced a rapid and smooth induction and recovery in llamas and alpacas. At 1 MAC ($1.05 \pm 0.17\%$), arterial blood pressure increased significantly from the baseline value in isoflurane-anesthetized llamas and alpacas. A trend of increase in heart rates was observed, although the values were not statistically significant. Respiratory rate and $PaCO_2$ remained unchanged during anesthesia [17]. A dose-dependent increase in heart rate and $PaCO_2$ and decrease in mean arterial blood pressure occurred when the concentration of isoflurane was increased up to two times of the MAC value [72]. The anesthetic effects of isoflurane, sevoflurane, and desflurane for maintenance were studied in sheep following induction of anesthesia with xylazine (0.1 mg/kg IM), ketamine (2 mg/kg IV), and midazolam (0.03 mg/kg IV). Buprenorphine (0.008 mg/kg IM) was administered to these sheep for additional analgesia [73]. All three inhalation anesthetics produced adequate and stable anesthesia during experimental orthopedic surgeries. There were no significant differences in heart rate and arterial blood pressures between anesthetics, and the values remained within normal ranges. Respiration was characterized by an irregular breathing pattern with intermittent rapid breaths followed by a short period of apnea. No significant difference was observed on the end-tidal CO_2, suggesting a similar ventilatory effect for the three anesthetics.

Considering the blood solubility of these anesthetics, the speed of recovery in theory from fastest to slowest should be in the order of desflurane > sevoflurane > isoflurane in the absence of other anesthetics. The result of this study showed that the time of recovery for sheep capable of keeping their head lifted for 5 minutes was fastest with desflurane (29.8 ± 11.5 minutes), slowest with sevoflurane (38.8 ± 16.6 minutes), and intermediate with isoflurane (32.8 ± 18.1 minutes). Two sheep receiving sevoflurane experienced rough recoveries, but all other sheep recovered uneventfully [73]. In lambs ranging from 3 to 6 weeks of age undergoing experimental spinal surgery, medetomidine (0.01 mg/kg IM) was administered to produce sedation, and anesthesia was induced with either isoflurane or sevoflurane. All lambs received meloxicam (0.6 mg/kg IV), morphine (0.5 mg/kg IV), a constant rate infusion of ketamine (loading dose, 1 mg/kg; infusion, 0.01 mg/kg IV), and atracurium (0.5 mg/kg IV) during surgery. In this study, lambs receiving sevoflurane maintained higher mean and diastolic arterial blood pressure than those receiving isoflurane. The duration from the end of anesthesia to the time the lambs were reunited with their ewes was shorter with sevoflurane [74]. In goats, the speed of recovery was faster for those receiving desflurane and sevoflurane than those receiving isoflurane [10]. Administration of injectable anesthetics to induce anesthesia, addition of supplemental analgesics to enhance analgesia during surgery, and the duration of anesthesia with inhalation anesthetics are very likely to affect the speed of recovery which explains the difference observed between studies.

Swine

Isoflurane and sevoflurane can be used to produce effective and safe anesthesia in pigs. Both anesthetics can be used for mask induction as no breath holding or coughing is observed when these anesthetics are used to anesthetize piglets for castration on the farm or in the field using a mask and a specially designed anesthetic inhaler [75]. Lerman *et al.* [76] reported that the heart rate decreased 19% and 31% and systolic arterial blood pressure decreased 43% and 36%, respectively, at 1.5 MAC of isoflurane and sevoflurane anesthesia in pigs when compared to awake values. Interestingly, isoflurane caused a 43% decrease in cardiac index (cardiac output/body weight in kg), but there was no difference observed with sevoflurane. It is apparent that sevoflurane depresses arterial blood pressure and cardiac output to a lesser degree than isoflurane in pigs [76]. Decreases in PaO_2 during inhalation anesthesia is a common complication, particularly in large adult commercial pigs. Depression of the medullary ventilator center, inhibition of hypoxic pulmonary vasoconstriction, and alteration of the distribution of pulmonary blood and thus a decrease in the PaO_2 value have been well documented during halothane anesthesia [77, 78]. In pigs with a preexisting gas exchange defect, sevoflurane may further impair pulmonary gas exchange, while isoflurane does not [79]. Therefore, close monitoring and efforts to maintain normal PaO_2 should be practiced when using sevoflurane in animals with pulmonary disease.

It seems that pig's age may have a great influence on the MAC value of sevoflurane. Different MAC values have been reported for different age groups of pigs such as 1.97% for 4–10 days of age, 2.5% for 12–13 weeks of age, 2.66% for 22–25 weeks of age, 3.5% for 9 weeks of age, and 4.4% for juvenile pigs [22, 76, 80–82]. In general, increasing age does not increase the anesthetic requirements or the MAC value for inhalation anesthetics in swine. Concurrent administration of preanesthetics, injectable anesthetics, or opioid analgesics and different types of stimulus such as electrical stimulation, tail clamping, or dewclaw clamping have been shown to change the requirement for inhalation anesthetic concentration.

All halogenated volatile anesthetics including isoflurane, sevoflurane, and desflurane are known triggering agents for malignant hyperthermia. Isoflurane has been reported to trigger malignant hyperthermia in susceptible pigs like Pietrain or Pietrain-mixed pigs [83]. Only one incidence of isoflurane-induced malignant hyperthermia has been reported in a potbellied pig [84]. Similarly, sevoflurane-induced malignant hyperthermia has been reported in purebred Poland China pigs [85]. Episodes of malignant hyperthermia induced by desflurane have been reported in Large White pigs, Pietrain pigs, and Pietrain-mixed pigs [83, 86]. Compared to well-documented halothane-induced malignant hyperthermia, the episodes induced by desflurane and isoflurane were reported to have a slower onset than halothane [83].

Successful general anesthesia with inhalation anesthetics requires experience with successful tracheal intubation and sophisticated anesthetic machines and accessories. A small animal anesthesia machine is usually adequate for newborn calves, small ruminants, potbellied pigs, and young camelids weighing less than 150 kg (Figure 5.3). A large animal machine will be required for adult cattle, camelids, and agricultural commercial pigs (Figure 5.4). Nevertheless, inhalation anesthesia has the advantage of maintaining steady levels of anesthesia even for lengthy surgical procedures or research experiments. The ease of adjusting the depth of the anesthetic level with inhalation anesthesia greatly improves patient survival, which is one of the major reasons for the advancement of complicated surgery techniques and research experiments in veterinary medicine in the last two decades.

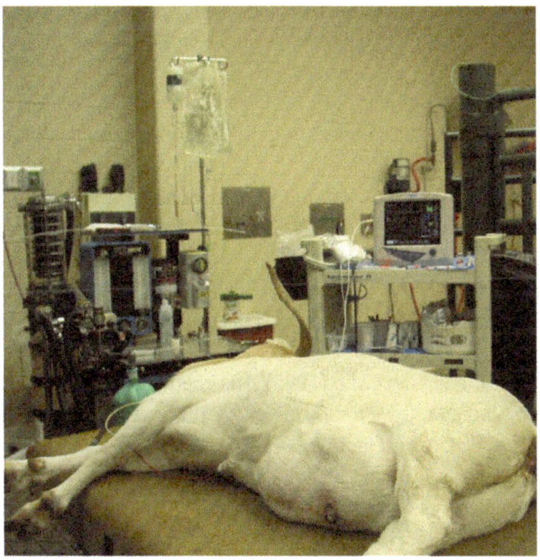

Figure 5.3 A goat anesthetized with isoflurane using small animal anesthesia machine.

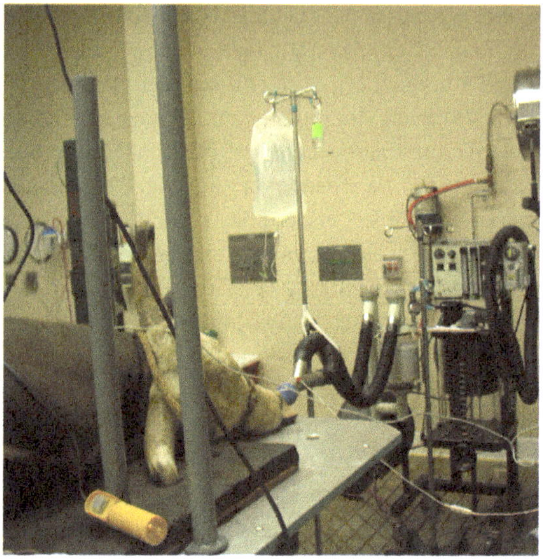

Figure 5.4 A bull anesthetized with isoflurane using large animal anesthesia machine.

References

1. Steffey, E. (2009) Inhalation anesthetics, in *Veterinary Pharmacology and Therapeutics*, 9th edn (eds J. Riviere and M. Papich), Wiley Blackwell, Ames, pp. 229–263.
2. Muir, W., Hubbell, J., Bednarski, R. and Skarda, R. (2007) Inhalation anesthesia, in *Handbook of Veterinary Anesthesia*, 4th edn, St. Louis, Mosby-Elsevier, pp. 164–194.
3. Stoelting, R. and Miller, R. (1989) Basic principles, in *Basics of Anesthesia*, 2nd edn, Churchill Livingstone, New York, pp. 9–23.
4. Stoelting, R. and Hillier, S. (2006) Inhaled anesthetics, in *Pharmacology & Physiology in Anesthetic Practice*, 4th edn, Lippincott Williams & Wilkins, A Wolters Kluwer Company, Philadelphia, pp. 42–86.
5. Hikasa, Y., Okuyama, K., Kakuta, T. *et al.* (1998) Anesthetic potency and cardiopulmonary effects of sevoflurane in goats: comparison with isoflurane and halothane. *Canadian Journal of Veterinary Research*, **62**, 299–306.
6. Stoelting, R. and Hiller, S. (2006) Pharmacokinetics and pharmacodynamics of injected and inhaled drugs, in *Pharmacology and Physiology in Anesthetic Practice*, 4th edn, Lippincott Williams & Wilkins, Philadelphia, pp. 3–41.
7. Steffey, E. and Mama, K. (2007) Inhalation anesthetics, in *Lumb & Jones' Veterinary Anesthesia and Analgesia*, 4th edn (eds W. Tranquilli, J. Thurmon and K. Grimm), Blackwell Publishing, Ames, pp. 355–393.
8. Riebold, T., Geiser, D. and Gable, D. (1995) Anesthetic agents and ancillary drugs, in *Large Animal Anesthesia*, 2nd edn, Iowa State University Press, Ames, IA, pp. 11–64.
9. Redua, M., Doherty, T., Castro-Queiroz, P. *et al.* (2004) Effect of intravenous lidocaine and ketamine on isoflurane minimum alveolar concentration in goats. American College of Veterinary Anesthesiology and Analgesia/Veterinary Academy of Pain Management/American Veterinary Anesthesia Technicians, 56.
10. Alibhai, H. (2001) *Aspects of inhalation anesthesia in the goat*. PhD thesis. University of London.

11. Alibhai, H., Clarke, K. and Hughes, G. (1994) Minimum alveolar concentration (MAC) in goats. International Congress of Veterinary Anaesthesia, 87.
12. Palahniuk, R., Shnider, S. and Eger, E. 2nd. (1974) Pregnancy decreases the requirements for inhaled anesthetic agent. *Anesthesiology*, **41**, 82–83.
13. Bernards, C., Kern, C. and Cullen, B. (1996) Chronic cocaine administration reversibly increase isoflurane minimum alveolar concentration in sheep. *Anesthesiology*, **85**, 91–95.
14. Lukasik, V., Nogami, W. and Morgan, S. (1998) Minimal alveolar concentration and cardiovascular effects of sevoflurane in sheep. *Veterinary Surgery*, **27**, 168.
15. Lukasik, V., Nogami, W. and Morgan, S. (1998) Minimal alveolar concentration and cardiovascular effects of desflurane in sheep. *Veterinary Surgery*, **27**, 167.
16. Brett, C., Teitel, D., Heymann, M. and Rudolph, A. (1987) The cardiovascular effects of isoflurane in lambs. *Anesthesiology*, **67**, 60–65.
17. Mama, K., Wagner, A., Parker, D. *et al.* (1999) Determination of minimum alveolar concentration of isoflurane in llamas. *Veterinary Surgery*, **28**, 121–125.
18. Grubb, T., Schlipf, J., Riebold, T. *et al.* (2003) Minimum alveolar concentration of sevoflurane in spontaneously breathing llamas and alpacas. *Journal of the American Veterinary Medical Association*, **223**, 1167–1169.
19. Grubb, T., Schlipf, J., Riebold, T. *et al.* (2006) Minimum alveolar concentration of desflurane in llamas and alpacas. *Veterinary Anaesthesia and Analgesia*, **33**, 351–355.
20. Eger, E., Johnson, B., Weiskopf, R. *et al.* (1988) Minimum alveolar concentration of I-653 and isoflurane in pigs: definition of a supramaximal stimulus. *Anesthesia and Analgesia*, **67**, 1174–1176.
21. Liu, X., Dingley, J., Elstad, M. *et al.* (2013) Minimum alveolar concentration (MAC) for sevoflurane and xenon at normothermia and hypothermia in newborn piglets. *Acta Anaesthesiologica Scandinavica*, **57**, 646–653.
22. Moeser, A., Blikslager, A. and Swanson, C. (2008) Determination of minimum alveolar concentration of sevoflurane in juvenile swine. *Research in Veterinary Science*, **84**, 283–285.
23. Eger, E. (1994) New inhaled anesthetics. *Anesthesiology*, **80**, 906–922.
24. Malan, T., DiNardo, J., Isner, R. *et al.* (1995) Cardiovascular effects of sevoflurane compared with those of isoflurane in volunteers. *Anesthesiology*, **83**, 918–928.
25. Weiskopf, R., Moore, M., Eger, E. *et al.* (1994) Rapid increase in desflurane concentration is associated with greater transient cardiovascular stimulation than with rapid increase in isoflurane concentration in humans. *Anesthesiology*, **80**, 1035–1045.
26. Ebert, T., Muzi, M. and Lopatka, C. (1995) Neurocirculatory responses to sevoflurane in humans: a comparison to desflurane. *Anesthesiology*, **83**, 88–95.
27. Muzi, M., Ebert, T., Hope, W. *et al.* (1996) Site(s) mediating sympathetic activation with desflurane. *Anesthesiology*, **85**, 737–747.
28. Weiskopf, R., Eger, E., Noorani, M. and Daniel, M. (1994) Fentanyl, esmolol, and clonidine blunt the transient cardiovascular stimulation induced by desflurane in humans. *Anesthesiology*, **81**, 1350–1355.
29. Yonker-Sell, A., Muzi, M., Hope, W. and Ebert, T. (1996) Alfentanil modifies the neurocirculatory responses to desflurane. *Anesthesia and Analgesia*, **82**, 162–166.
30. Stevens, W., Cromwell, T., Halsy, M. *et al.* (1971) The cardiovascular effects of a new inhalation anesthetic, forane, in human volunteers at constant arterial carbon dioxide tension. *Anesthesiology*, **35**, 8–16.
31. Philbin, D. and Lowenstein, E. (1976) Lack of beta-adrenergic activity of isoflurane in the dog: a comparison of circulatory effects of halothane and isoflurane after propranolol administration. *British Journal of Anaesthesia*, **48**, 1165–1170.

32. Mitchell, B. and Williams, J. (1976–1977) Respiratory function changes in sheep associated with lying in lateral recumbency and with sedation by xylazine. Great Britain and Ireland Association of Veterinary Anaesthetists, 30.
33. Klein, L. and Fisher, N. (1988) Cardiopulmonary effects of restraint in dorsal recumbency on awake cattle. *American Journal of Veterinary Research*, **49**, 1605–1608.
34. Torri, G. (2010) Inhalation anesthetics: a review. *Minerva Anestesiologica*, **75**, 215–228.
35. Yurino, M. and Kimura, H. (1992) Vital capacity breath technique for rapid anesthetic induction: comparison of sevoflurane and isoflurane. *Anaesthesia*, **47**, 946–949.
36. Gatecel, C., Losser, M. and Payen, D. (2003) The postoperative effects of halothane versus isoflurane on hepatic artery and portal vein blood flow in humans. *Anesthesia and Analgesia*, **96**, 740–745.
37. Frink, E., Morgan, S., Coetzee, A. *et al.* (1992) The effects of sevoflurane, halothane, enflurane, and isoflurane on hepatic blood flow and oxygenation in chronically instrumented greyhound dogs. *Anesthesiology*, **76**, 85–90.
38. Holmes, M., Weiskopf, R., Eger, E. *et al.* (1990) Hepatocellular integrity in swine after prolonged desflurane (I-653) and isoflurane anesthesia: evaluation of plasma alanine aminotransferase activity. *Anesthesia and Analgesia*, **71**, 249–253.
39. Eger, E., Johnson, B., Strum, D. and Ferrell, L. (1987) Studies of the toxicity of I-653, halothane, and isoflurane in enzyme-induced, hypoxic rats. *Anesthesia and Analgesia*, **66**, 1227–1229.
40. Cousins, M. and Mazze, R. (1973) Methoxyflurane nephrotoxicity. A study of dose response in man. *JAMA*, **225**, 1611–1616.
41. Mazze, R. and Jamison, R. (1995) Renal effects of sevoflurane. *Anesthesiology*, **83**, 443–445.
42. Holaday, D. and Smith, F. (1981) Clinical characteristics and biotransformation of sevoflurane in healthy human volunteers. *Anesthesiology*, **54**, 100–106.
43. Frink, E., Ghantous, H., Malan, T. *et al.* (1992) Plasma inorganic fluoride with sevoflurane anesthesia: correlation with indices of hepatic and renal function. *Anesthesia and Analgesia*, **74**, 231–235.
44. Newman, P., Quinn, A., Hall, G. and Grounds, R. (1994) Plasma inorganic fluoride ion levels following sevoflurane anaesthesia [Abstract]. *British Journal of Anaesthesia*, **72** (Suppl. 1), A166.
45. Shiraishi, Y. and Ikeda, K. (1990) Uptake and biotransformation of sevoflurane in humans: a comparative study of sevoflurane with halothane, enflurane, and isoflurane. *Journal of Clinical Anesthesia*, **2**, 381–386.
46. Smith, I., Ding, Y. and White, P. (1992) Comparison of induction, maintenance and recovery characteristics of sevoflurane-N_2O and propofol-sevoflurane-N_2O with propofol-isoflurane-N_2O anesthesia. *Anesthesia and Analgesia*, **74**, 253–259.
47. Kenna, J. and Jones, R. (1995) The organ toxicity of inhaled anesthetics. *Anesthesia and Analgesia*, **81**, S51–S66.
48. Bito, H. and Ikeda, K. (1994) Long-duration, low-flow sevoflurane anesthesia using two carbon dioxide absorbents: quantification of degradation products in the circuit. *Anesthesiology*, **81**, 340–345.
49. Bito, H. and Ikeda, K. (1994) Closed-circuit anesthesia with sevoflurane in humans: effects on renal and hepatic function and concentrations of breakdown products with soda lime in the circuit. *Anesthesiology*, **80**, 71–76.
50. Gonsowski, C., Laster, M., Eger, E. *et al.* (1994) Toxicity of compound A in rats. Effect of increasing duration of administration. *Anesthesiology*, **80**, 566–573.

51. Nakazawa, M., Miyano, K., Toriumi, K. and Tanifuzi, Y. (1994) Differential reactivities of three kinds of carbon dioxide absorbents with high concentration of sevoflurane. *Masui*, **43**, 1216–1220.
52. Foden, N., vanPelt, F. and Jones, R. (1994) Dose dependent degradation of sevoflurane to compound A [Abstract]. *Anesthesiology*, **81**, A432.
53. Munday, I., Foden, N., Ward, P. *et al.* (1994) Sevoflurane degradation in a circle system at 2 different fresh gas flow rates [Abstract]. *Anesthesiology*, **81**, A433.
54. Suzuki, Y., Miyasaka, K., Takata, M. *et al.* (1994) Concentration of sevoflurane breakdown products with soda lime [Abstract]. *Anesthesiology*, **81**, A571.
55. Versichelen, L., Bouche, M.-P., Rolly, G. *et al.* (2001) Only carbon dioxide absorbents free of both NaOH and KOH do not generate compound A during in vitro closed-system sevoflurane: evaluation of five absorbents. *Anesthesiology*, **95**, 750–755.
56. Morio, M., Fujii, K., Satoh, N. *et al.* (1992) Reaction of sevoflurane and its degradation products with soda lime. Toxicity of the byproducts. *Anesthesiology*, **77**, 1155–1164.
57. Iyer, R. and Anders, M. (1996) Cysteine congregate beta-lyase-dependent biotransformation of the cystein-s-conjugates of the sevoflurane degradation product compound A in human, non-human primate, and rat kidney cytosol and mitochondria. *Anesthesiology*, **85**, 1454–1461.
58. Neumann, M., Laster, M., Weiskopf, R. *et al.* (1999) The elimination of sodium and potassium hydroxides from desiccated soda lime diminishes degradation of desflurane to carbon monoxide and sevoflurane to compound A but does not compromise carbon dioxide absorption. *Anesthesia and Analgesia*, **89**, 768–773.
59. Martin, J., Dodge, M. and Pohl, L. (1994) Immunochemical detection of covalently modified kidney proteins in rats treated with the sevoflurane degradation product: compound A (sevo-olefin) [Abstract]. *Anesthesiology*, **81**, A436.
60. Kandel, L., Laster, M., Eger, E. *et al.* (1995) Nephrotoxicity in rats undergoing a one-hour exposure to compound A. *Anesthesia and Analgesia*, **81**, 559–563.
61. Frink, E., Green, W., Brown, E. *et al.* (1996) Compound A concentrations during sevoflurane anesthesia in children. *Anesthesiology*, **84**, 566–571.
62. Muir, W. and Gadawski, J. (1998) Cardiorespiratory effects of low-flow and closed circuit inhalation anesthesia, using sevoflurane delivered with an in-circuit vaporizer and concentrations of compound A. *American Journal of Veterinary Research*, **59**, 603–608.
63. Greene, S., Tyner, C., Morris, D. and Hartsfield, S. (1988) Comparison of cardiopulmonary effects of isoflurane and halothane after atropine-guaifenesin-thiamylal anesthesia for rumenotomy in steers. *American Journal of Veterinary Research*, **49**, 1891–1893.
64. Hirshman, C., Mccullough, R., Cohen, P. and Weil, J. (1977) Depression of hypoxic ventilatory response by halothane, enflurane and isoflurane in dogs. *British Journal of Anaesthesia*, **49**, 957–963.
65. Knill, R., Kieraszewicz, H., Dodgson, B. and Clement, J. (1983) Chemical regulation of ventilation during isoflurane sedation and anaesthesia in humans. *Canadian Anaesthetists' Society Journal*, **30**, 607–614.
66. Offinger, J., Meyer, H., Fischer, J. *et al.* (2012) Comparison of isoflurane inhalation anaesthesia, injection anaesthesia and high volume caudal epidural anaesthesia for umbilical surgery in calves; metabolic, endocrine and cardiopulmonary effects. *Veterinary Anaesthesia and Analgesia*, **39**, 123–136.
67. Keegan, R., Greene, S., Valdez, R. and Knowles, D. (2006) Cardiopulmonary effects of desflurane in mechanically ventilated calves. *American Journal of Veterinary Research*, **67**, 387–391.

68. Tendillo, F., Mascias, A., Santos, M. *et al.* (1997) Anesthetic potency of desflurane in the horse: determination of the minimum alveolar concentration. *Veterinary Surgery*, **26**, 354–357.
69. Lukasik, V., Nogami, W. and Morgan, S. (2005) Minimum alveolar concentration and cardiovascular effects of desflurane in sheep [Abstract]. *Veterinary Anaesthesia and Analgesia*, **32**, 237.
70. Hikasa, Y., Takase, K., Kondou, K. and Ogasawara, S. (1994) Sevoflurane anesthesia following administration of atropine-guaifenesin-thiopental in spontaneous breathing adult cattle. *The Journal of Veterinary Medical Science*, **56**, 613–616.
71. Sellers, G., Lin, H., Chamorro, M. and Walz, P. (2013) Comparison of isoflurane and sevoflurane anesthesia in Holstein calves for placement of portal and jugular vein cannulas. *American Journal of Animal and Veterinary Sciences*, **8**, 1–7.
72. Mama, K., Wagner, A. and Steffey, E. (2001) Circulatory, respiratory and behavioral responses in isoflurane anesthetized llamas. *Veterinary Anaesthesia and Analgesia*, **28**, 12–17.
73. Mohamadnia, A., Hughes, G. and Clarke, K. (2008) Maintenance of anaesthesia in sheep with isoflurane, desflurane or sevoflurane. *The Veterinary Record*, **163**, 210–215.
74. Vettorato, E., Schoffmann, G., Burke, J. *et al.* (2012) Clinical effects of isoflurane and sevoflurane in lambs. *Veterinary Anaesthesia and Analgesia*, **39**, 495–502.
75. Hodgson, D. (2007) Comparison of isoflurane and sevoflurane for short-term anesthesia in piglets. *Veterinary Anaesthesia and Analgesia*, **34**, 117–124.
76. Lerman, J., Oyston, J., Gallagher, T. *et al.* (1990) The minimum alveolar concentration (MAC) and hemodynamic effects of halothane, isoflurane, and sevoflurane in newborn swine. *Anesthesiology*, **73**, 717–721.
77. Johnson, D., Mayers, I. and To, T. (1990) The effect of halothane in hypoxic pulmonary vasoconstriction. *Anesthesiology*, **72**, 125–133.
78. Dueck, R., Young, I., Clausen, J. and Wagner, P. (1980) Altered distribution of pulmonary ventilation and blood flow following induction of inhalation anesthesia. *Anesthesiology*, **52**, 113–125.
79. Kleinsasser, A., Lindner, K., Hoermann, C. *et al.* (2001) Isoflurane and sevoflurane anesthesia in pigs with a preexistent gas exchange defect. *Anesthesiology*, **95**, 1422–1426.
80. Holmstrom, A. and Akeson, J. (2003) Cerebral blood flow at 0.5 and 1.0 minimum alveolar concentrations of desflurane or sevoflurane compared with isoflurane in normoventilated pigs. *Journal of Neurosurgical Anesthesiology*, **15**, 90–97.
81. Hecker, K., Baumert, J., Horn, N. *et al.* (2003) Minimum anesthetic concentrations of sevoflurane with different xenon concentrations in swine. *Anesthesia and Analgesia*, **97**, 1364–1369.
82. Manohar, M. and Parks, C. (1984) Porcine systemic and regional organ blood flow during 1.0 and 1.5 minimum alveolar concentrations of sevoflurane anesthesia without and with 50% nitrous oxide. *The Journal of Pharmacology and Experimental Therapeutics*, **231**, 640–648.
83. Wedel, D., Gammel, S., Milde, J. and Iaizzo, P. (1993) Delayed onset of malignant hyperthermia induced by isoflurane and desflurane compared with halothane in susceptible swine. *Anesthesiology*, **78**, 1138–1144.
84. Claxton-Gill, M., Cornick-Seahorn, J., Gamboa, J. and Boatright, B. (1993) Suspected malignant hyperthermia syndrome in a miniature pot-bellied pig anesthetized with isoflurane. *Journal of the American Veterinary Medical Association*, **203**, 1434–1436.
85. Shulman, M., Braverman, B., Ivankovich, A. and Gronert, G. (1981) Sevoflurane triggers malignant hyperthermia in swine. *Anesthesiology*, **54**, 259–260.
86. Bonome-Gonzales, C., Alvarez-Refojo, F., Fernandez-Goti, C. *et al.* (2001) Malignant hyperthermia in a pig anesthetized with desflurane. *Revista espanola de anestesiologia y reanimacion*, **48**, 81–84.

Chapter 6

Perioperative monitoring and management of complications

HuiChu Lin

Department of Clinical Sciences, College of Veterinary Medicine, Auburn University, USA

Perioperative monitoring

Anesthetized animals should be monitored closely and continuously throughout the anesthesia period. Routine variables to be monitored include heart rate and rhythm, pulse strength, respiratory rate and depth, arterial blood pressures, palpebral and corneal reflexes, eyeball rotation, capillary refill time, and mucous membrane color. Accurate assessment of the physical condition of an anesthetized patient and the depth of anesthesia of that patient are best accomplished using a combination of several parameters rather than relying on a single parameter. Presence of palpebral reflex, position of the eyeballs, and change in respiratory rate, heart rate, and arterial blood pressure are the most useful parameters and reliable indicators of the depth of anesthesia. These parameters should be evaluated and their values recorded periodically throughout the duration of anesthesia. Following induction of anesthesia, peripheral pulse should be palpable, and an electrocardiogram (ECG), if available, should be used at all times. Position of the eyeballs in anesthetized large ruminants correlates well with the depth of anesthesia. During the surgical plane of anesthesia, eyeballs rotate ventromedially with the cornea partially obscured by the lower eyelids. Palpebral reflex should be sluggish or just absent. As anesthetic depth deepens, eyeballs rotate to the central position with no palpebral reflex, diminished corneal reflex, and dilated cornea (Figure 6.1). Reducing the concentration of injectable or inhalation anesthetic delivered to the patient at this time may be warranted to avoid unnecessarily deepening the plane of anesthesia of the patient. If eyeballs are at the center position with strong palpebral and corneal reflexes, the depth of anesthesia may be inadequate and patients may be too light for surgical manipulation, and an increase in the anesthetic(s) concentration delivered is required. Eyeball rotation or position is not as reliable in small ruminants, camelids, and pigs as an indicator of anesthetic depth as it is in large ruminants. Changes in heart rate, respiratory rate,

Farm Animal Anesthesia: Cattle, Small Ruminants, Camelids, and Pigs, First Edition.
Edited by HuiChu Lin and Paul Walz.

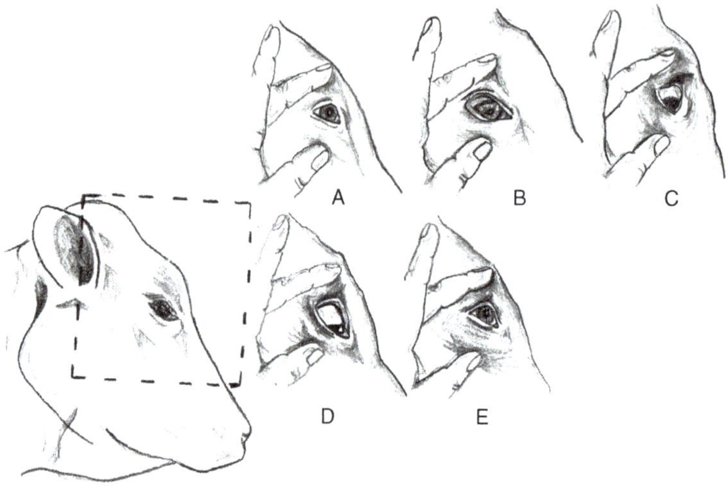

Figure 6.1 Changes in eyeball positions during anesthesia in cattle. A, Awake (strong palpebral reflex), B and C, light anesthesia, D, surgical plane of anesthesia, and E, deep anesthesia (absence of palpebral reflex). (Source: Illustration by Kim Crosslin.)

arterial blood pressures, and palpebral and corneal reflexes can be used to assess the depth of anesthesia in these animals. As a general rule, decrease in heart rate, respiratory rate, and arterial blood pressures, and absence of palpebral and corneal reflexes are more likely indicators of deep anesthesia.

Maintaining normal heart rate and stroke volume is the most important factor in maintaining normal cardiac output (cardiac output = heart rate × stroke volume) and normal arterial blood pressure (mean arterial blood pressure = cardiac output × systemic vascular resistance). ECG can be used to monitor heart rate and cardiac rhythm continuously throughout anesthesia. Abnormal cardiac rhythm and significant changes in heart rate have the potential to impact stroke volume, cardiac output, and thus O_2 delivery to the tissues. The most common method for ECG monitoring of ruminant patients requires placement of electrodes at left forelimb (LA), right forelimb (RA), and left hind limb (LL) of the patient. This simple technique generates three bipolar limb leads for evaluation of the cardiac rhythm. Lead I indicates the voltage difference between the RA and LA electrodes, lead II the voltage difference between the RA and LL electrodes, and lead III the voltage difference between the LA and LL electrodes. These electrodes are attached to a main cable that interfaces with a simple ECG monitor or a multiparameter monitor. The monitor then displays a real-time tracing of cardiac electrical activity using either one of the three leads of which the most commonly used for cardiac rhythm analysis is lead II, but the lead with largest amplitude should be used. The characteristic normal waveform composition includes a distinct P wave, QRS complex, and T wave [1]. Most ECG monitors also display heart rate. Tachycardia, bradycardia, and ventricular dysrhythmias such as premature ventricular contraction and ventricular tachycardia are the most commonly observed cardiac arrhythmias in farm animals undergoing anesthesia. Sinus tachycardia and atrial fibrillation, though rarely, have also been observed in these animals. The ECG only shows the electrical activity of the myocardium; it does not provide information of the arterial blood pressure or pulse strength. Digital palpation of a peripheral artery for pulse strength should always be incorporated with the data from the ECG rhythm.

Arterial blood pressure can be measured either by indirect or direct methods. Indirect arterial blood pressures can be measured using an oscillometric blood pressure machine with an inflatable blood pressure cuff placed on the coccygeal or dorsal metatarsal artery. The cuff is inflated automatically to a suprasystolic pressure, and the air is gradually released until the characteristic arterial oscillation is detected by an electronic sensor. The computer then interprets the oscillation and displays measured values of systolic, mean, and diastolic blood pressures. For accurate measurement, the width of the cuff should be approximately 40% of the circumference of the extremity around which the cuff is placed. Too small a cuff tends to overestimate the blood pressure, whereas too big a cuff tends to underestimate it. Direct arterial blood pressure measurement is achieved using a catheter placed in a superficial artery such as auricular artery or metatarsal artery. The catheter is connected to an electronic resistance-type transducer via a semirigid saline-filled arterial blood pressure tubing. The transducer is then connected to a cable that interfaces with a simple sphygmomanometer or a multiparameter monitor. Sphygmomanometer provides mean arterial blood pressure, whereas multiparameter monitor displays systolic, mean, and diastolic arterial blood pressures as well as heart rate. Both indirect and direct methods provide continuous monitoring and reading of the arterial blood pressures. Changes in arterial blood pressures can be detected immediately and treatment can be instituted if needed [1, 2]. Sophisticated multiparameter monitor may not be practical in field settings; simple auscultation of the heart and lung, continuous recording of the heart rate and respiratory rate, digital palpation of the pulse strength, and close monitoring of the eye reflexes should be sufficient for routine patient monitoring during field anesthesia. Significant changes in heart rate, cardiac rhythm, respiratory rate, and breathing pattern should provide sufficient information regarding the depth of anesthesia and the condition of the patient.

The use of capnogram and pulse oximetry to evaluate end-tidal CO_2 ($ETCO_2$) and arterial O_2 saturation (SpO_2), respectively, has become part of the routine monitoring accessories to ensure adequate ventilation, efficient gas exchange, and appropriate oxygenation of an anesthetized patient (Figure 6.2). The alveolar ventilation (V_A) to eliminate overall systemically produced CO_2 determines the arterial partial pressure of CO_2 ($PaCO_2$). While CO_2 production remains stable under normal conditions, $PaCO_2$ varies inversely with the changes in V_A. The ability of the lung to remove $PaCO_2$ indicates the effectiveness of ventilation. When an anesthetized patient is healthy and has no preexisting diffusion disturbance in the pulmonary tissues, $ETCO_2$ is usually closely related to alveolar CO_2 and $PaCO_2$. Therefore, $ETCO_2$ can be used to estimate $PaCO_2$ and to assess the adequacy of ventilation. Capnography allows continuous monitoring of the adequacy of ventilation during anesthesia. The amount of alveolar CO_2 and thus $ETCO_2$ measured in the exhaled gas at the end of expiration is determined by infrared absorption. Samples for measurement of $ETCO_2$ are collected

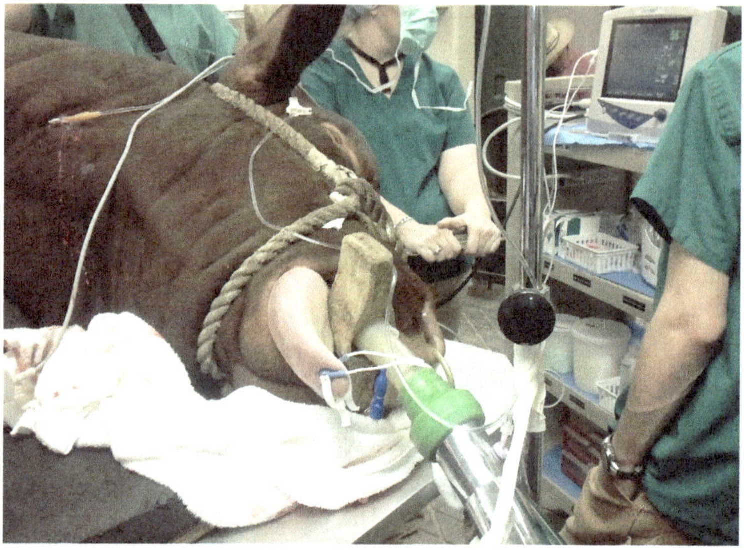

Figure 6.2 Placement of $ETCO_2$ sample collection line and SpO_2 probe on an adult cattle.

directly at the connecting point between the Y piece of the breathing system of an anesthesia machine and the end of an endotracheal tube (Figure 6.2). In awake, unsedated cattle, normal $PaCO_2$ is reported to be between 38 and 43 mm of Hg [3]. $ETCO_2$ is usually lower than $PaCO_2$ by 10–15 mm of Hg due to a slight degree of ventilation/perfusion (*V*/*Q*) mismatch even in the awake state [4]. Most anesthetics depress respiratory function resulting in hypoventilation and a significant increase in $PaCO_2$ with subsequent respiratory acidosis [5–12]. Severe hypoventilation with $PaCO_2$ greater than 60 mm of Hg is common in anesthetized, recumbent farm animals, particularly in adult cattle. Furthermore, a greater difference between $ETCO_2$ and $PaCO_2$ is also expected because of the increased *V*/*Q* mismatch in anesthetized, recumbent large animals, with the greatest difference occurring during dorsal recumbency (Figure 6.3) [13]. In halothane-anesthetized horses, a significantly greater difference between $ETCO_2$ and $PaCO_2$ occurred when they were anesthetized longer than 90 minutes as compared to that recorded at 60 minutes or less. But this increased difference with time between $ETCO_2$ and $PaCO_2$ did not occur in isoflurane-anesthetized horses [14]. Though there is no similar study reported in farm animals, increase in the difference between $ETCO_2$ and $PaCO_2$ as a result of prolonged duration of isoflurane anesthesia has not been observed in anesthetized adult cattle. The measurement of $ETCO_2$ does not reflect the true value of $PaCO_2$; clinical experience shows that monitoring of $ETCO_2$ can be used as an indicator to predict the direction of the change of $PaCO_2$ during anesthesia. However, it is important to remember that the difference between $ETCO_2$ and $PaCO_2$ is affected by the efficiency of the ventilation during anesthesia and the position of the patient required for surgery [4].

Adequate tissue oxygenation is essential for patient survival following anesthesia. Tissue O_2 delivery is determined by the blood flow and arterial blood O_2 content

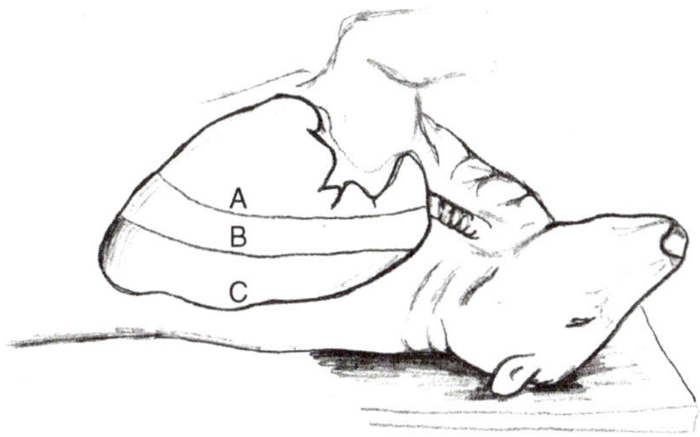

Figure 6.3 *V/Q* mismatch during dorsal recumbency in adult cattle. A, $V/Q > 1$, B, $V/Q \approx 1$, and C, $V/Q < 1$. (Source: Illustration by Kim Crosslin.)

(CaO_2) in that tissue. When O_2 diffuses into the blood, 98% of that is bound to hemoglobin and only 1–2% is dissolved in the plasma. The O_2-bound hemoglobin is represented by the measurement of O_2 saturation (SaO_2), and the amount dissolved in the plasma is represented as the partial pressure of arterial O_2 (PaO_2). Although PaO_2 only constitutes a small fraction of total CaO_2, its well-defined relationship with SaO_2 in the arterial blood is demonstrated by the O_2 dissociation curve. Therefore, SaO_2 can be used to estimate PaO_2. A pulse oximeter uses the difference in the ability in absorbing infrared light of saturated and desaturated hemoglobin to calculate the amount of O_2 bound to the hemoglobin (SpO_2) [15]. This technique is noninvasive with the sensor clip or probe placed on a superficial pulsating artery either on the lingual artery in the tongue, on the auricular artery in light-colored ears, or occasionally on the mucous membrane of the rectum of the animal (Figure 6.2). In normal, healthy patients, SpO_2 readings are reliable estimates of SaO_2, ranging from 80 to 100% [16]. Normal hemoglobin SaO_2 should always be near 98–100% which correlates to a PaO_2 of 95–100 mm of Hg when breathing room air with 21% O_2. During anesthesia, when a patient is breathing 100% O_2, PaO_2 can range from 60 to 500 mm of Hg. Using the O_2 dissociation curve, PaO_2 can be estimated by subtracting 30 from the SpO_2 value when the SpO_2 is in the range of 60–90%. For example, PaO_2 is estimated to be 60 mm of Hg when the SpO_2 reading is 90% [17]. Factors that alter pulse strength of a peripheral artery such as hypotension, hypothermia, and vasoconstriction affect the ability of pulse oximeter to accurately estimate the SpO_2 [1, 4]. Increased $ETCO_2$ and decreased SpO_2 imply inadequate ventilation and severe *V/Q* mismatch which oftentimes are the result of abnormal positioning of the animal and deep anesthesia. Decrease delivery of anesthetics and assisted or controlled ventilation should be instituted immediately to improve ventilation. Measurements of $ETCO_2$ and SpO_2 require appropriate pulmonary perfusion and pulsating peripheral arterial blood flow from adequate myocardial contractility and cardiac output. Sudden dramatic decrease in $ETCO_2$ and SpO_2 is the first indication of impending cardiac arrest. Gradual and persistent increase in $ETCO_2$ may indicate the beginning of a malignant hyperthermia episode.

Table 6.1 The body temperature, heart rate, respiratory rate, and arterial blood pressures for farm animals.

Species	Temp (°F)	Heart rate (beats/minute)	Respiratory rate (breaths/minute)	Arterial blood pressure (mm of Hg)
Cattle [18]	101–103	70–90	20–30	SAP: 120–150 MAP: 90–120 DAP: 80–110
Camelids [19]	100–102	60–80	10–30	SAP: 60–135 MAP: 70–100 DAP: 45–95
Goats [20]	102–104	70–95	15–30	SAP: 80–120 MAP: 75–100 DAP: 60–80
Sheep [20]	102–104	70–80	20–30	SAP: 80–120 MAP: 75–100 DAP: 60–80
Pigs [21] (adult)	101–104	70–110	20–30	SAP: 95–126 MAP: 68–83 DAP: 44–77
Pigs [21] (weaning)	102	80–100	25–30	SAP: 83–114* MAP: 58–76* DAP: 40–51*

SAP, systolic arterial pressure; MAP, mean arterial pressure; DAP, diastolic arterial pressure.
*Lin, H.C. Clinical observation.

Table 6.1, Table 6.2, Table 6.3, Table 6.4, Table 6.5, and Table 6.6 provide normal values of commonly monitored physiological parameters (body temperature, heart rate, respiratory rate, and systolic, mean, and diastolic arterial blood pressures), hematology, and blood chemistry for cattle, goats, sheep, camelids, and pigs.

Supportive fluid therapy

Supportive fluid therapy during anesthesia is not absolutely necessary in healthy animals undergoing short-term surgery. However, if the animal is fasted and water is withheld for 24 hours or longer prior to anesthesia, a balanced electrolyte solution should be administered. In large ruminants, a 12- or 14-gauge needle or 5¼-in. Teflon indwelling catheter can be placed in the jugular vein for fluid administration and, if needed, for administration of emergency drugs. A 14- or 16-gauge, 3–5¼-inch indwelling catheter is usually used for small ruminants and camelids. Normal maintenance fluid therapy in healthy patients during anesthesia is 4–8 ml/kg/hour, but 10–25 ml/kg/hour may be required to correct hypotension in compromised patients. Ruminants salivate copiously during anesthesia, but administration of balanced electrolyte solution for replacement of fluid loss through salivation usually is not required

Table 6.2 Normal values for hematology and blood chemistry of cattle.

Hematology*		**Blood chemistry***	
Hematocrit (%)	24–46	Blood urea nitrogen (mg/dl)	7–17
Hemoglobin (g/dl)	8–15	Creatinine (mg/dl)	1–3
Red blood cells (10^6/μl)	5–10	Total protein (g/dl)	5.8–8.5
Mean corpuscular hemoglobin (MCH, pg)	14–19	Albumin (g/dl)	3–4.8
Mean corpuscular hemoglobin concentration (MCHC, g/dl)	30–36	Bilirubin(mg/dl)	0.2–4
Mean corpuscular volume (MCV, fl)	40–65	Glucose (mg/dl)	48–70
White blood cells (10^3/μl)	5–17	Calcium (mg/dl)	8.5–10.3
Seg. neutrophils (10^3/μl)	0.6–4	Phosphorus (mg/dl)	2.4–7.9
Band neutrophils (10^3/μl)	0–0.1	Sodium (mEq/l)	137–151
Lymphocytes (10^3/μl)	2.5–7.5	Potassium (mEq/l)	2.5–5.9
Basophils (10^3/μl)	0–0.1	Chloride (mEq/l)	98–107
Monocytes (10^3/μl)	0.025–0.85	Magnesium (mg/dl)	1.9–2.7
Eosinophil (10^3/μl)	0–1.6	Bicarbonate (mmol/l)	16–40
Reticulocytes (10^3/μl)	0.001–0.008	Anion gap (mmol/l)	10–27
Platelets (10^3/μl)	0.1–0.8	Osmolality (mmol/kg)	270–350
Fibrinogen (mg/dl)	100–600	Creatine kinase (CK, U/l)	40–264
		Aspartate aminotransferase (AST (SGOT), U/l)	69–112
		γ-Glutamyl transferase (GGT, U/l)	3.7–31
		Sorbitol dehydrogenase (SDH (SGOT), U/l)	4.5–18

*Reference data from Clinical Pathology Laboratory, Auburn University.

CHAPTER 6

Table 6.3 Normal values for hematology and blood chemistry of goats.

Hematology*		**Blood chemistry***	
Hematocrit (%)	22–38	Blood urea nitrogen (mg/dl)	10–20
Hemoglobin (g/dl)	8–12	Creatinine (mg/dl)	1–1.82
Red blood cells (10^6/μl)	8–18	Total protein (g/dl)	6.4–7
MCH (pg)	5.2–8	Albumin (g/dl)	2.7–3.9
MCHC (g/dl)	30–36	Bilirubin (mg/dl)	0.10–1.71
MCV (fl)	16–25	Glucose (mg/dl)	50–75
White blood cells (10^3/μl)	4–13	Calcium (mg/dl)	8.9–11.7
Seg. neutrophils (10^3/μl)	1.2–7.2	Phosphorus (mg/dl)	4.2–9.1
Band neutrophils (10^3/μl)	0	Sodium (mEq/l)	142–155
Lymphocytes (10^3/μl)	2–9	Potassium (mEq/l)	3.5–6.7
Basophils (10^3/μl)	0–0.3	Chloride (mEq/l)	99–110.3
Monocytes (10^3/μl)	0–0.05	Magnesium (mg/dl)	2.8–3.6
Eosinophil (10^3/μl)	0.05–0.65	Bicarbonate (mmol/l)	N/A
Platelets (10^3/μl)	0.3–0.6	Anion gap (mmol/l)	N/A
Fibrinogen (g/l)	100–400	CK (U/l)	0.8–9
		AST (SGOT, U/l)	167–513
		GGT (U/l)	20–56
		SDH (SGOT, U/l)	14–23.6

*Adapted from Reference [22].

Table 6.4 Normal values of hematology and blood chemistry of sheep.

Hematology*		**Blood chemistry***	
Hematocrit (%)	27–45	Blood urea nitrogen (mg/dl)	8–20
Hemoglobin (g/dl)	9–15	Creatinine (mg/dl)	1.2–1.9
Red blood cells (10^6/μl)	9–15	Total protein (g/dl)	6–7.5
MCH (pg)	8–12	Albumin (g/dl)	2.4–3
MCHC (g/dl)	31–34	Bilirubin(mg/dl)	0.1–0.5
MCV (fl)	28–40	Glucose (mg/dl)	50–80
White blood cells (10^3/μl)	4–12	Calcium (mg/dl)	11.5–12.8
Seg. neutrophils (10^3/μl)	0.7–6	Phosphorus (mg/dl)	5–7.3
Band neutrophils (10^3/μl)	0	Sodium (mEq/l)	139–152
Lymphocytes (10^3/μl)	2–9	Potassium (mEq/l)	3.9–5.4
Basophils (10^3/μl)	0–0.3	Chloride (mEq/l)	95–103
Monocytes (10^3/μl)	0–0.75	Magnesium (mg/dl)	2.2–2.8
Eosinophil (10^3/μl)	0–1	Bicarbonate (mmol/l)	20–25
Platelets (10^3/μl)	0.21–0.71	CK (U/l)	8–13
Fibrinogen (mg/dl)	100–500	AST (SGOT, U/l)	60–280
		GGT (U/l)	20–52
		SDH (SGOT, U/l)	5.8–27.9

*Adapted from Reference [22].

Table 6.5 Normal values for hematology and blood chemistry of camelids.

Hematology*		**Blood chemistry***	
Hematocrit (%)	34 ± 4.0	Blood urea nitrogen (mg/dl)	29.0 ± 6.1
	25–46		9–34
Hemoglobin (g/dl)	15.3 ± 1.7	Creatinine (mg/dl)	2.5 ± 0.5
	11.5–19.5		1.4–3.2
Red blood cell (10^6/μl)	10.88 ± 1.1	Total protein (g/dl)	5.9 ± 0.5
	9.9–17.7		5.1–7.8
MCH (pg)	11.2	Albumin (g/dl)	3.6 ± 0.6
	9.8–12.7		3.1–5.2
MCHC (g/dl)	43.3	Bilirubin (mg/dl)	0.2 ± 0.2
	37.7–49		0–0.2
MCV (fl)	26	Glucose (mg/dl)	134.2 ± 36.0
	22–30.1		74–154
White blood cell (10^3/μl)	8.0–23.3	Calcium (mg/dl)	9.0 ± 0.7
	7.5–20.0		7.4–10.4
Seg. neutrophils (10^3/μl)	4.18–14.87	Phosphorus (mg/dl)	5.8 ± 2.2
			2.6–7.3
Band neutrophils (10^3/μl)	0–0.13	Sodium (mEq/l)	149.4 ± 5.4
	0–169		148–158
Lymphocytes (10^3/μl)	0.96–7.64	Potassium (mEq/l)	3.8 ± 0.9
	0.7–4.9		3.7–6.1
Basophils (10^3/μl)	0–0.3	Chloride (mEq/l)	115.9 ± 4.8
			102–120
Monocytes (10^3/μl)	0.0–1.34	Magnesium (mg/dl)	1.9 ± 0.3
	0.0–1.0		
Eosinophil (10^3/μl)	0.07–5.83	Bicarbonate (mmol/l)	N/A
	0.16–4.5		
		Total CO_2 (mm/l)	13–31
Reticulocytes (10^3/μl)	12–79	CK (U/l)	81.8 ± 110
			8–77
Platelets (10^3/μl)	200–600	AST (SGOT, U/l)	216–378
			166–447
Fibrinogen (g/l)	300 ± 114	GGT (U/l)	7–29
	100–500		9–27
		SDH (U/l)	1–17
			1–5

*Adapted from (a) Oregon State University Veterinary Diagnostic Laboratory; (b) Reference [23]; (c) Reference [24].

[27, 28]. Camelids do not handle the administration of large amount of fluid in a short period of time well. Hypoproteinemia and subsequent pulmonary edema may develop and thus impair gas exchange within the alveoli. As a result, respiratory distress and death may occur [29].

Intravenous (IV) catheterization for perioperative fluid therapy in pigs is difficult and often impossible, particularly in potbellied pigs, because of lack of visible superficial

Table 6.6 Normal values for hematology and blood chemistry of pet pigs.

Hematology*,†		**Blood chemistry*,†**	
Hematocrit (%)	32–50	Blood urea nitrogen (mg/dl)	10–25
	(30–50)		(9.2–29.2)
Hemoglobin (g/dl)	10–16	Creatinine (mg/dl)	0.5–1.7
			(1.2–2)
Red blood cells ($10^6/\mu l$)	5–8	Total protein (g/dl)	6.2–9.3
			(6.1–8.9)
MCH (pg)	17–21	Albumin (g/dl)	3.1–4.3
			(3.9–5.6)
MCHC (g/dl)	30–34	Bilirubin (mg/dl)	0.5–1
			(0–0.3)
MCV (fl)	50–56	Glucose (mg/dl)	31–77
			(36.4–123.2)
White blood cells ($10^3/\mu l$)	11–22	Calcium (mg/dl)	8.3–10.4
	(6.6–18.6)		(9.6–11.6)
Seg. neutrophils ($10^3/\mu l$)	3.2–10	Phosphorus (mg/dl)	4.9–9.1
			(5.1–8.1)
Band neutrophils ($10^3/\mu l$)	0–0.8	Sodium (mEq/l)	135–153
Band neutrophils (%)	(0.0–1.2)		(144–152.6)
Lymphocytes ($10^3/\mu l$)	4.5–13	Potassium (mEq/l)	3.9–6
Lymphocytes (%)	(19.2–72)		(4–5.2)
Basophils ($10^3/\mu l$)	0–2	Chloride (mmol/l)	92–117
Basophils (%)	(0–2.5)		(94.4–114)
Monocytes ($10^3/\mu l$)	0.25–2	Magnesium (mg/dl)	2.7–3.7
Monocytes (%)	(1.1–13.9)		
Eosinophil ($10^3/\mu l$)	0.05–2	Bicarbonate (mmol/l)	21–31
Eosinophil (%)	(0–10)		
Platelets ($10^3/\mu l$)	130–950	Anion gap (mmol/l)	14–23
	(201–679)		
Fibrinogen (mg/dl)	100–500	CK (U/l)	77–256
			(48–288)
		AST (SGOT, U/l)	53–162
			(10.4–56)
		SDH (U/l)	1–5.8
		GGT (U/l)	11–39

*Values in parenthesis for Yucatan miniature pigs.
†Adapted from (a) Reference [25]; (b) Reference [26].

CHAPTER 6

veins. An ear vein can be used for placement of IV catheter if the pig cooperates. This may be easier to accomplish in a large farm (agricultural) pig, while it can be quite difficult in an awake potbellied pig but easier when done during anesthesia. Ear veins especially lateral auricular veins are common sites because they are superficial and easily accessible. An 18- or 20-gauge, 1–1½-in. hypodermic needle, indwelling catheter, or butterfly catheter can be used for large adult pigs, while 21- or 23-gauge is suitable for smaller-sized pigs and pigs with small ears. Intramedullary cannulation has been used for fluid and drug administration when no other vascular access can be established. An 18-gauge cannula can be placed into the greater tubercle of the humerus or the trochanteric fossa of the femur for intramedullary administration. This technique can be performed in immature pigs, but the administration rate of drug solution or fluid may be limited in older pigs due to the presence of fat and fibrosis of the medullary canal [30]. Please refer to Chapter 10 for detailed discussion on fluid therapy in farm animals.

Positioning

Improper positioning of the patient can result in postanesthetic neuromyopathy in cattle and camelids, similar to that seen in horses. Uneven distribution of the body weight of the animal and inadequate surface padding such as would occur on gravel, concrete, or a metal table surface without foam padding where the animal was placed during anesthesia are examples of improper positioning. Myopathy does not occur as readily in large ruminants, but nerve paralysis due to improper positioning has occurred in adult cattle and camelids following anesthesia. Adult cattle should be placed on a 10-cm-thick high-density foam pad, whereas a 5-cm-thick foam pad is sufficient for calves, small ruminants, camelids, and pigs. When placed in dorsal recumbency, veterinarian should make sure that the animal is balanced squarely on its back with gluteal areas bearing equal weight. All limbs should be flexed and relaxed. While in lateral recumbency, an automotive inner tube (valve stem pointed down) can be placed under the elbow of the dependent forelimb. The inner tube can be placed directly under the shoulder (Figure 6.4a) or through the dependent forelimb and under the shoulder (Figure 6.4b). Duct tape or other nonelastic tape can be placed on the part of the inner tube that is not under the shoulder (opposite of valve stem) (Figure 6.4c), which prevents collapsing of the

(a)

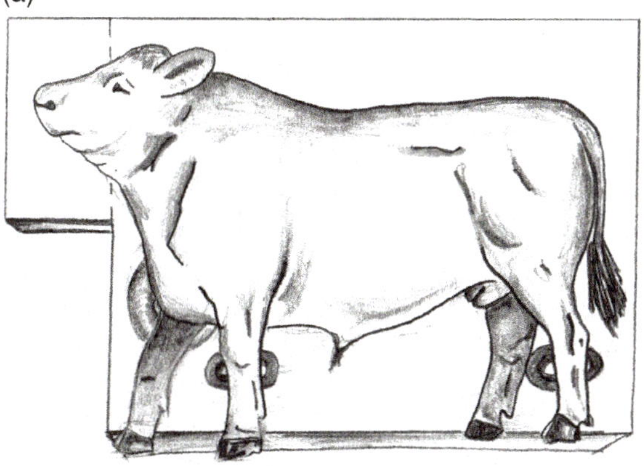

Figure 6.4 (a) Placement of an inner tube under the shoulder during lateral recumbency in an adult cattle.

CHAPTER 6

(b)

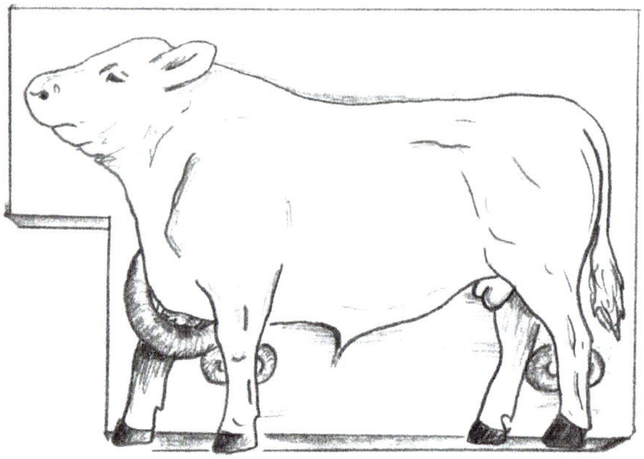

(c)

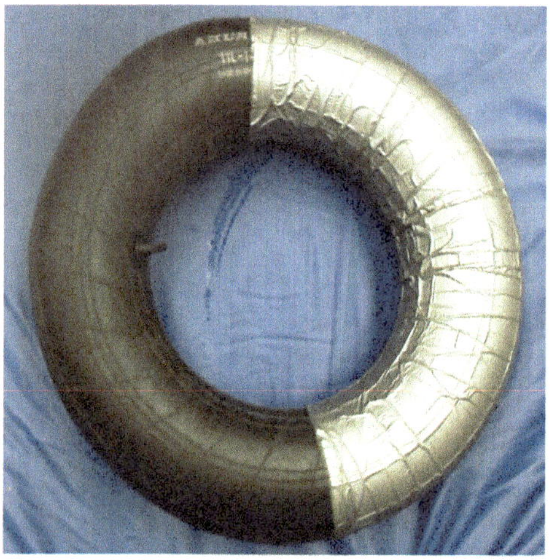

Figure 6.4 (b) Placement of an inner tube through the dependent forelimb under the shoulder during lateral recumbency in an adult cattle. (c) Taped inner tube. (Source: Illustration by Kim Crosslin.)

inner tube under the animal and, at the same time, limits the expansion of the inner tube that is not under the animal. Once the inner tube is in place, pulling the dependent forelimb anteriorly will help to distribute the weight of the thorax on the triceps rather than on the humerus. Upper forelimb and hind limb should be positioned perpendicularly to the table surface and both uppermost limbs elevated and parallel to the table surface (Figure 6.5). These techniques minimize the pressure on the radial or femoral/peroneal nerve of the dependent limb and prevent nerve paralysis [28]. The head and neck should be at a slightly extended position. If possible, the head should be slightly lower than the neck, which will allow draining of the saliva and ruminal contents if regurgitation occurs. Apply ophthalmic ointment in the eyes and make sure the dependent eye is closed to minimize the risk of a corneal ulcer [2, 28].

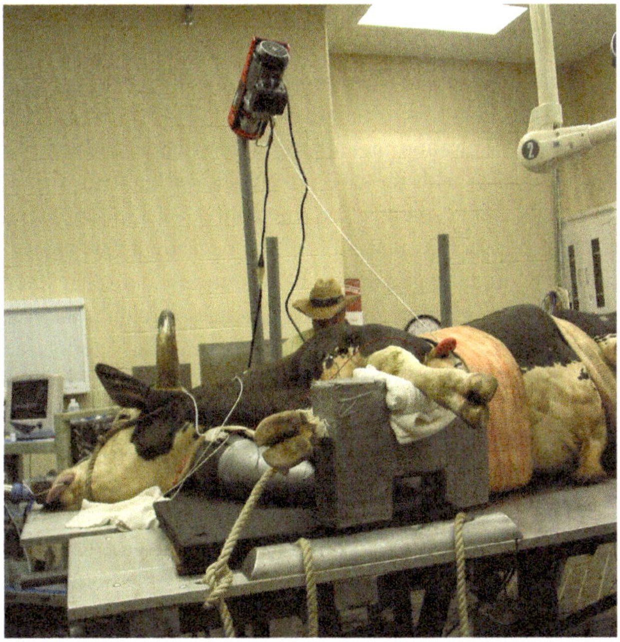

Figure 6.5 Anesthetized adult cattle in lateral recumbency position.

Recovery

Ruminants and camelids usually recover from anesthesia smoothly but gradually. Emergence delirium and premature attempts to stand seldom occur in these animals. They should be placed in sternal recumbency with support during the recovery period. If regurgitation occurred during anesthesia, the oral cavity and pharynx should be lavaged to prevent aspiration of ruminal materials and subsequent aspiration pneumonia. The endotracheal tube with the cuff still inflated should be left in place until the animal regains its chewing and coughing reflexes. The tube should be removed with the cuff inflated. Pigs can be placed in either lateral or sternal recumbency for recovery as long as adequate ventilation is ensured. Deflate the cuff of the endotracheal tube after the pigs are disconnected from the anesthesia machine and remove the tube when swallowing and coughing reflexes return.

Perioperative complications

Regurgitation and aspiration pneumonia

Regurgitation can occur during light (active regurgitation) and deep (passive regurgitation) anesthesia in ruminants in spite of preoperative fasting and withholding of water. Active regurgitation is a reflexive, protective mechanism of the body, intent on rejecting unwanted materials from the pharynx, upper airway, and upper digestive tract. Active regurgitation is characterized by explosive discharge of large quantities of ruminal materials.

Passive regurgitation occurs when the esophageal muscles and transluminal pressure gradients relax as a result of the anesthetic effect. Aspiration pneumonia or, in most severe cases, death can occur if the airway is not protected, and a large amount of ruminal materials can be aspirated into the airway and reach small airways. Please refer to Chapter 1 for detailed discussion on aspiration pneumonia. Preanesthetic feed and water withholding and endotracheal intubation with the cuff adequately inflated are recommended in all anesthetized ruminants and camelids for prevention of aspiration pneumonia [31]. Preventive measurements such as elevation of the neck by a sandbag or a rolled towel as well as avoiding vigorous manipulation of the rumen and other internal abdominal organs during surgery help minimizing the occurrence of regurgitation. If regurgitation occurs prior to intubation and protection of the trachea, the veterinarian should either quickly lower the animal's head or place the endotracheal tube in the esophagus and inflate the cuff to allow ruminal contents to flow out of the mouth while another endotracheal tube is placed in the trachea [2]. IV aminophylline (2–4 mg/kg over a period of 5 minutes or 11 mg/kg over a period of 20 minutes) or other bronchodilators along with 100% O_2 can be administered to relieve bronchospasm at the time of aspiration. If the animal survives the initial insult, corticosteroids and broad-spectrum antibiotics are indicated for the treatment of pneumonia. If regurgitation occurs after the endotracheal tube is in place, make sure the cuff is properly inflated and then lavage the mouth, nares, and pharynx with water to minimize the risk of aspiration of the regurgitated materials upon extubation. Always pull the endotracheal tube with the cuff inflated, so the remainder of the ruminal materials accumulated around the trachea cephalad to the cuff can be removed along with the endotracheal tube. Other methods that can be used to decrease the risk of perioperative regurgitation include positioning the animal in left lateral or sternal recumbency if possible to reduce pressure on the rumen and avoiding vigorous manipulation of the rumen and intestinal tracts during surgery [2, 28].

Airway obstruction

Airway obstruction can occur in ruminants from aspiration of ruminal contents during induction (active regurgitation) or during maintenance (passive regurgitation) of anesthesia. Ruminal contents contain more solid materials than gastric contents of monogastric animals. Liquid ruminal contents tends to drain out from the mouth, while solid materials are easily lodged at the larynx and can be aspirated into the airway and result in airway obstruction. If the cause of the obstruction is from active regurgitation, treatment should include rapidly increasing the depth of anesthesia and placement of an endotracheal tube. For an animal with an endotracheal tube already in place, removal of regurgitated materials from the buccal cavity either manually or by lavaging the buccal cavity with water or irrigation saline should be performed prior to the removal of the endotracheal tube as the animal recovers from anesthesia [2]. Improper positioning of the head and malposition of an anesthetic machine during anesthesia can result in kinking of the endotracheal tube and, subsequently, airway obstruction. Airway obstruction can also result from inflation of the cuff on an esophageal placement of the endotracheal tube and overinflation of the cuff on a correctly placed endotracheal tube; either cause may lead to collapsing of the tube. Observe the movement of the chest wall and/or the movement of the rebreathing bag of an anesthesia machine to confirm correct placement of the endotracheal tube to prevent dyspnea and apnea due to accidental airway obstruction.

Dorsal displacement of the soft palate following extubation of an endotracheal tube in camelids results in the soft palate to be situated dorsally to the epiglottis and thereby subsequently hindering the airflow into the larynx. This is a serious condition because camelids are obligate nasal breathers, and the obstruction, if not corrected immediately, can lead to dyspnea and eventually cardiac arrest. If the animal is awake enough at the time of extubation and the swallowing reflex has returned, then the problem can be corrected by initiating a swallowing reflex to allow the soft palate to return to its normal position and thus remove the source of airway obstruction. However, if the swallowing reflex has not yet returned, then the animal needs to be reintubated until the swallowing reflex returns [31]. Prolonged duration of dorsal recumbency in camelids often results in severe nasal edema and congestion. Upper airway obstruction sometimes occurs following extubation during recovery. Placing the animal in sternal recumbency, keeping the head high, administering nasal spray containing phenylephrine, and insufflation of 100% O_2 should be instituted until the nasal edema diminishes and adequate airflow in and out of the nasal cavity resumes.

Pigs are more difficult to intubate and several attempts are sometimes required to place the endotracheal tube successfully. Repeated attempts at intubation may provoke laryngeal edema and laryngospasm which may result in airway obstruction in lightly anesthetized pigs. Application of topical lidocaine to the larynx and an adequate plane of anesthesia aid in a smooth and successful intubation and minimize trauma to the larynx. Because of the long soft palate of pigs engaging the larynx, dorsal displacement of soft palate may result in airway obstruction, and suffocation has been reported in swine [32]. This complication can occur following extubation and also in pigs that are not intubated during anesthesia. In sows receiving spinal anesthesia and placed in lateral recumbency for cesarean section, restraining the head with rope may be necessary to prevent head movement. Care should be taken not to place the head in extension to avoid dorsal displacement of the soft palate. Noisy respiration after extubation indicates possible laryngeal spasm or upper airway obstruction and should be investigated immediately [33].

Ruminal tympany/bloat

Ruminal tympany or bloating can occur during anesthesia as a result of anesthetic-induced decreased gastrointestinal motility, accumulation of gas produced by fermentation of ingesta, and the animal's inability to eructate. Consequently, intra-abdominal pressure increases which pushes the diaphragm cranially and ventrally. Therefore, functional residual capacity of the lungs decreases resulting in severe hypoventilation accompanied by hypercapnia and hypoxemia. Placing the animal in sternal recumbency immediately after anesthesia helps to eliminate the accumulated gas in the rumen. However, decompression of the rumen may need to be performed while the surgery is in progress and the animal is still anesthetized. Passage of a stomach tube or, alternatively, insertion of a 12-gauge needle through the abdominal wall allows an outflow for the accumulated gas and reduces the pressure in the abdomen and on the diaphragm, thereby improving the ventilation of the patient. Trocarization to relieve bloating should only be performed as a last resort due to the potential for peritoneal cavity contamination and peritonitis. Preanesthetic fasting may reduce gas production, but it does not prevent continuous fermentation of the ingesta during anesthesia. In addition, most anesthetics, particularly α_2 agonists (e.g., xylazine) and opioid agonists (e.g., morphine), decrease gastrointestinal motility. Fortunately, there are antagonists available to reverse the gastrointestinal effect of an α_2 agonist or an opioid agonist in order to treat the ruminal tympany if necessary. Preoperative fasting is strongly recommended in ruminants and camelids to reduce the amount of gas produced from fermentable food materials and thereby decrease the chance for development of perioperative ruminal tympany and bloating [31].

Salivation

A ruminant normally produces copious quantities of saliva (i.e., 50 l/day for cattle, 6–16 l/day for sheep) [34, 35] that continue to flow even after the induction of anesthesia and loss of swallowing reflex. Older inhalation anesthetics such as halothane have been reported to decrease salivation in dogs and humans [36, 37]. Compared to ether and chloroform, salivation in cattle was reduced from 78 and 33.9 ml/minute, respectively, to 24 ml/minute during halothane anesthesia [38]. It is reasonable to expect that isoflurane and sevoflurane, like halothane, are capable of reducing salivation to some extent in ruminants. In the past, atropine had been administered routinely to ruminants prior to induction of anesthesia to reduce salivation. However, atropine does not completely inhibit salivation. More importantly, atropine decreases the water content of the saliva which causes the saliva to be more viscous and more difficult to clean out of the trachea, particular in neonates [39]. Today, atropine is only administered for treatment of bradycardia and for emergency situations when needed. Positioning of an anesthetized ruminant and camelid to elevate the neck in order to avoid pooling of saliva and regurgitated materials [2, 28] has been described in section "Positioning."

Hypoventilation

Placing an anesthetized animal in lateral or dorsal recumbency is required for most surgical procedures requiring general anesthesia. This alteration of the animal's normal position often results in cranial shift of the abdominal organs and the diaphragm and, as a result, decreases functional residual lung capacity of the animal. Awake animals may respond to decreased functional residual capacity by increasing respiratory rate and tidal volume. However, this response may be obtunded by the anesthetics administered, and respiratory depression develops. Severe hypercapnia and hypoxemia characterized by a significant increase in $PaCO_2$ and decrease in PaO_2 resulting from significant *V*/*Q* mismatch and eventually right-to-left shunting due to abnormal body position required by surgery and anesthetic-induced respiratory depression are common complications during anesthesia. In conscious sheep, lateral recumbency alone induces significant hypoxemia [40]. When cows were placed in dorsal recumbency either in an awake state or sedated with intramuscular (IM) xylazine (0.22 mg/kg) while breathing room air, PaO_2 decreased to a dangerous level of 45–60 mm of Hg. Returning these cows into sternal recumbency, PaO_2 values greatly improved [28, 41]. Assisted or controlled ventilation by simply squeezing the rebreathing bag or using a mechanical ventilator with positive pressure set at 20–25 cm of H_2O for small ruminants and camelids and 25–30 cm of H_2O for large ruminants can be used to minimize hypercapnia and/or hypoxemia during inhalation anesthesia. Supplemental O_2 without an anesthesia machine can be provided to sedated animals through an orotracheal or endotracheal tube by using an O_2 demand valve during recumbency, particularly if xylazine is part of the anesthetic regimen. Occasionally, apnea may occur and persist throughout anesthesia. Veterinarians should always make sure the animal is under an adequate plane of anesthesia, not deeply anesthetized, before instituting any drug treatment. Doxapram, a respiratory stimulant, can be administered at 0.1–0.5 mg/kg IV to initiate respiration. If the apnea persists, doxapram can be administered as a continuous IV infusion (5–10 μg/kg/minute) [42]. Doxapram is not effective in stimulating respiration if the cause of apnea is deep anesthesia. Doxapram does not just stimulate the respiratory center in the medulla; it is in fact a generalized central nervous system stimulator. Therefore, administration of doxapram may result in movement and awakening of the animal during the surgery.

Cardiac arrhythmias

Severe cardiac arrhythmias rarely occur in anesthetized farm animals. However, premature ventricular contractions have been observed in animals with preexisting electrolyte imbalance and severe hypercapnia or during light anesthesia. Bigeminal premature ventricular contractions have been associated with the administration of xylazine in adult cattle, especially in more excitable ones. Xylazine is known to sensitize myocardium to circulating catecholamines and lower the arrhythmogenic threshold for cardiac arrhythmias. Isoflurane and sevoflurane do not sensitize the myocardium to circulating catecholamines. Anesthetic-induced cardiac arrhythmias caused by xylazine have not been a major concern in anesthetized farm animals. However, in case of severe premature ventricular contraction, especially when cardiac output and arterial blood pressures are affected, lidocaine is the drug of choice for treatment. A single dose of lidocaine (1–2 mg/kg IV) is effective for treatment of premature ventricular contractions. Premature ventricular contractions may return, and continuous infusion of lidocaine (40–60 μg/kg/minute) may be instituted for longer-lasting effect [28]. Atrial fibrillation, a consequence of gastrointestinal disease or obstruction, and the resultant metabolic disturbances in cattle, is often resolved when the primary cause is surgically corrected. Physical restraint combined with local anesthesia provides adequate analgesia and is often used to perform standing abdominal surgery in these animals [2]. In goats with experimentally induced urethral obstruction, hyperkalemia often with profound increases in serum potassium concentration has been associated with sinus arrhythmias with occasional premature ventricular contraction. Though no drug treatments are often necessary except administration of IV 0.9% sodium chloride, goats should be under close monitoring and a light plane of anesthesia throughout the surgical period (personal observation).

Traction or pressure on the eyeball causes bradycardia as a result of oculocardiac reflex mediated through trigeminal and vagal nerves. Enucleation-induced bradycardia is frequently observed in horses. Similarly, manipulation and traction of the abdominal organs such as ovary also induce vagal stimulation and bradycardia. Relieving the traction or pressure on the eyeball or ovary usually returns the heart rate back to within baseline range. Atropine (0.06–0.12 mg/kg IV) can be administered if bradycardia persists and cardiac output and arterial blood pressure are affected [28]. Camelids tend to be more sensitive to vagal stimulation caused by tracheal intubation or painful surgical stimulation, and atropine (0.02 mg/kg IV or 0.04 mg/kg IM) has been administered for treatment of bradycardia [2].

Preanesthetic fasting for 48 hours has been reported to cause bradycardia in cattle [43]. It is believed that increased vagal tone and/or decreased sympathetic tone is responsible for the bradycardia since there are vagal afferent nerve fibers located throughout the gastrointestinal tract with receptors that can be activated by changes in pH (gastric chemoreceptors), stretch (gastric mechanoreceptors), or other chemical mediators associated with food withdrawal [44, 45]. Clinical experience of the author suggests that there are no significant hemodynamic changes or detrimental effects associated with preanesthetic withholding of feed and water for 48 and 24 hours, respectively, in cattle. Nevertheless, one should be aware that pain-induced sympathetic stimulation during light plane of anesthesia and the subsequent increase in heart rate may be masked by the bradycardia resulting from deprivation of feed so that the heart rate of the animal may appear to be lower than normal or within normal ranges [44].

Hypotension

In horses, hypotension with a mean arterial blood pressure below 60 mm of Hg persisting for long periods during anesthesia has been associated with increased incidence of postanesthetic neuromyopathy. However, hypotension is rarely observed in anesthetized adult cattle unless these animals are under excessive deep anesthesia [46]. Thus, adult cattle may not be as prone to develop postanesthetic neuromyopathy as horses. On occasion, postanesthetic neuromyopathy does occur, particularly nerve paralysis, due to inappropriate positioning and anesthetic-induced severe cardiovascular depression and hypotension. Xylazine-induced cardiovascular depression has been shown to result in hypotension [47]. Lateral and dorsal recumbencies in adult cattle have been associated with hypotension as a result of the compression of the vena cava caused by the pressure from the abdominal cavity, which in turn decreases venous return, cardiac output, and arterial blood pressures. The primary goals of anesthetic management for anesthetized animals are to maintain reasonable depth of anesthesia and normal cardiovascular function. For mild hypotension during anesthesia, reducing anesthetic concentration administered and initiating IV infusion of a balanced electrolyte solution and calcium borogluconate (23% solution) may be sufficient to return arterial blood pressure back to acceptable ranges. Calcium is an essential electrolyte for adequate muscle contraction including skeletal muscles, vascular smooth muscles, and myocardial muscles. The administration of calcium borogluconate enhances myocardial contractility and thus indirectly increases cardiac output and arterial blood pressure. However, ruminants tend to be more sensitive to calcium and bradycardia, and further decreases in cardiac output and arterial blood pressure may negate the usefulness of calcium borogluconate [2]. If decreasing anesthetic concentration in hypotensive patients doesn't return blood pressure back to within the normal range without the patient awakening from anesthesia, then treatment with a sympathomimetic drug, such as dobutamine, dopamine, phenylephrine, or ephedrine should be instituted. Dobutamine is a β_1 agonist. When administered at a low dosage (1–5 μg/kg/minute), dobutamine increases cardiac output and arterial blood pressure by increasing myocardial contractility. Dobutamine seldom increases heart rate except in animals suffering hypovolemia or when the drug is administered at high doses [48]. Dopamine is a dose-dependent dopaminergic α and β agonist. When administered at a low infusion rate of 1–2 μg/kg/minute, dopamine increases renal perfusion by stimulating renal dopaminergic receptors. Increasing the infusion rate to 2–10 μg/kg/minute results in stimulation of β_1 receptors and subsequently increases heart rate. Vasoconstriction and an increase in arterial blood pressure mediated by stimulation of α_1 receptors are not evident until a high infusion rate of greater than 10 μg/kg/minute is administered [49]. Phenylephrine is a pure α_1 agonist, and it increases arterial blood pressure by its effect on peripheral vasoconstriction. Phenylephrine can be administered as a bolus at 2–4 mg/kg IV, or it can be administered as a continuous infusion at 0.2–0.4 μg/kg/minute for a longer-lasting effect. Ephedrine is a mixed α_1 and β_1 agonist (22–66 μg/kg IV), and it increases arterial blood pressure by improving cardiovascular functions with only a small increase in heart rate but without significant vasoconstriction [50]. Though either one of the four aforementioned drugs is useful in treatment of hypotension, the most effective treatment for hypotension during anesthesia is maintaining an adequate plane of anesthesia.

Hypothermia

Decreased heat production and increased heat loss are the primary causes for the significant decrease in body temperature observed during anesthesia and surgery [51]. Hypothermia is a common anesthetic complication in small companion animals, but it is rarely an issue for adult cattle and camelids because of their large body mass to surface area ratio and, in camelids, thick hair coat. The body temperature of adult cattle and camelids seldom drops more than 0.5°C unless a major body cavity is opened during anesthesia. However, hypothermia can be a significant problem for small ruminants and pigs, especially in pediatric patients. Hypothermia can result in a significant reduction in anesthetic requirement and prolonged recovery [52]. Although often obese, pigs lack an insulating hair coat, thus are prone to hypothermia, and must be protected from extreme temperature and insensible heat loss during anesthesia [21]. An average decrease of 2.8 ± 0.6 C (5.04 ± 1.08 F) in body temperature was reported in pigs weighing 46–109 kg (101.2–239.8 lb) that underwent experimental magnetic resonance imaging guided convection enhanced drug delivery. These pigs were premedicated with azaperone (2 mg/kg IM) and ketamine (10 mg/kg IM), and anesthesia was induced with propofol (1.87 ± 0.6 mg/kg IV, to effect) and maintained with isoflurane. The average duration of anesthesia (from injection of propofol to the time of extubation) was 304 ± 55 minutes. Peripheral vasodilation, depression of thermoregulatory center, cool ambient temperature, and long duration of anesthesia were most likely the contributing factors of hypothermia in the pigs of this study [53]. In a pediatric potbellied pig, a long duration of anesthesia (4 hours) even with supplemental heat still resulted in significant hypothermia with body temperature of 33.3°C (92°F) and a prolonged recovery (personal observation). Therefore, supplemental heat with circulating warm air or warm water blanket, heating pad, or, at the very least, latex gloves or plastic bottles filled with warm water can be placed around the animal to minimize the decrease in body temperature and prevent severe hypothermia during anesthesia.

Malignant hyperthermia

Malignant hyperthermia, also referred to as "porcine stress syndrome," is a genetic disorder with mutation on the ryanodine receptors (ryr-1 locus) of the calcium channels in the skeletal muscles [54–56]. Detailed descriptions of the mechanism and causes of malignant hyperthermia have been discussed in Chapters 1 and 5. The clinical signs of malignant hyperthermia syndrome are manifested as sudden and dramatic increases in body temperature and $ETCO_2$ followed by excessive muscle fasciculation, muscle rigidity, tachypnea, tachycardia, arrhythmias, myoglobinuria, metabolic acidosis, renal failure, and, often times, death. Sudden increases in $ETCO_2$ and muscle rigidity are the early indication of an imminent malignant hyperthermia episode. If recognized very early and treatments instituted immediately, survival rates improve, and the prognosis is more favorable that if treatment is delayed. However, prognosis is often poor once the episode is initiated in spite of aggressive treatments. Halogenated inhalation anesthetics are known triggers for malignant hyperthermia, and halothane seems to be the most potent trigger and has been most frequently reported in pigs [57]. The newer inhalation anesthetics, isoflurane, sevoflurane, and desflurane, have also been reported to trigger malignant hyperthermia in Pietrain, Pietrain-mixed, Poland China, and Large White pigs [58–60]. Compared to halothane-induced malignant hyperthermia, the malignant hyperthermia episodes induced by desflurane and isoflurane were reported to have a slower onset than halothane [58]. Only one incidence of isoflurane-induced malignant hyperthermia has been reported in a potbellied pig [61]. There are no reports of isoflurane- or sevoflurane-induced malignant hyperthermia in cattle. Even though there are few reports on isoflurane- and sevoflurane-induced malignant hyperthermia in farm animal species other than pigs, these two anesthetics are nonetheless potent triggering agents to warrant caution when anesthetizing animals susceptible to malignant hyperthermia.

Treatments for malignant hyperthermia are primarily symptomatic. Early recognition of symptoms, such as muscle rigidity, sudden rise in body temperature, and $ETCO_2$, and aggressive treatments, such as immediate discontinuation of inhalation anesthetic and institution of ice packs and alcohol baths, are the keys to a more favorable prognosis. Controlled ventilation should also be instituted at early stage to remove excessive CO_2 and maintain normal blood pH and acid–base status. Dantrolene sodium has been shown to be effective for treatment (1–3 mg/kg IV) and prophylaxis (5 mg/kg PO) of malignant hyperthermia episodes [30]. In 1981, McGrath *et al.* [62] reported that acepromazine at 1.1 and 1.65 mg/kg IM reduced the incidence of malignant hyperthermia by 40% and 73%, respectively. A lower dose of 0.55 mg/kg IM was only able to delay the onset but did not prevent the episode. Azaperone at doses of 0.5–2.0 mg/kg IM has been shown to offer 100% protection against malignant hyperthermia in susceptible Pietrain pigs [63].

Postanesthetic neuromyopathy

Ruminants are not as susceptible to postanesthetic myositis or nerve paralysis as are horses. Fortunately, postanesthetic localized or generalized myositis like that observed in horses has not been reported in adult cattle and camelids. However, inadequate padding and/or positioning combined with severe hypotension during anesthesia has resulted in temporary radial nerve paralysis in adult cattle and llamas when placed in lateral recumbency. Affected animals stood but were not able to bear weight on the affected limb. The condition improved within 24 hours and recovery with full motor function returned in 2–3 days. Affected animals should be treated symptomatically which may include maintaining circulating blood volume by infusion of balanced electrolyte solutions, administration of anti-inflammatory drugs to relieve inflammation, analgesics to relieve pain, diazepam to reduce anxiety and provide muscle relaxation, and sodium bicarbonate (350–500 mEq/450 kg (990 lb) IV) for correction of metabolic acidosis. During anesthesia, preventive measures should include the following: maintaining light anesthesia, reducing the dose of anesthetics that produce profound cardiovascular depression, close monitoring, maintaining cardiovascular function with infusion of balanced electrolytes and vasoactive and inotropic drugs (dobutamine, dopamine, ephedrine), ensuring adequate padding of the surgical table, even distribution of the body weight of the anesthetized animal, proper means to protect radial and femoral nerves, support of the upper front and hind legs, and minimizing the duration of anesthesia [42].

Cardiovascular collapse

During anesthesia, significant and prolonged decrease in pulse pressure, hypotension, increased capillary refill time, pale mucous membranes, bradycardia, and/or tachycardia can lead to cardiovascular collapse. Causes of perioperative collapse include significant endotoxin-induced peripheral vasodilation, severe systemic disease, extreme hypovolemia due to dehydration and/or blood loss, and excessive deep anesthesia resulting in profound myocardial depression. Treatment of impending cardiovascular failure should begin with correction of the causative disease status, rapid administration of supportive fluid (90 ml/kg), and reduction or even cessation of anesthesia. Additional symptomatic treatments include vasoactive drugs (e.g., dopamine, phenylephrine, ephedrine) for hypotension, inotropic drugs (e.g., dobutamine) for myocardial depression, chronotropic drugs (e.g., atropine, glycopyrrolate) for bradycardia, and antiarrhythmic drugs (e.g., lidocaine) for ventricular arrhythmias such as ventricular tachycardia or premature ventricular contractions [42].

Prolonged untreated cardiovascular collapse may result in cardiac arrest and death. Cardiopulmonary resuscitation (CPR) should follow the general *ABC technique*. A is opening of the *a*irway by endotracheal intubation; *B* is the initiation of controlled *b*reathing by squeezing an Ambu bag or using the rebreathing bag of an anesthesia machine (12–20 breaths/minute); and *C* is the establishment of artificial *c*irculation by cardiac compression (80–100 compressions/minute). After CPR has been instituted, an IV catheter should be placed if one is not already in place. If the attempts at IV catheterization is unsuccessful, emergency drugs may be administered intratracheally through the endotracheal tube at 2–2.5 times the IV dose after dilution with sterile water or saline to a volume of 5–10 ml. Absorption of the drugs from the lung is sometimes significant enough to be more effective than IV administration through a peripheral vein [42]. Emergency drugs and products frequently used during CPR include 100% O_2, balanced electrolyte solutions, atropine, lidocaine, and epinephrine. Depending on the animal's condition, the vasoactive drugs mentioned previously can be administered in conjunction with emergency drugs. Electrical defibrillation is the most effective treatment for conversion of ventricular fibrillation, but it is not practical in field situations or effective in large animals. Epinephrine (10 μg/kg IV) is usually the drug of choice for treatment of ventricular fibrillation. Epinephrine induces peripheral vasoconstriction and increases arterial diastolic blood pressure, intracranial and coronary blood flow, coarseness of ventricular fibrillation, and positive inotropic effect by stimulating α and β adrenoceptors. Potential side effects of epinephrine include increased myocardial and cerebral O_2 demand, postresuscitation arrhythmia, and tachycardia. A bolus injection of lidocaine (0.5–2 mg/kg IV) may be used to treat postresuscitation ventricular arrhythmia. Chemical defibrillation with IV potassium chloride (1 mg/kg) and acetylcholine (6 mg/kg) followed by administration of 10% calcium chloride (1 ml/10 kg (22 lb)) has been recommended for treatment of ventricular fibrillation. Although it is ineffective in defibrillation, this technique usually converts fibrillation to asystole [42]. A normal sinus rhythm is actually easier to initiate from asystole than from fibrillation. In general, the best treatment for perioperative complications is prevention, which requires a devoted and vigilant anesthetist. Careful preanesthetic evaluation and preparation, proper use of anesthetic regimens, and adjustment of the dosages of the anesthetics used can prevent most anesthetic-related complications. Close monitoring and attention to details allow the anesthetist to recognize potentially dangerous situations quickly and institute corrective measures at an early stage. Always keep in mind that "there are no safe anesthetics; there are no anesthetic techniques, there are only safe anesthetists."

References

1. Haskins, S. (2011) Patient monitoring, in *Essentials of Small Animal Anesthesia and Analgesia*, 2nd edn (eds K. Grimm, W. Tranquilli and L. Lamont), Wiley-Blackwell, Ames, pp. 197–239.
2. Riebold, T. (2007) Ruminants, in *Lumb and Jones' Veterinary Anesthesia and Analgesia*, 4th edn (eds W. Tranquilli, J. Thurmon and K. Grimm), Blackwell Publishing, Ames, pp. 731–746.
3. McDonnell, W. and Kerr, C. (2007) Respiratory system, in *Lumb and Jones' Veterinary Anesthesia and Analgesia*, 4th edn (eds W. Tranquilli, J. Thurmon and K. Grimm), Blackwell Publishing, Ames, pp. 117–151.
4. Hubbell, J. and Muir, W. (2009) Monitoring anesthesia, in *Equine Anesthesia: Monitoring and Emergency Therapy*, 2nd edn, Saunders/Elsevier, St. Louis, pp. 149–170.
5. Hodgson, D., Dunlop, C., Chapman, P. and Smith, J. (2002) Cardiopulmonary effects of xylazine and acepromazine in pregnant cows in late gestation. *American Journal of Veterinary Research*, **63**, 1695–1699.
6. Greene, S., Tyner, C., Morris, D. and Hartsfield, S. (1988) Comparison of cardiopulmonary effects of isoflurane and halothane after atropine-guaifenesin-thiamylal anesthesia for rumenotomy in steers. *American Journal of Veterinary Research*, **49**, 1891–1893.

7. deMoor, A. and Desmet, P. (1971) Effect of rompun on acid–base-equilibrium and arterial O_2 pressure in cattle. *Veterinary Medicine Research*, **213**, 163–169.
8. Gavier, D., Kittleson, M., Fowler, M. *et al.* (1988) Evaluation of a combination of xylazine, ketamine, and halothane for anesthesia in llamas. *American Journal of Veterinary Research*, **49**, 2047–2055.
9. Mama, K., Wagner, A. and Steffey, E. (2001) Circulatory, respiratory and behavioral responses in isoflurane anesthetized llamas. *Veterinary Anaesthesia and Analgesia*, **28**, 12–17.
10. Tulamo, R.-M., Raekallio, M. and Ekblad, A. (1995) Cardiovascular effects of medetomidine-ketamine anaesthesia in sheep, with and without 100% oxygen and its reversal with atipamezole. *Journal of Veterinary Anaesthesia*, **22**, 9–14.
11. Aziz, M. and Carlyle, S. (1978) Cardiopulmonary and respiratory effects of xylazine in sheep. *Zentralbl Veterinarmed A*, **25**, 173–180.
12. Hikasa, Y., Okuyama, K., Kakuta, T. *et al.* (1998) Anesthetic potency and cardiopulmonary effects of sevoflurane in goats: comparison with isoflurane and halothane. *Canadian Journal of Veterinary Research*, **62**, 299–306.
13. Cribb, P. (1988) Capnographic monitoring during anesthesia with controlled ventilation. *Veterinary Surgery*, **17**, 48–52.
14. Meyer, R. and Short, C. (1985) Arterial to end-tidal CO_2 tension and alveolar dead space in halothane- or isoflurane-anesthetized ponies. *American Journal of Veterinary Research*, **46**, 597–599.
15. Wright, B. and Hellyer, P. (1996) Respiratory monitoring during anesthesia: pulse oximetry and capnography. *The Compendium on Continuing Education for the Practicing Veterinarian*, **18**, 1083–1097.
16. White, G., Matthews, N., Walker, M. and Slater, M. (1994) Pulse oximetry for estimation of oxygenation in dogs with experimental pneumothorax. *Journal of Veterinary Emergency and Critical Care*, **4**, 69–76.
17. Jones, J. (1996) Noninvasive monitoring techniques in anesthetized animals. *Veterinary Medicine*, **91**, 326–336.
18. Matthews, N., Gleed, R. and Short, C. (1986) Cardiopulmonary effects of general anesthesia in adult cattle. *Modern Veterinary Practice*, **67**, 618–620.
19. Mama, K., Wegner, A., Parker, D. *et al.* (1999) Determination of the minimum alveolar concentration of isoflurane in llamas. *Veterinary Surgery*, **28**, 121–125.
20. Snyder, J. and Wolff, P. (2009) Small ruminant tips for small animal practice. *North American Veterinary Community Conference*, 331–337.
21. Wolff, P. (2009) Pet pig problems. *North American Veterinary Community Conference*, pp. 416–419.
22. Christian, J. and Pugh, D. (2012) Reference intervals and conversions. (Appendix 2), in *Sheep and Goat Medicine*, 2nd edn (eds. D.G. Pugh and A.N. Baird), Elsevier-Saunders, Maryland Heights, pp. 596–600.
23. Jain, N. (1993) *Essential of Veterinary Hematology*, Lea & Febiger, Philadelphia, pp. 54–71.
24. Fowler, M. and Zinkl, J. (1989) References ranges for hematologic and serum biochemical values in llamas (Lama glama). *American Journal of Veterinary Research*, **50**, 2049–2053.
25. van Amstel, S. (2008) Aspects of the treatment and management of pet pigs. *North American Veterinary Community Conference*, pp. 361–368.
26. Radin, N., Weiser, M. and Fettman, M. (1986) Hematologic and biochemical values for Yucatan miniature swine. *Laboratory Animal Science*, **36**, 425–427.
27. Riebold, T. (1996) Ruminants, in *Lumb & Jones' Veterinary Anesthesia*, 3rd edn (eds J. Thurmon, W. Tranquilli and G. Benson), Lea & Febiger, Baltimore, pp. 610–626.

28. Thurmon, J. and Benson, G. (1993) Anesthesia in ruminants and swine, in *Current Veterinary Therapy: Food Animal Practice*, 3rd edn (ed J. Howard), WB Saunders, Philadelphia, pp. 58–76.
29. Marqués, F. (2008) Fluid therapy: general practical recommendations for camelids. *Large Animal Veterinary Rounds (Western College of Veterinary Medicine, University of Saskatchwan)*, **8** (1), 1–6.
30. Anderson, D. and St Jean, G. (2012) Anesthesia and surgical procedures in swine, in *Diseases of Swine*, 10th edn (eds J. Zimmerman, L. Karriker, A. Ramirez *et al.*), Ames, Wiley-Blackwell, pp. 119–140.
31. Steffey, E. (1986) Some characteristics of ruminants and swine that complicate management of general anesthesia. *The Veterinary Clinics of North America. Food Animal Practice*, **2**, 507–516.
32. Benson, G. (1986) Anesthetic management of ruminants and swine with selected pathophysiologic alterations. *The Veterinary Clinics of North America. Food Animal Practice*, **2**, 677–691.
33. Ko, J., Thurmon, J., Tranquilli, W. *et al.* (1993) Problems encountered when anesthetizing potbellied pigs. *Veterinary Medicine*, **88**, 435–440.
34. Somers, M. (1958) Comparison of the salivary secretion of both parotid glands in a sheep. *Nature*, **182**, 400.
35. Kay, R. (1960) The rate of flow and composition of various salivary secretion in sheep and calves. *The Journal of Physiology*, **150**, 515–537.
36. Raventos, J. and Goodall, R. (1956) The action of fluothane: a new volatile anesthetic. *British Journal of Pharmacology*, **11**, 394–410.
37. Brennan, H., Hunter, A. and Johnstone, M. (1957) Halothane: a clinical assessment. *Lancet*, **273**, 453–457.
38. Jennings, S. (1971) General anesthesia of ruminants and swine, in *Textbook of Veterinary Anesthesia* (ed L. Soma), Williams & Wilkins, Baltimore, pp. 344–358.
39. Short, C. (1986) Preanesthetic medications in ruminants and swine. *The Veterinary Clinics of North America. Food Animal Practice*, **2**, 553–566.
40. Mitchell, B. and Williams, J. (1976–1977) Respiratory function changes in sheep associated with lying in lateral recumbency and with sedation by xylazine. *Great Britain and Ireland Association of Veterinary Anaesthetists*, 30.
41. Klein, L. and Fisher, N. (1988) Cardiopulmonary effects of restraint in dorsal recumbency on awake cattle. *American Journal of Veterinary Research*, **49**, 1605–1608.
42. Kruse-Elliott, K. (1996) Management and emergency intervention during anesthesia. *The Veterinary Clinics of North America. Food Animal Practice*, **12**, 563–578.
43. McGuirk, S., Bednarski, R. and Clayton, M. (1990) Bradycardia in cattle deprived of food. *Journal of the American Veterinary Medical Association*, **196**, 894–896.
44. Longhurst, J., Spilker, H. and Ordway, G. (1981) Cardiovascular reflexes elicited by passive gastric distension in anesthetized cats. *American Journal of Physiology*, **240**, H539–H545.
45. Longhurst, J., Ashton, J. and Iwamoto, G. (1980) Cardiovascular reflexes resulting from capsaicin-stimulated gastric receptors in anesthetized dogs. *Circulation Research*, **46**, 780–788.
46. Dugdale, A. (2010) Ruminants: local and general anaesthesia, in *Veterinary Anaesthesia: Principle to Practice* (ed A. Dugdale), Wiley-Blackwell, Ames, pp. 279–298.
47. Campbell, K., Klavano, P., Richardson, P. and Alexander, J. (1979) Hemodynamic effects of xylazine in the calf. *American J ournal of Veterinary Research*, **40**, 1777–1780.
48. Daunt, D. (1990) Supportive therapy in the anesthetized horse. *The Veterinary Clinics of North America*, **6**, 557–574.

49. Riebold, T., Geiser, D. and Goble, D. (1995) Anesthetic emergencies, in *Large Animal Anesthesia: Principles and Techniques*, 2nd edn, Iowa State University Press, Ames.
50. Tranquilli, W. and Greene, S. (1987) Cardiovascular medications and the autonomic nervous system, in *Principle and Practice of Veterinary Anesthesia* (ed C. Short), Williams & Wilkins, Baltimore, pp. 426–454.
51. Haskins, S. (2007) Monitoring anesthetized patients, in *Lumb and Jones' Veterinary Anesthesia and Analgesia*, 4th edn (eds W. Tranquilli, J. Thormon and K. Grimm), Blackwell Publishing, Ames, pp. 533–557.
52. Hall, L. and Clarke, K. (1983) Accident and emergencies associated with anesthesia, in *Veterinary Anaesthesia*, 8th edn (eds L. Hall and K. Clarke), Baillière Tindall, London, pp. 367–388.
53. Jones, A., Bienemann, A., Barua, N. *et al.* (2012) Anaesthetic complications in pigs undergoing MRI guided convection enhanced drug delivery to the brain: a case series. *Veterinary Anaesthesia and Analgesia*, **39**, 647–652.
54. Fujii, J., Otsu, K., Zorzato, F. *et al.* (1991) Identification of a mutation in porcine ryanodine receptor associated with malignant hyperthermia. *Science*, **253**, 448–451.
55. Geers, R., Decanniere, C., Ville, H. *et al.* (1992) Identification of halothane gene carriers by use of an in vivo 3IP nuclear magnetic resonance spectroscopy in pigs. *American Journal of Veterinary Research*, **53**, 1711–1714.
56. Houde, A., Pomnier, S. and Roy, R. (1993) Detection of the ryanodine receptor mutation associated with malignant hyperthermia in purebred swine populations. *Journal of Animal Science*, **71**, 1414–1418.
57. Hildebrand, S. (1987) Hyperthermia, malignant hyperthermia, and myopathy, in *Principle & Practice of Veterinary Anesthesia* (ed C. Short), Williams & Wilkins, Baltimore, pp. 517–532.
58. Wedel, D., Gammel, S., Milde, J. and Iaizzo, P. (1993) Delayed onset of malignant hyperthermia induced by isoflurane and desflurane compared with halothane in susceptible swine. *Anesthesiology*, **78**, 1138–1144.
59. Bonome-Gonzales, C., Alvarez-Refojo, F., Fernandez-Goti, C. *et al.* (2001) Malignant hyperthermia in a pig anesthetized with desflurane. *Revista Espanola de Anestesiologia y Reanimacion*, **48**, 81–84.
60. Shulman, M., Braverman, B., Ivankovich, A. and Gronert, G. (1981) Sevoflurane triggers malignant hyperthermia in swine. *Anesthesiology*, **54**, 259–260.
61. Claxton-Gill, M., Cornick-Seahorn, J., Gamboa, J. and Boatright, B. (1993) Suspected malignant hyperthermia syndrome in a miniature pot-bellied pig anesthetized with isoflurane. *Journal of the American Veterinary Medical Association*, **203**, 1434–1436.
62. McGrath, C., Rempel, W., Addis, P. and Crimi, A. (1981) Acepromazine and droperidol inhibition of halothane-induced malignant hyperthermia (porcine stress syndrome) in swine. *American Journal of Veterinary Research*, **42**, 195–198.
63. McGrath, C., Lee, J. and Ashen, M. (1984) Azaperone (Stresnil) in malignant hyperthermia (MH) susceptible swine: determination of protective effects to halothane challenge and toxicity (Abstract). *Veterinary Surgery*, **14**, 75.

Chapter 7

Local and regional anesthetic techniques

Misty A. Edmondson

Department of Clinical Sciences, College of Veterinary Medicine, Auburn University, USA

Local and regional anesthesia are commonly used in farm animals as they are considered both safe and effective. Many surgical procedures are performed using a physical restraint, mild sedation, and/or local or regional anesthesia. Local anesthetic techniques are typically simple to perform and inexpensive and provide a reversible loss of sensation to a distinct area of the body. Local and regional anesthesia also provides some advantages over general anesthesia. These advantages include lower risk of toxic effects, decrease in the risks associated with placing animals in recumbency, and the need for less equipment.

Local anesthetics

Numerous local or regional anesthetics have been used for surgery in cattle. These anesthetics have been used to prevent pain during surgery and act locally or regionally with acceptable onset times and predictable duration. These drugs vary in their potency, duration, toxicity, and cost [1, 2]. Two percent lidocaine hydrochloride and 2% mepivacaine hydrochloride have become two of the most widely used local anesthetic drugs used in cattle due to the limited toxicity and low cost. Lidocaine hydrochloride has a duration of 90–180 minutes, is three times more potent than procaine, and diffuses into tissues more widely [3, 4]. The addition of a vasoconstrictor, such as epinephrine (5 µg/ml), to the local anesthetic solution (0.1 ml of epinephrine (1:1000) to 20 ml of local anesthetic) increases the potency and duration of activity of both regional and epidural anesthesia. However, local anesthetics containing epinephrine (1:200,000) should not be used in wound edges or in the subarachnoid space due to the risk of causing tissue necrosis and spinal cord ischemia [3]. In cattle, procaine (1–2%) is expected to have a slower onset of anesthesia when compared to lidocaine and a shorter duration of action at no more than 60 minutes.

Farm Animal Anesthesia: Cattle, Small Ruminants, Camelids, and Pigs, First Edition.
Edited by HuiChu Lin and Paul Walz.

Alternatively, mepivacaine (1–2%) is expected to have a similar time of onset of anesthesia but longer duration of activity at 120–180 minutes when compared to lidocaine. Bupivacaine (0.25–0.5%) is a long-acting local anesthetic of up to 360 minutes of duration of activity. However, bupivacaine can be toxic to cattle if it is given intravenously. Hence, bupivacaine is not recommended for routine clinical use because of the risk of inadvertent intravenous injection [1].

It is imperative that toxicity be considered and preventative measures taken to ensure that overdosage does not occur. This is especially important when local anesthesia is being performed in a large area, such as for a cesarean section. The maximum safe dose of lidocaine hydrochloride in cattle is 10 mg/kg of body weight. Small ruminants are much more sensitive to anesthetics with a maximum safe dose of lidocaine hydrochloride of 4 mg/kg [1]. In some instances where more volume is necessary, the standard 2% lidocaine hydrochloride may be diluted to 1% with sterile saline.

Anesthesia for dehorning

The cornual nerve block is one of the most common techniques used for dehorning cattle. The horn and skin around the base of the horn are innervated by the cornual branch of the lacrimal or zygomaticotemporal nerve, which is part of the ophthalmic division of the trigeminal nerve. The cornual nerve passes through the periorbital tissues dorsally and runs along the frontal crest to the base of the horns. Approximately 5–10 ml of local anesthetic is administered subcutaneously and relatively superficially midway between the lateral canthus of the eye and the base of the horn along the zygomatic process (Figure 7.1A). Complete anesthesia occurs within 10 minutes following the administration of local anesthetic. Larger cattle with large, well-developed horns may require additional anesthetic infiltration along the caudal aspect of the horn, in the form of a partial ring block, to desensitize subcutaneous branches of the second cervical nerve [4–6].

Because of anatomical differences, the cornual nerve block in goats requires at least two injection sites per horn versus the aforementioned one site in cattle. In goats, the cornual nerve is a branch of the zygomaticotemporal nerve and lies halfway between the lateral canthus of the eye and the lateral base of the horn. The horn base in goats is also heavily innervated by the cornual branches of the infratrochlear nerve which exits the orbit at or in close proximity to the medial canthus. Because of the widespread branching, the nerve is best blocked using a line block midway between the medial canthus of the eye and the medial horn base (Figure 7.2) [7]. Alternatively, a ring block around the base of the horn may also be used for anesthesia for dehorning.

Nasal anesthesia

The infraorbital nerve block may be used for the surgical repair of nasal lacerations and the placement of a nose ring. The infraorbital nerve is the continuation of the maxillary branch of the fifth cranial nerve after it enters the infraorbital canal. The infraorbital nerve has only sensory function and emerges on the face as a flat band

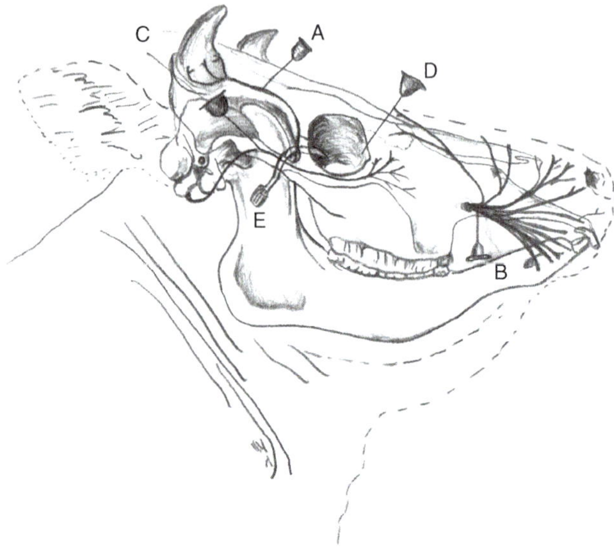

Figure 7.1 Facial nerve blocks in cattle: (A) cornual nerve block for dehorning, (B) infraorbital nerve block, (C) auriculopalpebral nerve block, (D) local infiltration of the eyelids, and (E) injection site for Peterson eye block. (Source: Illustration by Kim Crosslin.)

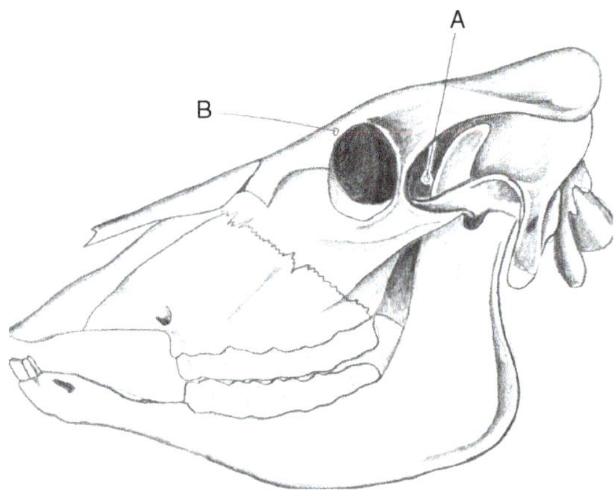

Figure 7.2 Cornual branch of the zygomaticotemporal (A) nerve block and infratrochlear (B) nerve blocks for dehorning in goats. (Source: Illustration by Kim Crosslin.)

through the infraorbital foramen where it is covered by the levator nasolabialis muscle [4]. The infraorbital nerve is blocked as it emerges from the infraorbital canal. The nerve is difficult to palpate but is located rostral to the facial tuberosity on a line extending from the nasomaxillary notch to the second upper premolar. A total of 20–30 ml of local anesthetic is injected deep into the levator nasolabialis muscle with an 18-gauge, 3.8-cm needle (Figure 7.1B). The injection should be repeated on the opposite side [8].

Anesthesia of the eye

The globe, conjunctiva, nictitating membrane, and most of the eyelids are supplied by the ophthalmic branch of the trigeminal nerve. The extraocular muscles of the eye are innervated by the trochlear nerve, the abducens nerve, and the oculomotor nerve. The eyelids are innervated by the auriculopalpebral nerve. Topical and regional analgesia techniques are necessary for surgery of the eye and its associated structures, most commonly for squamous cell carcinoma; removal of foreign bodies from the cornea; and subconjunctival injections [9].

Eyelid

Anesthesia of the eyelid is accomplished by performing a line block of the eyelid or by blocking the auriculopalpebral branch of the facial nerve. A line block is performed by using a 20- or 22-gauge, 2.5-cm needle to inject 10 ml of local anesthetic at multiple sites 0.5 cm apart on a line approximately 0.5 cm from the margin of the eyelid [9]. The auriculopalpebral nerve block is performed by using an 18- or 20-gauge, 2.5-cm needle placed subcutaneously approximately 5–7.5 cm lateral to the zygomatic arch. A total of 5–10 ml of local anesthetic is then injected (Figure 7.1C) [4]. Because the auriculopalpebral nerve block only blocks the lower eyelid, desensitization of the upper eyelid with a line block is also required if the surgical procedure involves upper eyelid.

Eye and orbit

Anesthesia of the eye and orbit and immobilization of the globe that is necessary for such procedures as enucleation may be accomplished by performing a retrobulbar eye block or Peterson eye block.

Retrobulbar eye block

The retrobulbar eye block is used for enucleation of the eye or for surgery of the cornea and when properly performed, causes analgesia of the cornea, mydriasis, and proptosis. Adequate restraint of the head is necessary when performing this procedure. The sites for needle placement for retrobulbar injection are the medial and lateral canthus or the upper and lower eyelids (Figure 7.3) [10]. An 18-gauge, 15-cm needle is used and may be bent slightly to facilitate passage around the globe once it has been introduced through the eyelid or canthus at the orbital rim. The surgeon's finger is used to deflect the globe to protect it from the point of the needle. Approximately 15 ml of local anesthetic is injected in small increments as the needle is advanced slowly toward the back of the orbit. The advantage of the retrobulbar eye block is that it is considered a much easier technique to perform. Some possible adverse effects of retrobulbar injections include penetration of the globe, orbital hemorrhage, damage to the optic nerve, cardiac dysrhythmias caused by initiation of the oculocardiac reflex, and injection of the local anesthetic into the optic nerve meninges [4].

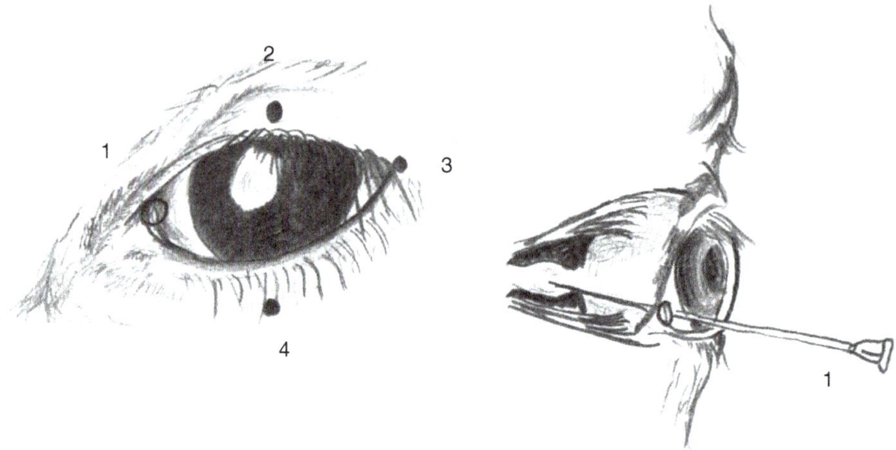

Figure 7.3 Retrobulbar eye block, (1) medial canthus, (2) dorsal eyelid, (3) lateral canthus, and (4) ventral eyelid in cattle. (Source: Illustration by Kim Crosslin.)

Peterson eye block

The Peterson eye block requires significantly more skill to perform than the retrobulbar eye block but is considered safer and more effective if performed correctly. There is also less edema and inflammation associated with the Peterson eye block than with infiltration of local anesthetics into the eyelids and orbit (Figure 7.1D-E). The Peterson eye block desensitizes the nerves (oculomotor, trochlear, abducent, and trigeminal nerves) responsible for sensory and motor function of all structures of the eye except the eyelid [4]. An auriculopalpebral nerve block can be performed to anesthetize the eyelid. The landmark for needle placement for the Peterson eye block is the notch that is created by the supraorbital process cranially, the zygomatic arch ventrally, and the coronoid process of the mandible caudally. Approximately 5 ml of local anesthetic is injected subcutaneously at this site using a 22-gauge, 2.5-cm needle. A 14-gauge, 2.5-cm needle serves as a cannula and is placed through the anesthetized area as far anterior and ventral as possible in the notch. A straight or slightly curved 18-gauge, 10- to 12-cm needle is inserted into the cannula and directed horizontally and slightly caudally until it comes into contact with the coronoid process of the mandible at approximately 2.5 cm below the skin. The needle is then gently manipulated rostrally until its point passes medially around the coronoid process. It is then advanced to the pterygopalatine fossa rostral to the solid bony plate that is in close proximity to the orbital foramen at a depth of 7.5–10 cm (Figure 7.1E). Penetration of the nasopharynx and turbinates should be avoided. Aspiration ensures that the ventral maxillary artery has not been penetrated [4, 9]. Approximately 15 ml of local anesthetic is then injected. Both the retrobulbar block and the Peterson eye block prevent blinking for several hours [9]. The cornea must be kept moist if these blocks are used for procedures other than enucleation. Caution must also be used with animals that are transported immediately following these procedures. A lubricating eye ointment can be applied to the cornea, or the eyelids may be sutured together until motor function of the eyelids returns.

Anesthesia for laparotomy

Anesthesia of the paralumbar fossa and abdominal wall can be achieved by several techniques. These techniques include the proximal paravertebral nerve block, the distal paravertebral nerve block, the inverted-L block, and infusion of the incision or line block. These anesthetic techniques are commonly used for such procedures as surgery of the digestive tract (abomasopexy, omentopexy, rumenotomy, or volvulus), cesarean section, ovariectomy, and liver and kidney biopsy.

Proximal paravertebral nerve block

The proximal paravertebral nerve block desensitizes the dorsal and ventral nerve roots of the last thoracic (T13) and first and second lumbar (L1 and L2) spinal nerves as they emerge from the intervertebral foramina. To facilitate proper needle placement of anesthetic, the skin at the cranial edges of the transverse processes of L1, L2, and L3 and at a point 2.5–5 cm off the dorsal midline can be desensitized by injecting 2–3 ml of local anesthetic using an 18-gauge, 2.5-cm needle. A 14-gauge, 2.5-cm needle is used as a cannula or guide needle to minimize skin resistance during insertion of an 18-gauge, 10- to 15-cm spinal needle. Approximately 5 ml of local anesthetic may be placed through the cannula to anesthetize the needle tract for further needle placement.

To desensitize T13, the cannula needle is placed through the skin at the anterior edge of the transverse process of L1 at approximately 4–5 cm lateral to the dorsal midline. The 18-gauge, 10- to 15-cm spinal needle is passed ventrally until it contacts the transverse process of L1. The needle is then walked off of the cranial edge of the transverse process of L1 and advanced approximately 1 cm to pass slightly ventral to the process and into the intertransverse ligament. A total of 6–8 ml of local anesthetic is injected with little resistance to desensitize the ventral branch of T13. The needle is then withdrawn 1–2.5 cm above the fascia or just dorsal to the transverse process, and 6–8 ml of local anesthetic is infused to desensitize the dorsal branch of the nerve.

To desensitize L1 and L2, the needle is inserted just caudal to the transverse processes of L1 and L2. The needle is walked off of the caudal edges of the transverse processes of L1 and L2, at a depth similar to the injection site for T13, and advanced approximately 1 cm to pass slightly ventral to the process and into the intertransverse ligament. A total of 6–8 ml of local anesthetic is injected with little resistance to desensitize the ventral branches of the nerves. The needle is then withdrawn 1–2.5 cm above the fascia or just dorsal to the transverse processes, and 6–8 ml of local anesthetic is infused to desensitize the dorsal branch of the nerves (Figure 7.4).

Evidence of a successful proximal paravertebral nerve block includes increased temperature of the skin; analgesia of the skin, muscles, and peritoneum of the abdominal wall of the paralumbar fossa; and scoliosis of the spine toward the desensitized side. Advantages of the proximal paravertebral nerve block include small doses of anesthetic, wide and uniform area of analgesia and muscle relaxation, decreased intra-abdominal pressure, and absence of the local anesthetic at the margins of the surgical site. Disadvantages of the proximal paravertebral nerve block include scoliosis of the spine, which may make closure

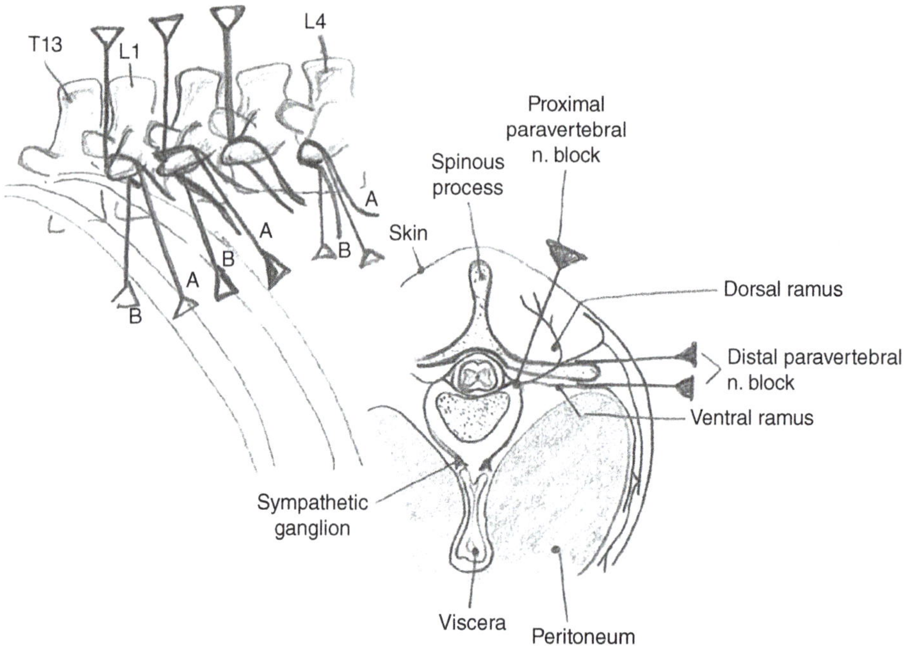

Figure 7.4 Proximal and distal paravertebral nerve blocks in cattle. (Source: Illustration by Kim Crosslin.)

of the incision more difficult; difficulty in identifying landmarks in obese and heavily muscled animals; and more skill or practice required for consistent results [4, 9, 11].

Distal paravertebral nerve block

The distal paravertebral nerve block desensitizes the dorsal and ventral rami of the spinal nerves T13, L1, and L2 at the distal ends of the transverse processes of L1, L2, and L4, respectively. An 18-gauge, 3.5- to 5.5-cm needle is inserted ventral to the transverse process, and 10 ml of local anesthetic is infused in a fan-shaped pattern. The needle can then be removed completely and reinserted or redirected dorsal to the transverse process, in a caudal direction, where 10 ml of local anesthetic is again infused in a fan-shaped pattern. This procedure is repeated for the transverse processes of the second and fourth lumbar vertebrae (Figure 7.4). Advantages of the distal paravertebral nerve block compared with the proximal paravertebral nerve block include lack of scoliosis, it is easier to perform, and it offers more consistent results.

Disadvantages of the distal paravertebral nerve block compared with the proximal paravertebral nerve block include larger doses of local anesthetic required and variations in efficiency caused by variation in anatomical pathways of the nerves [4, 9, 11].

Inverted-L block

The inverted-L block is a nonspecific regional block that locally blocks the tissue bordering the caudal aspect of the 13th rib and the ventral aspect of the transverse processes of the lumbar vertebrae [11]. An 18-gauge, 3.8-cm needle is used to inject up to a total of 100 ml

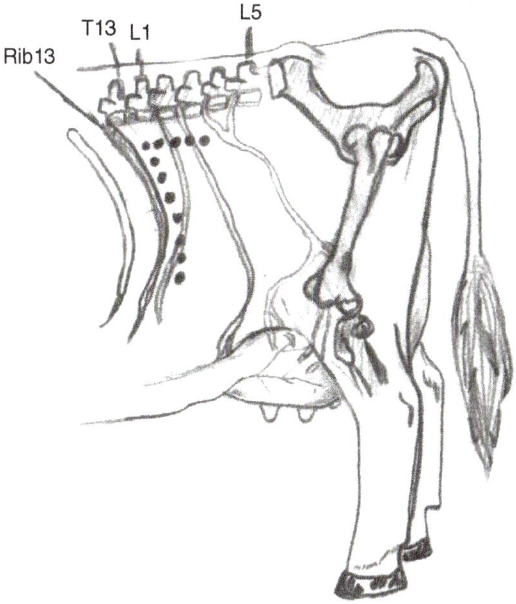

Figure 7.5 Inverted-L block in cattle. (Source: Illustration by Kim Crosslin.)

of local anesthetic solution in multiple small injection sites into the tissues bordering the dorsocaudal aspect of the 13th rib and ventrolateral aspect of the transverse processes of the lumbar vertebrae (Figure 7.5). This creates an area of anesthesia under the inverted-L block. Advantages of the inverted-L block include that the block is simple to perform, it does not interfere with ambulation, and deposition of the local anesthetic away from the incision site minimizes incisional edema and hematoma [3]. Disadvantages include incomplete analgesia and muscle relaxation of the deeper layers of the abdominal wall (particularly in obese animals), possible toxicity from the administration of larger doses of local anesthetic, and increased cost because of larger doses of local anesthetic required [3].

Line block

Infusion of local anesthetic into the incision site or a line block may be used to desensitize a selected area of the paralumbar fossa (Figure 7.6). An 18-gauge, 3.8-cm needle is used to infuse multiple, small injections of 10 ml of local anesthetic solution subcutaneously and into the deep muscle layers and peritoneum. Pain of successive injections may be alleviated by placing the edge of the needle into the edge of the previously desensitized area at an approximately 20°–30° angle [9]. In heavily muscled or overweight cattle, it may be necessary to use an 18-gauge, 7.5-cm needle to penetrate through the large amount of subcutaneous fat to reach the deep muscle layers. The amount of local anesthetic needed to acquire adequate anesthesia depends on the size of the area to be desensitized. Adult cattle weighing 450 kg (990 lb) can safely tolerate 250 ml of a 2% lidocaine hydrochloride solution [9]. Delayed healing of the incision site is a possible complication of infiltration of local anesthetic at the surgical site.

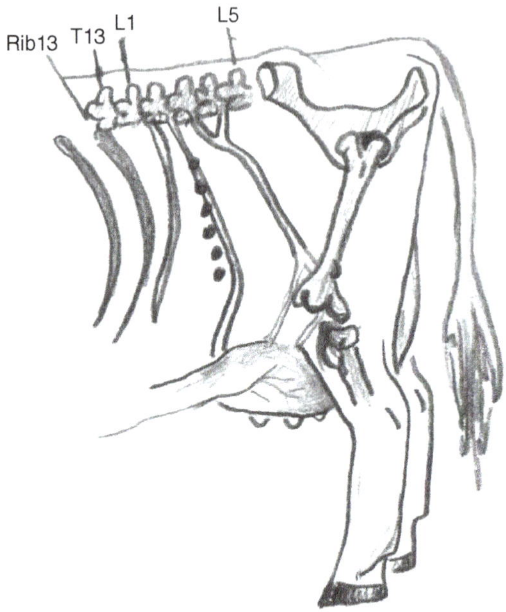

Figure 7.6 Line block in cattle. (Source: Illustration by Kim Crosslin.)

Anesthesia for reproductive procedures

Caudal epidural anesthesia

Caudal epidural anesthesia is an easy and inexpensive method of analgesia that is commonly used in cattle and other ruminants for obstetrical manipulations or replacement of prolapses. A high caudal epidural at the sacrococcygeal space (S5–Co1) desensitizes sacral nerves S2, S3, S4, and S5. The low caudal epidural at first coccygeal space (Co1–Co2) desensitizes sacral nerves S3, S4, and S5; as the anesthetic dose increases, nerves cranial to S2 may also become affected [12]. If possible, the hair should be clipped and the skin scrubbed and disinfected. Standing alongside the cow, the tail should be moved up and down to locate the fossa between the last sacral vertebra and the first coccygeal vertebra (first freely moveable space) or between the first and second coccygeal vertebrae. An 18-gauge, 3.8-cm needle (with no syringe attached) is directed perpendicular to the skin surface. Once the skin is penetrated, place a drop of local anesthetic solution in the hub of the needle (hanging drop technique). The needle should then be advanced slowly until the anesthetic solution is drawn into the epidural space by negative pressure. The syringe may then be attached to the needle, and the anesthetic solution slowly injected with no resistance (Figure 7.7). The dose of local anesthetic to be used is 0.5 ml per 45 kg (99 lb) of body weight.

Sheep with severely docked tails can be difficult to perform a caudal epidural technique (Figure 7.8). Thus, a lumbosacral epidural technique may be the only option in these animals. In goats, the tail should be pumped up and down to identify the most cranial

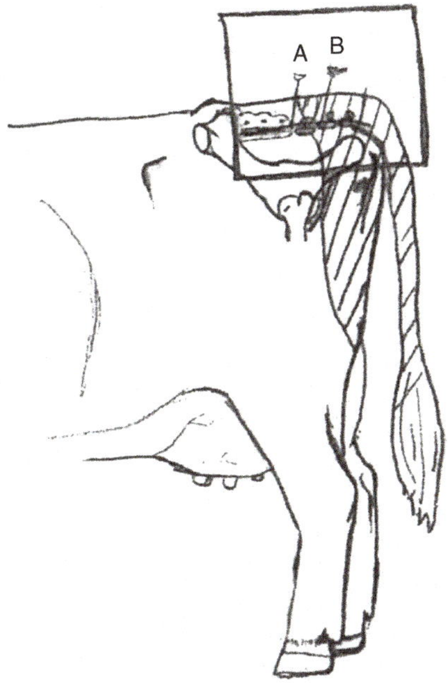

Figure 7.7 Caudal epidural nerve block in cattle, (A) intersacrococcygeal space (S_4 and Co_1) and (B) intercoccygeal space (Co_1 and Co_2). (Source: Illustration by Kim Crosslin.)

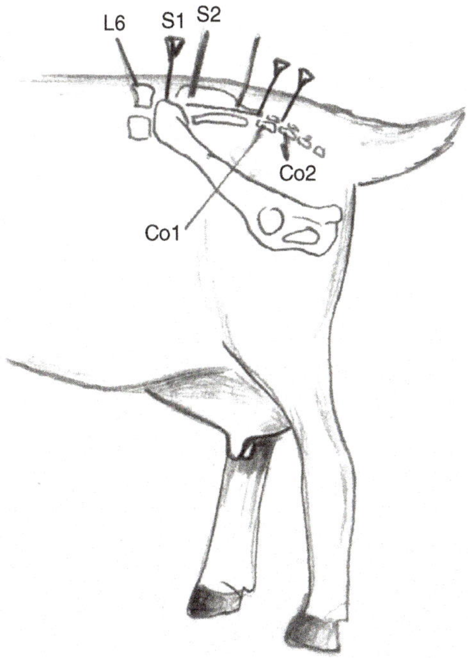

Figure 7.8 Caudal epidural and lumbosacral epidural nerve blocks in goats. (Source: Illustration by Kim Crosslin.)

moveable space into which the needle is inserted at a 45° angle to the vertebrae. The hanging drop technique, which was previously described, is used to ensure correct placement of the anesthetic into the epidural space. In small ruminants, the dose of 2% lidocaine hydrochloride ranges from 1 ml/50 kg (110 lb) to 1 ml/15 kg (33 lb) [7].

For tail docking of sheep, an epidural or local ring block just proximal to the site of docking may be used, although it appears that the local ring block was more beneficial than an epidural anesthesia [7].

Continuous caudal epidural anesthesia

Continuous caudal epidural anesthesia is used in cattle with chronic rectal and vaginal prolapse that experience continuous straining after the initial epidural anesthesia. This procedure is performed by placing a catheter into the epidural space for intermittent administration of local anesthetic. A 17-gauge, 5-cm spinal needle (Tuohy needle) with stylet in place is inserted into the epidural space at Co1 to Co2 with the bevel directed craniad. The stylet is removed, and 2 ml of local anesthetic is injected to determine if the needle is in the epidural space. A catheter is inserted into the needle and advanced cranially for 2–4 cm beyond the needle tip. The needle is then withdrawn while the catheter remains in place (Figure 7.9). An adapter is placed on the end of the catheter and the catheter secured to the skin on the dorsum. Local anesthetic solution may then be administered as needed [9].

More recently, α_2 agonists (xylazine, detomidine, medetomidine, and romifidine) and opioids (morphine, fentanyl, and buprenorphine) either alone or in combination with

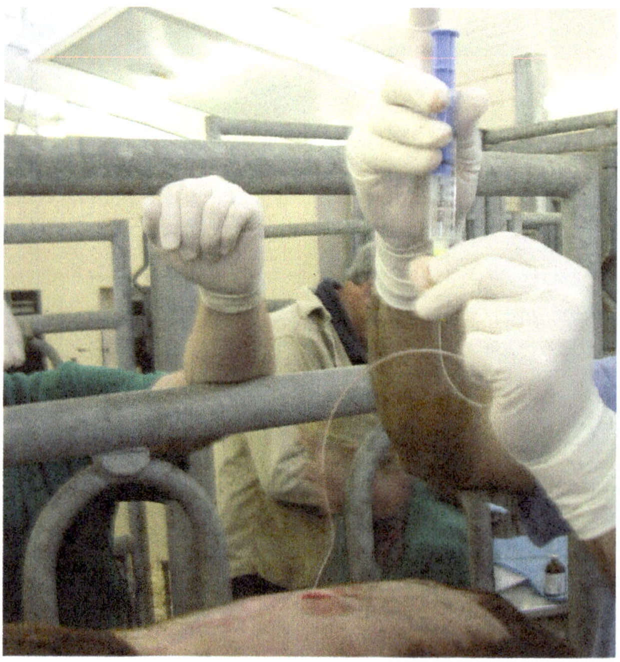

Figure 7.9 Caudal epidural catheterization in cattle.

local anesthetic solution have been used for epidural anesthesia. Epidural administration of xylazine hydrochloride (0.05 mg/kg) diluted in 5–12 ml of sterile saline or xylazine hydrochloride (0.3 mg/kg) added to 5 ml of 2% lidocaine hydrochloride combinations offers similar anesthesia to lidocaine. Although the duration of anesthesia is prolonged (4–5 hours) using these combinations, systemic effects (sedation, salivation, and ataxia) may also occur [3]. Epidural administration of an opioid, such as morphine (0.1 mg/kg) diluted in 20 ml of sterile saline, is used to provide analgesia for a prolonged period (approximately 12 hours) without interfering with motor function. Disadvantages of using opioids for epidural anesthesia are that the analgesia is not as potent as lidocaine and the maximum effect from epidural administration of morphine may not occur for 2–3 hours. Caudal epidural administration of morphine may be used to help alleviate pain in the perineal area and straining [6].

Lumbosacral epidural anesthesia

The lumbosacral epidural anesthesia is a relatively easy and commonly used technique in sedated pigs for cesarean section, repair of hernias (umbilical and inguinal), prolapses (rectal, vaginal, and uterine), and surgery of the rear limbs, penis, and prepuce. It is important to remember that epidural anesthesia is contraindicated in pigs with cardiovascular disease, bleeding disorders, or toxemic shock due to potential sympathetic blockade resulting in significant reduction in blood pressure. The 14-gauge needle can be used to guide and stabilize the spinal needle. The spinal needle needed varies according to the size of the pig with a 20-gauge, 6- to 8-cm needle appropriate for pigs weighing 10–20 kg (22–44 lb) and an 18-gauge, 10- to 16-cm needle for pigs weighing over 100 kg (220 lb). The site for needle placement is on the midline immediately caudal to the spinous process of the last lumbar (L6) vertebra (Figure 7.10). The injection site is felt as a palpable depression slightly caudal to a transverse line between the cranial prominences of the wing of the ilium on either side (0.5–1.5 cm in pigs weighing 10–50 kg (22–110 lb) and 1.5–2.5 cm in pigs weighing 50 kg (110 lb) or more). If the wings of the ilium are not palpable in larger pigs, a vertical line through the patella may be used as a guide to locate the lumbosacral space 2.0–3.0 cm caudal to the vertical

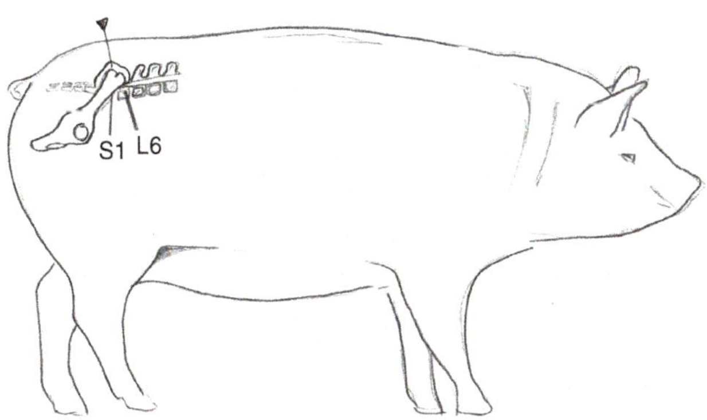

Figure 7.10 Lumbosacral epidural nerve block in pigs. (Source: Illustration by Kim Crosslin.)

line [3]. The spinal needle and stylet with the bevel of the needle directed cranially are inserted into the lumbosacral space using a 20° caudovertical angle. The depth of penetration of the needle depends on the size and condition of the pig. The depth may be up to 2–4 cm in pigs weighing between 10 and 20 kg (22–44 lb) and 4–10 cm in pigs weighing between 20 and 100 kg (44 and 220 lb). The needle will meet resistance as it encounters the interarcuate ligament. Penetration through the ligament often feels like slight pop and is associated with sudden movements indicating entrance into the vertebral canal. The lumbosacral aperture in the pig is relatively large (1.5 × 2.5 cm) and allows for some margin of error [3]. The dose of anesthetic needed to provide anesthesia caudal to the umbilicus is 1.0 ml of 2% lidocaine hydrochloride per 4.5 kg (10 lb) of body weight at a rate of 1.0 ml per 2–3 seconds. Anesthesia should occur within 10 minutes and recovery within 2 hours. A smaller dose has been utilized with similar results by using 1.0 ml per 7.5 kg (16.5 lb) for pigs weighing up to 50 kg (110 lb) and an additional 1.0 ml for every 10 kg (22 lb) increase in body weight. A maximum dose of 20 ml of 2% lidocaine hydrochloride is suggested as the upper limit: for standing castrations, 4 ml per 100 kg (220 lb), 6 ml per 200 kg (440 lb), and 8 ml per 300 kg (660 lb) of body weight and for cesarean sections, 10 ml per 100 kg (220 lb), 15 ml per 200 kg (440 lb), and 20 ml per 300 kg (660 lb) of body weight [3].

The lumbosacral space in small ruminants can be accessed by palpating the space caudal to the dorsal vertebral process of the sixth lumbar vertebrae between the wings of the ilium (Figure 7.8). Typically, an 18- or 20-gauge, 3.8-cm needle is sufficient. Llamas and animals that are overconditioned may require an 8.4-cm spinal needle for the lumbosacral space. The needle is advanced on the midline of the animal perpendicular to the vertebrae until a pop is felt. A drop of 2% lidocaine hydrochloride placed into the hub of the needle should be drawn into the needle if in the epidural space. Injection of the anesthetic should not have any resistance. The injection should be given slowly over 60–90 seconds to prevent rapid cranial migration of the anesthetic [7].

Sacral paravertebral nerve block

Sacral paravertebral anesthesia is used to relieve rectal tenesmus associated with rectal prolapse without affecting the sciatic nerve and the animal's ability to stand or tail function. The sacral paravertebral nerve block is used to provide analgesia to the pudendal nerve (pudic nerve), medial hemorrhoidal nerve (pelvic splanchnic nerve), and caudal hemorrhoidal nerve (caudal rectal nerve) by blocking S3, S4, and S5 as they branch off of the spinal cord. This block provides analgesia to the anus, vulva, and vagina [3, 13]. In bulls, S3 supplies motor function to the retractor penis muscles. Physical restraint in a squeeze chute and/or sedation may be beneficial as to prevent lateral movement of the animal during the procedure. In addition, a caudal epidural anesthesia may be helpful if the animal is fractious. The skin over the dorsal sacrum should be clipped of hair and surgically prepared for the procedure. The paired S5 foramina are 1–2 cm lateral to the sacral coccygeal joint. The S4 foramina are about 3–4 cm cranial and more lateral to the S5 foramina. The S3 foramina are an additional 3–4 cm cranial to the S4 foramina. A stab incision can be made dorsal to each foramen to aid in the introduction of a 5- to 7-cm,

18-gauge needle. The foramina can be palpated rectally with a finger placed in or over the ring which allows for identification of the foramen and ensures correct needle placement. Once the needle has entered the osseous ring, inject 2–3 ml of 2% lidocaine hydrochloride; this should be repeated for each foramen [13]. The use of a lidocaine/alcohol mixture has also been described to manage tenesmus following chronic cervicovaginal prolapse or rectal prolapse. A mixture of 1 ml of 2% lidocaine hydrochloride and 2 ml of 95% ethyl alcohol has been used effectively [13].

The sacral paravertebral nerve block can also be utilized in sheep and goats by using an 18-gauge, 7.5-cm needle. This block in small ruminants uses the same technique described for cattle with a reduced volume of 1– 2 ml of 2% lidocaine hydrochloride per injection site [3].

Internal pudendal nerve block

The procedure for bilateral internal pudendal (pudic) nerve block was first described by Larson to facilitate relaxation of the bull's penis without causing locomotor impairment [14]. The internal pudendal nerve block can be used in the standing bull for penile relaxation and analgesia distal to the sigmoid flexure and examination of the penis. In the standing female, the internal pudendal nerve block can be used to relieve straining caused by chronic vaginal prolapse. This technique may also be used for surgical procedures of the penis, such as repair of prolapses, removal of peripenile tumors, and removal of penile papillomas or warts, and other minor surgeries of the penis and prepuce.

This procedure involves desensitizing the internal pudendal nerve and the anastomotic branch of the middle hemorrhoidal nerve using an ischiorectal approach. The internal pudendal nerve consists of fibers originating from the ventral branches of the third and fourth sacral nerves (S3 and S4) and the pelvic splanchnic nerves. The skin at the ischiorectal fossa on both sides is clipped, disinfected, and desensitized with approximately 2 ml of local anesthetic. A 14-gauge, 1.25-cm needle is inserted through the desensitized skin at the ischiorectal fossa to serve as a cannula. An 18-gauge, 10- to 15-cm spinal needle is then directed through the cannula to the pudendal nerve. The operator's left hand is placed into the rectum to the level of the wrist and the fingers directed laterally and ventrally to identify the lesser sacrosciatic foramen. The lesser sciatic foramen is first identified by rectal palpation as a soft depression in the sacrosciatic ligament. The internal pudendal nerve can be readily identified lying on the ligament immediately cranial and dorsal to the foramen and approximately one finger's width dorsal to the pudendal artery passing through the foramen. The internal pudendal artery can be readily palpated a finger's width ventral to the nerve. The spinal needle is held in the operator's right hand and introduced through the cannula in the ischiorectal fossa. The spinal needle is directed medial to the sacrosciatic ligament and directed cranioventrally (Figure 7.11). The needle is not felt until it has been introduced approximately 5–7 cm and can then be repositioned to the nerve. Once at the pudendal nerve, 20 ml of local anesthetic is deposited at the nerve. The needle is then partially withdrawn and redirected 2–3 cm more caudodorsally where an additional 10 ml of local

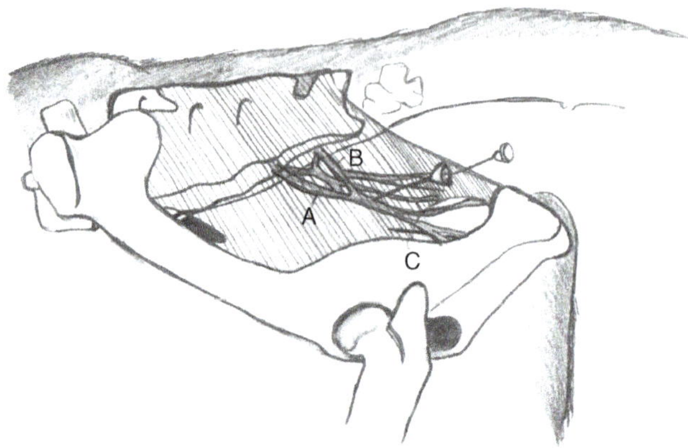

Figure 7.11 Internal pudendal nerve on left pelvis of cattle: (A) internal pudendal nerve, (B) pelvic splanchnic nerve, and (C) pudendal artery. (Source: Illustration by Kim Crosslin.)

anesthetic is deposited at the cranial aspect of the foramen to desensitize the muscular branches and the middle hemorrhoidal nerve. The needle is then removed and the sites of deposition are massaged to aid in dispersal of the local anesthetic. This procedure is then repeated on the opposite side of the pelvis. Relaxation of the penis varies and may take as long as 30–40 minutes for full effect. Effectiveness of the block can be assessed by firmly squeezing the tail of the epididymis of each testicle. The bull's inability to lift or retract the testicle signifies adequate analgesia. The duration of the internal pudendal nerve block lasts from 2 to 4 hours [13].

Dorsal penile nerve block

The dorsal nerve of the penis may be desensitized at a location just proximal to the surgical site. With the bull restrained, the penis should be manually extended, and a towel clamp should then be placed under the dorsal apical ligament. Alternatively, a gauze tourniquet may be placed around the free portion of the penis to aid in penile extension. With the dorsal aspect of the penis thoroughly cleansed, 2–4 ml of 2% lidocaine hydrochloride should be infused subcutaneously across the dorsum of the penis proximal to the lesion [15].

Alternatively, the dorsal nerve of the penis may also be desensitized as it passes over the ischial arch for penile anesthesia and relaxation. The skin associated with the penile body and located 10 cm ventral to the anus and 2.5 cm from midline is infiltrated with 2–4 ml of 2% lidocaine hydrochloride using a small-gauge needle (22–25 gauge). A 20-gauge, 4-cm needle is then inserted through the desensitized skin and advanced for 5–7 cm to contact the pelvic floor. Aspiration ensures that the needle is not in the dorsal artery of the penis. The needle is then withdrawn approximately 1 cm, and the area infiltrated with 20–30 ml of 2% lidocaine hydrochloride. The procedure is then repeated on the opposite side of the penis. Analgesia and paralysis of the penis will occur within 20 minutes and should last for 1–2 hours [3].

Castration

Castration of bulls is a very common surgical procedure in general practice. Historically, castration was often performed with minimal or no anesthesia. However, anesthesia for castration is more commonly practiced today because calves benefit from anesthesia with improved feed consumption and rate of gain. Depending on the age and size of the animal, the surgery is usually performed with chemical and/or regional anesthesia (scrotum and testicles). Depending on the size of the calf, the proposed line of incision for removal of the distal aspect of the scrotum should be subcutaneously infiltrated with 5–10 ml of 2% lidocaine hydrochloride. In bulls and boars, a 16- to 18-gauge, 3.8- to 7.5-cm needle is inserted at an angle (30°–45°) into the center of the testicle, and 10–15 ml of local anesthetic per 200 kg (440 lb) of body weight is injected into the parenchyma of each testicle. The anesthetic quickly enters the lymphatics and desensitizes the sensory fibers in the spermatic cord. For smaller animals or calves, a smaller needle (20 gauge, 2.5 cm) may be used to administer 2–10 ml of 2% lidocaine hydrochloride [3].

Another method involves using 10 ml of 2% lidocaine hydrochloride subcutaneously along the circumference of the neck of the scrotum followed by the placement of 5 ml of 2% lidocaine hydrochloride into each spermatic cord [16].

In bull calves, rams, and bucks, a 20-gauge, 2.5- to 3.8-cm needle is used to inject 2% lidocaine hydrochloride into the center of the testicle (Figure 7.12). The dose varies from 2 to 10 ml depending on the size of the animal [3]. Castration of camelids is typically delayed until the animals are mature and, thus, requires general anesthesia.

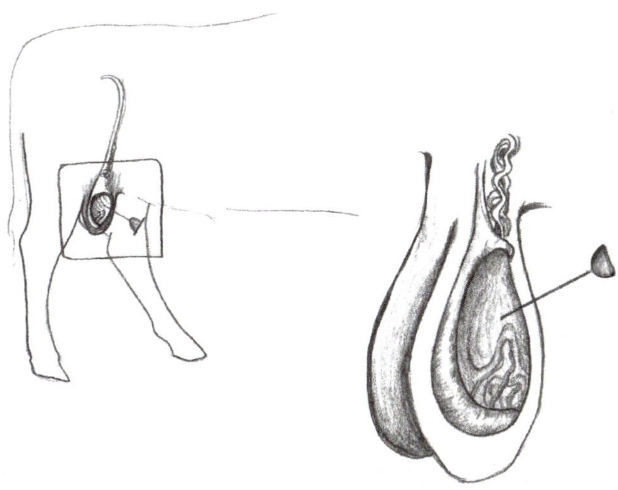

Figure 7.12 Injection site for intratesticular anesthesia for castration in cattle. (Source: Illustration by Kim Crosslin.)

Teat anesthesia

Inverted-V block

The inverted-V block has been principally used for focal lesions of the teat such as a teat laceration or wart. Using a 25-gauge, 1.5-cm needle, 5 ml of anesthetic is injected into the skin and musculature of the teat immediately dorsal to the surgical site in an inverted-V pattern (Figure 7.13A) [8].

Ring block

The ring block has been commonly used to anesthetize the teat for surgeries. A 25-gauge, 3.8-cm needle is used to inject 5 ml of local anesthetic into the skin and musculature circumscribing the base of the teat (Figure 7.13B) [8].

Infusion of teat cistern

The teat cistern may be infused with local anesthetic for surgical procedures, such as removal of polyps, which involve only the mucous membranes. Prior to infusing the teat, the cistern should be stripped of milk and the orifice thoroughly cleaned with alcohol. A tourniquet (rubber band) may then be placed at the base of the teat to prevent leakage of local anesthetic into the udder from the teat cistern. A sterile teat cannula is then used to instill 10 ml of local anesthetic into the teat (Figure 7.13C). It is important to remember

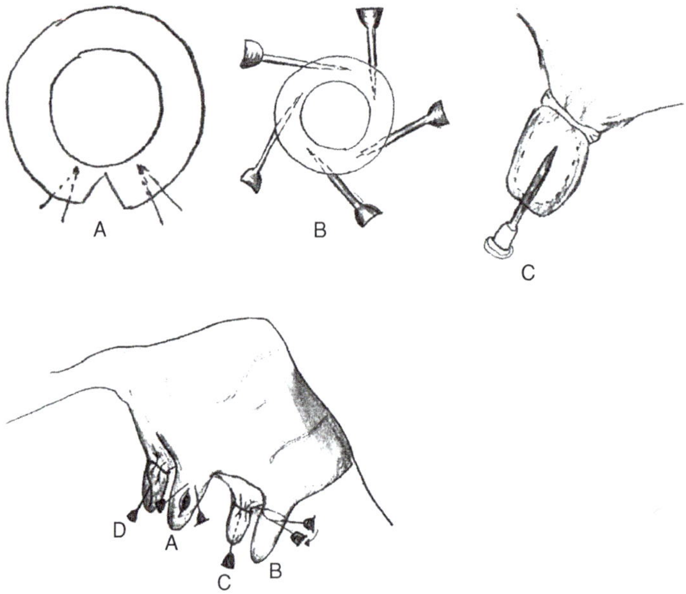

Figure 7.13 Teat blocks for cattle: (A) inverted-V block, (B) teat ring block, (C) teat cistern infusion, and (D) intravenous regional teat block. (Source: Illustration by Kim Crosslin.)

that the musculature and the skin are not desensitized using this technique. The teat cannula is removed from the teat, and the remaining anesthetic is milked out. Once the surgery is performed, the tourniquet is removed [8].

Anesthesia of the distal limb

Intravenous regional anesthesia (Bier block) of the foot is regularly performed and is often the favored technique for surgery of the foot. A tourniquet is placed proximal to the fetlock just before injection of local anesthetic when the vein is maximally distended. In the thoracic limb, intravenous regional analgesia can be performed using the dorsal metacarpal vein, the plantar metacarpal vein, and the radial vein (Figure 7.14). In the pelvic limb, the lateral saphenous vein or lateral plantar digital vein may be used for injection. Approximately 20 ml of local anesthetic is injected intravenously as close to the surgical site as possible using a 20-gauge, 3.3-cm needle or 21-gauge butterfly catheter. It is only necessary to administer anesthetic into one vein to provide anesthesia to the entire area distal to the tourniquet. The tourniquet can be safely left on for up to 1 hour to provide hemostasis during surgical procedures of the foot. Anesthesia of the foot occurs within 5–10 minutes. Once the surgical procedure is complete, the tourniquet is released [8].

It is difficult to use the dorsal digital vein or the palmar (plantar) digital veins in small ruminants as commonly as in large ruminants. However, some have found the Bier block easier in small ruminants when the tourniquet was placed either above the elbow in the forelimb or below the tarsus in the hind limb. This allows the use of the larger cephalic and recurrent tarsal veins, respectively. Using 3–4 ml of 2% lidocaine hydrochloride in small goats usually results in limb anesthesia for as long as the tourniquet is in place [7].

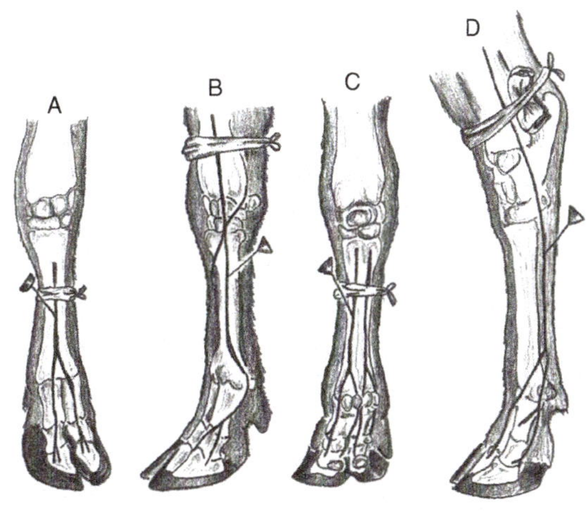

Figure 7.14 Injection sites for regional intravenous anesthesia (Bier block) in cattle: (A) common dorsal metacarpal vein of the forelimb, (B) lateral palmar digital vein of the forelimb, (C) lateral palmar metacarpal vein of the forelimb, and (D) lateral saphenous vein of the hind limb. (Source: Illustration by Kim Crosslin.)

References

1. Anderson, D. and Edmondson, M. (2013) Prevention and management of surgical pain in cattle. *Veterinary Clinics of North America: Food Animal Practice*, **29**, 157–184.
2. Broom, D. (2000) The evolution of pain. *Vlaams Diergeneeskundig Tijdschrift*, **69**, 385–411.
3. Skarda, R. (2007) Local and regional anesthetic techniques: ruminants and swine, in *Lumb and Jones' Veterinary Anesthesia and Analgesia*, 4th edn (eds W. Tranquilli, J. Thurmon and K. Grimm), Blackwell Publishing, Oxford, pp. 731–746.
4. Edwards, B. (2001) Regional anesthesia techniques in cattle. *In Practice*, **23**, 142–149.
5. Elmore, R. (1980) Food animal regional anesthesia, bovine blocks: cornual. *Veterinary Medicine, Small Animal Clinician*, **75**, 1610–1612.
6. Navarre, C. (2006) Numbing: nose to tail. *Annual Convention of the American Association of Bovine Practitioners*, pp. 53–55.
7. Plummer, P. and Schleining, J. (2013) Assessment and management of pain in small ruminants and camelids. *Veterinary Clinics of North America: Food Animal Practice*, **29**, 185–208.
8. Edmondson, M. (2008) Local and regional anesthesia in cattle. *Veterinary Clinics of North America: Food Animal Practice*, **24**, 211–226.
9. Skarda, R. (1986) Techniques in local analgesia in ruminants and swine. *Veterinary Clinics of North America: Food Animal Practice*, **2**, 621–663.
10. Skarda, R. (1996) Local and regional anesthesia in ruminants and swine. *Veterinary Clinics of North America: Food Animal Practice*, **12**, 579–626.
11. Noordsy, J. and Ames, N. (2006) Local and regional anesthesia, in *Food Animal Surgery*, 4th edn (eds J. Noordsy and N. Ames), Veterinary Learning Systems, Yardley, pp. 21–42.
12. Noordsy, J. and Ames, N. (2006) Epidural anesthesia, in *Food Animal Surgery*, 4th edn (eds J. Noordsy and N. Ames), Veterinary Learning Systems, Yardley, pp. 43–55.
13. Hopper, R., King, H., Walters, K. and Christiansen, D. (2012) Management of urogenital surgery and disease in the bull: the scrotum and its contents. *Clinical Theriogenology*, **4**, 332–338.
14. Larson, L. (1953) The internal pudendal (pudic) nerve block for anesthesia of the penis and relaxation of the retractor penis muscle. *Journal of the American Veterinary Medical Association*, **123**, 18–27.
15. Wolfe, D., Beckett, S. and Carson, R. (1999) Acquired conditions of the penis and prepuce, in *Large Animal Urogenital Surgery*, 2nd edn (eds D. Wolfe and D. Moll), Williams and Wilkins, Baltimore, pp. 237–272.
16. Rust, R., Thomson, D. and Loneragan, G. (2007) Effect of different castration methods on growth performance and behavioral responses of postpubertal beef bulls. *The Bovine Practitioner*, **41**, 116–118.

Chapter 8

Anesthetic management for specific procedures

Benjamin Newcomer and Paul Walz
Department of Pathobiology, College of Veterinary Medicine, Auburn University, USA

Selection and implementation of anesthetic protocols in farm animals are largely influenced by the species of animal, particular procedure to be performed, individual knowledge and experience of the veterinarian with respect to inhalant or injectable anesthesia agents, economics, and the facilities and personnel available for support. The purpose of this chapter is not to present an in-depth discussion of surgical procedures, as details on the surgical approaches and procedures are well documented in other texts [1–3]. Rather, this section presents anesthetic techniques utilized routinely for the procedures described. The authors recognize that many alternatives and personal preferences exist for anesthetic management of various conditions in farm animals.

Because of the docile nature of ruminant patients and capability for physical restraint in a chute, most standing surgical procedures in field settings can be performed using local anesthetics alone or utilizing combinations of chemical restraint with local or regional anesthesia. Chemical restraint can also be utilized for procedures where recumbence is preferred. Although the term "balanced" anesthesia is not often associated with field anesthesia in farm animals, the reality is that most surgical procedures involving ruminants can be accomplished using this method, where combinations of two or more classes of drugs including sedatives, tranquilizers, analgesics, and local anesthetics are utilized to provide sedation, analgesia, and muscle relaxation. The advantage of utilizing multiple classes of drugs in an anesthetic plan is safety, as smaller doses of two or more agents are considered safer than the usual large dose of a single agent. Swine are less tolerant of physical restraint; therefore, deep sedation or general anesthesia is often necessary to perform even minor surgical procedures.

For surgical procedures where recumbence is preferred or where a procedure requires an extended period of immobility or high level of analgesia, general anesthesia offers optimal restraint, ability for aseptic surgical conditions, proper handling of tissues, and hemostasis. Location for performing the general anesthesia, positioning of the patient,

Farm Animal Anesthesia: Cattle, Small Ruminants, Camelids, and Pigs, First Edition.
Edited by HuiChu Lin and Paul Walz.

and preparing for regurgitation, rumen tympany, and salivation are important considerations prior to induction (Chapter 1). The choice of injectable or inhalation maintenance general anesthesia often depends on the availability of gas anesthetic equipment and personal experience. Since depth of anesthesia can be easily and rapidly adjusted with inhalation anesthetics (e.g., isoflurane, sevoflurane, and desflurane), inhalation anesthesia is preferred over injectable anesthesia for lengthy procedures or for patients considered higher anesthetic risk because of systemic illness. If general anesthesia is utilized, anesthetic protocols should be individually designed, especially with respect to critically ill patients, neonates, and other animals where anesthetic risk is considered high. Prior to anesthesia, patients should be evaluated by physical examination with or without clinical pathologic examination to assess their risk associated with anesthesia and surgery. Heart defects and pulmonary dysfunction can be identified during careful auscultation of the thorax, and evidence of cardiovascular compromise can be subjectively assessed by mucous membrane color and capillary refill time. Complete blood counts and biochemistry panels should be evaluated in cases where inflammatory disease or vital organ dysfunction is suspected. Classification of animals by physical status 1–5 has been proposed to aid in determining anesthetic risk, with higher physical status having greater risk of complications associated with anesthesia [4]. Apparently healthy animals undergoing an elective surgical procedure can be classified as physical status 1. For simple elective surgical procedures in young, apparently healthy animals, preoperative laboratory evaluation is not usually necessary. An animal with a slight to moderate systemic disturbance that does not interfere with function is physical status 2, and examples include mild dehydration, obesity, umbilical hernias, poor body condition, and simple fractures. Physical status 3 animals are those with slight to moderate systemic disturbances that do interfere with normal function, and examples include heart defects, severe electrolyte imbalances, oxygen exchange problems such as pneumonia, moderate to severe dehydration, and compound fractures. Physical status 4 animals are those with uncompensated systemic disturbances or life-threatening conditions where surgical intervention is deemed lifesaving. Finally, physical status 5 animals are those in moribund condition. If at all possible, assessing clinical pathology and stabilizing body systems by provision of fluid and electrolyte therapy are important in physical status 3–5 animals. Packed cell volume and total protein measurements are screening tests which are easily performed and can provide information that can influence preparation for anesthesia and surgery. For physical status 4 and 5 animals, anesthesia and surgery are often performed without the luxury of time and presurgical stabilization. Monitoring of high-risk patients during anesthesia is important and should continue throughout the recovery phase. Anesthetic deaths can occur during the recovery phase.

Umbilical hernias

Umbilical hernias in calves occur with relative frequency and may be hereditary or acquired in origin. General anesthesia is recommended, particularly for large hernias or those with associated abscessation that requires additional dissection and extended surgical times. Surgical success is enhanced when patient movement is minimized throughout the procedure. Intravenous (IV) administration of ketamine (2–3 mg/kg) and xylazine (0.1–0.2 mg/kg) is a commonly used induction protocol and will usually provide

20–30 minutes of anesthesia. The duration of anesthesia can be extended by intubation and maintenance with inhalant anesthetics such as isoflurane, or in field situations, by additional dosage of injectable anesthetics. Redosing with ⅓ to ½ of the induction dose of ketamine and xylazine or ketamine alone (1–2 mg/kg given slowly to effect) will provide an additional 15 minutes of anesthesia in most cases. Induction and maintenance with xylazine alone induces a decrease in heart rate, and for this reason, the addition of ketamine to injectable anesthesia protocols is preferred. In one study, calves undergoing umbilical hernia repair were more likely to experience hypoxemia and had a greater intraoperative response to surgical stimulation when maintained on injectable anesthesia than when maintained on isoflurane after induction [5]. Periumbilical infusions of local anesthetic (described in the following paragraph) are recommended for use in conjunction with general anesthetic protocols.

Heavy sedation in conjunction with local and regional anesthetic techniques has also been used successfully for umbilical hernia repair in calves. A ring block with local anesthetic is performed at the periphery of the surgical site. A subcutaneous (SC) ring block can be followed by deposition of 2–5 ml of local anesthetic at approximately 1–2-cm intervals deep to the SC block to desensitize the underlying muscle layers. Alternatively, high-volume caudal epidural anesthesia has been shown to be an acceptable protocol for umbilical surgery [5]. High-volume caudal epidurals are administered at the standard caudal epidural site but, as the name implies, involve the administration of lidocaine in much larger volumes (1 ml per 5 kg (11 lb) of body weight) than typically given for perineal anesthesia. One study reported no adverse health effects when using a higher dose of 1 ml per 2 kg (4.4 lb) of body weight [6]. Recumbency and loss of hind limb motor control last for 4–6 hours following epidural administration, and proper postoperative care must be taken for the safety and welfare of the patient. Intramuscular (IM) xylazine sedation (0.1 mg/kg) has been used in conjunction with a lumbosacral epidural of 2% lidocaine (0.18–0.24 ml/kg) and xylazine (0.05 mg/kg) for umbilical hernia repair but without perfusion of local anesthetic was insufficient for adequate analgesia [7].

In swine, general anesthesia, either with inhalation or injectable anesthetics, is commonly used for umbilical hernia repair when surgical correction is pursued. As in calves, periumbilical infusions of local anesthetic are recommended for maximum analgesia. Alternatively, a lumbosacral epidural (Chapter 7) can provide adequate analgesia for umbilical surgery. Desensitization of the area caudal to the umbilicus is achieved with a dose of 1 ml of 2% lidocaine per 4.5 kg (9.9 lb) of body weight. The anesthetic should be infused at a rate of 1 ml per 2–3 seconds and provides approximately 2 hours of anesthesia. Alternatively, similar results are seen at a dose of 1 ml per 7.5 kg (16.5 lb) for pigs up to 50 kg (110 lb); for larger pigs, 1.0 ml of lidocaine is added for every additional 10 kg (22 lb) of body weight.

Wounds, lumps, bumps, and abscesses

Wound management

Appropriate anesthetic techniques for wound management will be determined by the extent of the wound(s) and the attitude of the patient. Adequate restraint for a thorough examination is essential, and sedation may be necessary for extended examinations or in patients that are fractious or aggressive. Xylazine is the most frequently used drug for sedation in large animals. General anesthesia may be required to appropriately examine small ruminants that suffer a severe predator attack and also may be useful for the performance of ancillary diagnostic tests such as imaging techniques to determine the extent of internal injuries.

Regional anesthetic techniques are desirable whenever possible as local anesthetics can delay wound healing. Additionally, when injected at the wound site, lidocaine can result in cell injury due to its acidic nature. The additional cell injury not only delays healing but acts as an additional painful stimulus to the animal. Buffering 2% lidocaine with 8.4% sodium bicarbonate in a 10:1 ratio will decrease the pain and discomfort of SC lidocaine injection without decreasing analgesic efficacy. When regional techniques are impossible or impractical, local injections should be made through the wound to avoid the abundant pain receptors located within the epidermis. Use of longer needles allows deposition of the local anesthetic farther away from the wound margin and minimizes its negative effect on wound healing. Epinephrine, a potent vasoconstrictor, is sometimes added to lidocaine to enhance the efficacy and duration of action of the injection; this is contraindicated when providing analgesia around wound edges due to the risk of tissue necrosis.

Ocular squamous cell carcinoma

Ocular squamous cell carcinoma is the most common indication for surgery of the periocular tissues in cattle. The surgical procedure utilized and the anesthetic techniques performed will be influenced by the surgeon's preference and the size, location, and involvement of local structures of the lesion. Local anesthetic techniques are almost always sufficient for routine cases; sedation with acepromazine (0.01 mg/kg IV, 0.1 mg/kg IM) or other sedatives can be of use when adequate restraint is not available, the animal is unusually agitated, or the lesion is extremely involved. Topical anesthetic can be applied to the cornea as desired. Local infusion of lidocaine around the lesion using an 18- or 20-gauge needle is recommended for removal of small lesions of the eyelids and conjunctiva by sharp dissection. When cryosurgery is the procedure of choice, the surgical area can be blocked using topical or local anesthetics. The nictitating membrane can be desensitized by injecting lidocaine directly into the base of the third eyelid using a 2.5-cm, 22- to 24-gauge needle.

Enucleation

Enucleation, or more commonly orbit exenteration, is commonly performed in farm animals to correct extensive inflammatory or neoplastic lesions of the eye or orbital structures. General anesthesia may be beneficial for fractious animals or those with extensive lesion involvement. However, the procedure is commonly performed using physical restraint and local anesthetic techniques. Sedation with acepromazine (0.01 mg/kg IV, 0.1 mg/kg IM) or xylazine (0.05 mg/kg IV, 0.1 mg/kg IM) prior to the procedure is recommended. An SC ring block is performed approximately 5 cm from the eyelid margins. The globe is desensitized by use of the Peterson block or retrobulbar technique (Chapter 7) according to the surgeon's preference. The author prefers a four-point retrobulbar injection using an 18-gauge, 15-cm needle. The needle may be bent manually to mimic the curvature of the globe before insertion through the eyelid or canthus at the orbital rim. Local anesthetic is injected in small increments as the needle is advanced, with 10–15 ml deposited at the back of the globe when the needle is fully inserted.

Entropion

Correction of mild cases of entropion in young ruminants is often performed without the use of sharp dissection and may not require anesthesia; infusion of a small amount of lidocaine locally can be performed if desired. When cases require more invasive techniques, general anesthesia is recommended. This is indicated most commonly in overweight potbellied pigs. In field situations, combinations of xylazine and ketamine (2 mg/kg and 11 mg/kg IM, respectively) or **TKX-P** (Chapter 4) generally work well. The **TKX-P** is a combination of tiletamine, zolazepam, ketamine, and xylazine formed by reconstituting one 500-mg vial of Telazol with 250 mg (2.5 ml) of ketamine and 250 mg of xylazine (2.5 ml). The resulting combination is dosed at 1 ml/35–75 kg (77–165 lb) in commercial pigs or 1 ml/75–140 kg (165–308 lb) in potbellied pigs. Alternatively, general anesthesia may be maintained with inhalation anesthetics when the adequate equipment is available and circumstances warrant.

Abscess removal

Lymph node abscessation in cases of caseous lymphadenitis in small ruminants is the most common indication for surgical extirpation of lymph nodes in farm animals. Removal of the abscess *in toto* decreases environmental contamination and is frequently performed in valuable animals or on farms with strict biosecurity/biocontainment programs. General anesthesia is recommended for the procedure as complicated surgical dissection is often required due to the proximity to vital structures of the most commonly involved lymph nodes. Maintenance of anesthesia with inhalation anesthetics is preferred, but injectable anesthetic protocols may be suitable for some cases. Specific protocols are discussed previously (Chapters 4 and 5); selection should be based on the surgeon's preferences and the location of the targeted lymph nodes. Inhalant anesthetic protocols are recommended when removing lymph nodes in closer proximity to vital structures (e.g., carotid arteries, esophagus).

Surgical disorders of the abdomen

Laparotomy

Abdominal surgery (laparotomy, celiotomy) is the most common major surgical procedure performed by farm animal veterinarians. Laparotomy is used to access the abdominal cavity during diagnostic exploration, cesarean section, ovariectomy, rumenotomy, urolithiasis with or without ruptured urinary bladder, intestinal accidents, abomasal displacements and volvulus, biopsy of abdominal organs, large intestinal disorders, and renal disease. Surgical exploration of the abdomen should not be considered only for therapy but is also a cost- and time-efficient diagnostic tool. Many surgical approaches exist for entering the abdominal cavity. Because of the large size of the cattle abdomen, it is advantageous to enter the abdomen as close to the lesion or target as possible which necessitates a thorough physical examination to determine the optimal approach for success. The main approaches for a laparotomy in cattle are the right paralumbar fossa, the left paralumbar fossa, the ventral midline, right paracostal, and paramedian. The standing approaches are preferred for exploratory laparotomy because the internal organs are in their normal position as compared to the approaches utilizing lateral or dorsal recumbency. The standing right paralumbar fossa laparotomy using local/regional anesthesia with or without sedation is a very common approach in adult cattle and can be utilized for exploration of the abdomen and therapy for conditions which include cecal dilatation and dislocation, enterotomies, displaced abomasum, small intestinal accidents, surgery of the colon, nephrectomy, and physiologic mastectomy.

In general, most cattle, especially dairy cattle, are docile and calm enough that most abdominal surgeries can be performed in the standing animal under local or regional anesthesia alone. Anesthesia of the paralumbar fossa and abdominal wall for standing laparotomies can be achieved by local infiltration of anesthetic or several different regional anesthetic techniques described in Chapter 7. The standing laparotomy is preferred for many conditions and reduces problems associated with bloat, regurgitation, and nerve or muscle damage. In fractious and aggressive cattle, mild sedation with xylazine (0.015–0.025 mg/kg IV or IM) can be utilized to assist with performing the regional anesthetic technique. In this use, xylazine will provide sedation but should not be relied on for significant analgesia when the injections of local or regional anesthetics are made. The onset of IV administration is rapid and the duration of sedation is dose dependent. Quiet cattle require less of a dose for standing sedation than anxious or unruly cattle [8]. Using the IV dose (0.01 mg/kg) in an IM or SC route xylazine can produce mild sedation with a lower risk of recumbency. For extremely agitated or aggressive cattle, xylazine sedation can also be utilized, but higher doses are necessary for sedation (0.02–0.05 mg/kg IV), and the potential for recumbency increases. For this reason, many clinicians have utilized a **Ketamine Stun** technique, which is the addition of a small dose of ketamine to an injectable chemical restraint technique [8]. The **Ketamine Stun** can be given IV, IM, or SC; however, the SC route is preferred for a standing paralumbar fossa laparotomy. A combination of butorphanol (0.01 mg/kg), xylazine (0.02 mg/kg), and ketamine (0.04 mg/kg) is given SC, with onset of activity occurring in 5–10 minutes. This protocol has been referred to as the 5–10–20 technique, because for a 500-kg (1100-lb) cow, 5 mg of butorphanol, 10 mg of xylazine, and 20 mg of ketamine are used. Morphine can be substituted for butorphanol at a dose of 0.05–0.06 mg/kg, thus converting the 5–10–20 technique to a 25–10–20 technique (25 mg of morphine for a 500-kg (1100-lb) cow). The purpose of the **Ketamine Stun** for a standing laparotomy is to calm the patient; local or regional anesthetic techniques are still necessary to perform the laparotomy. Duration of activity is approximately 60–90 minutes. If the duration of the procedure dictates extending the **Ketamine Stun**, xylazine and ketamine can be administered subcutaneously at 25–50% of the initial doses. Including butorphanol in the redosing regimen has been associated with a greater likelihood of recumbency.

Although laparotomy is performed at a greater frequency in adult cattle, camelids, small ruminants, calves, and swine occasionally require a laparotomy. Laparotomy is often performed in the recumbent small ruminant or calf patient, because most will lie down during the procedure if a standing procedure is attempted. Sheep, goats, and calves should be heavily sedated combined with local/regional anesthesia or preferably placed under general anesthesia. Llamas and alpacas that require a laparotomy are best placed under general anesthesia. While combinations of xylazine at 0.25 mg/kg and ketamine at 2–5 mg/kg can be used for minor dental procedures, wound care, etc., their duration of activity and depth of anesthesia are often unsatisfactory for laparotomy in camelids. For pigs, the most common indication for a laparotomy is cesarean section which is described later in this chapter.

Disorders of the forestomachs

Disorders of the forestomach in ruminants can result from a variety of causes, including those that are dietary, inflammatory, and/or mechanical. Acute lactic acidosis (grain overload, acute carbohydrate engorgement) is an example of a dietary forestomach disease resulting from consumption of large amounts of rapidly fermentable concentrate feeds. If in the acute stage of the disease, a rumenotomy can be performed to remove as much of the offending feedstuff as possible. This procedure can also be performed for lead toxicity or other conditions where removal of feed material from the reticulorumen is warranted. The rumen is apposed against the left body wall, which makes this location an ideal portal to access the rumen, reticulum, and reticulo-omasal canal. The surgical procedure is ideally performed in the standing patient with the approach being the left paralumbar fossa. Regional anesthesia alone is the preferred method of anesthesia, although mild sedation can be added. Most cases of acute lactic acidosis have some degree of depression and metabolic abnormalities, so choice of sedative and dose is important.

Rumenotomy can also be performed to diagnose ruminal–reticular diseases (rumenitis, parakeratosis), remove foreign material (bags, plastic, placenta), remove impacted ingesta, and as part of the treatment for traumatic reticuloperitonitis (hardware disease). Traumatic reticuloperitonitis is a disease primarily of cattle because of their indiscriminate eating behavior. Metal linear foreign bodies, that is, wire and nails, perforate the cranial aspect of the reticulum, resulting in an inflammatory reaction, forestomach stasis, localized or generalized peritonitis, a perireticular abscess, and adhesions or vagal indigestion. The foreign body can also continue to migrate resulting in pericarditis or myocarditis. For traumatic reticuloperitonitis, a standing left paralumbar fossa laparotomy and rumenotomy can be utilized for therapeutic and diagnostic purposes. The left paralumbar fossa is anesthetized using local or regional anesthetic techniques with or without sedation as described for laparotomy. In cattle too weak to stand for the lengthy procedure, sedation combined with local/regional anesthesia or general anesthesia can be used with the patient positioned in right lateral recumbency. Although small ruminants and camelids rarely get hardware disease, a rumenotomy is occasionally necessary for removal of toxic ingesta or foreign bodies. Placement of the animal in right lateral recumbency using general anesthesia is recommended.

Displacements and volvulus of the abomasum

Left displaced abomasum is one of the most common digestive tract conditions in dairy cattle and is associated with significant economic losses from both decreased milk production and increased culling rates. Several minimally invasive closed procedures along with several surgical techniques have been described to correct abomasal displacement in dairy cattle [9]. Minimally invasive closed procedures include rolling, blind tack, toggle pin, and laparoscopy-assisted toggle pin. For all but laparoscopy, the procedure is of short duration (<15 minutes) and can be accomplished by casting the animal using ropes or using a rapid-acting, short-duration sedative, with xylazine (0.05–0.1 mg/kg IV) most commonly used since it can be reversed with yohimbine (0.125 mg/kg IM) or tolazoline (2.0 mg/kg IM) after the procedure has been completed.

Laparoscopic correction of abomasal displacements has been described using either a one-step or two-step approach. Laparoscopy is a minimally invasive technique that permits the observation of the abdominal organs. Minimal invasion of the abdominal cavity with this technique is therapeutically beneficial with quick return to normal activity. The one-step approach involves either a left paralumbar fossa incision or ventral paramedian incision, while the two-step approach involves both incisions [10]. Anesthesia for the left paralumbar incision is provided by local or regional anesthesia. For the ventral paramedian incision, xylazine (0.05–0.1 mg/kg IV) sedation combined with local or regional anesthetic techniques is used.

Conventional open surgical procedures for correction of a displaced abomasum include standing right paralumbar fossa omentopexy or pyloropexy, standing left paralumbar fossa abomasopexy, or dorsal recumbent paramedian abomasopexy. For abomasal volvulus, the standing right flank paralumbar fossa approach or dorsal recumbency paramedian approach is used. For the standing procedures, anesthesia is usually accomplished with local/regional anesthetic techniques alone or with mild sedation. For the dorsal recumbent paramedian abomasopexy, the cow is often placed in dorsal recumbency using casting ropes, but for fractious cattle, sedation can be provided to assist with casting and placement in dorsal recumbency. Xylazine (0.05–0.1 mg/kg IV) is the most frequently used sedative for this purpose; however, acepromazine (0.025–0.075 mg/kg IV) or butorphanol (0.0025–0.005 mg/kg IV) can also be used.

Small intestine disorders (intussusception, intestinal volvulus, intestinal obstruction)

The prevalence of surgical conditions requiring anesthesia for small intestinal disorders is much less than for the forestomach or abomasum in cattle. Obstructive lesions of the small intestine are more common in cattle than in small ruminants and swine. In cattle, most obstructive lesions occur in the distal jejunum. Ileus, sequestration of fluid, colic, abdominal distension, and scant or absent fecal production are clinical signs observed. Careful physical examination, along with clinical pathologic examination and abdominocentesis, is important to determine if a surgical disease is present. Intussusception is the invagination of one portion of intestine into the lumen of adjacent bowel, often creating an intestinal obstruction. Laparotomy is indicated for intussusception and intestinal obstruction, and the right paralumbar fossa approach provides the best exposure to the small and large intestine. A standing right paralumbar fossa laparotomy can be performed using mild sedation and local/regional anesthesia previously described; however, resection and anastomosis of intestine is difficult in the standing patient. Manipulation of the bowel and mesentery often results in pain and recumbency in the patient. In the authors' experience, general inhalation anesthesia with the patient positioned in left lateral recumbency is preferred for resection and anastomosis. The cow with abdominal distension and placement in lateral recumbency is at greater risk for regurgitation of rumen contents, so the head should be tilted downward and a cuffed endotracheal tube should be securely placed during the procedure. Injectable anesthesia protocols are usually for short-duration procedures but can be utilized in surgical correction of intestinal disorders. Surgical time must be considered. Injectable anesthesia protocols usually involve double drip (ketamine added to 5% guaifenesin at 1 mg/ml) or **Bovine Triple Drip** (ketamine at 1 mg/ml and xylazine at 0.1 mg/ml added to 5% guaifenesin). The use of xylazine in compromised ruminant patients, which many cases of intestinal accidents are, is risky because of the cardiovascular-depressant effects. Double drip or **Bovine Triple Drip** is slowly administered to effect to induce anesthesia. Anesthesia can be maintained by constant rate infusion of double drip or **Bovine Triple Drip** at 2.6 ml/kg/hour.

Intestinal volvulus can involve either segmental volvulus of the jejunoileum or torsion of the mesenteric root. The distal jejunum and ileum have a longer mesentery, often referred to as the distal flange, and this section of intestine is more mobile and prone to volvulus. Cattle affected by the segmental volvulus will present with clinical findings very similar to those with an intussusception. Torsion of the mesenteric root is a very dramatic and painful condition of cattle. Animals with torsion of the mesenteric root have bilateral abdominal distension and are very difficult to examine because of the pain associated with the condition, and epidural administration of xylazine (0.05–0.07 mg/kg) can be used to assist with examination. Both intestinal volvulus conditions require surgical intervention. While performing the surgery standing has the advantage of the bowel being suspended in the abdominal cavity making manipulation easier, the pain associated with manipulation of distended bowel usually results in recumbency. For this reason, general anesthesia is much preferred with placement of the animal in left lateral recumbency.

Urolithiasis and ruptured urinary bladder

Obstructive urolithiasis is the most common urinary tract disease of small ruminants. Males, especially castrated males, are most commonly affected. Urolithiasis is a multifactorial disease process with diet, water intake, and urinary pH all providing contributing roles to the formation of uroliths. Complete physical examination and evaluation of clinical pathology are important to perform prior to anesthesia. Ruminants with ruptured urinary bladder often have severe hemoconcentration and acid–base and electrolyte abnormalities that can result in cardiac arrhythmias during anesthesia. Numerous surgical techniques are available for treatment of obstructive urolithiasis and involve either surgery of the urethra or the urinary bladder. Surgical procedures involving the urethra include urethral process amputation, penile amputation, perineal or ischial urethrostomy, or urethrotomy. Most of these procedures can be performed in the standing patient under local and/or caudal epidural anesthesia or in the recumbent patient using a lumbosacral epidural (2 ml of 2% lidocaine per 10-kg (22-lb) body weight) or general anesthesia. If rupture of the urinary bladder is confirmed by abdominal ultrasound or abdominocentesis, then urinary bladder surgery is often warranted. In addition, when dealing with breeding livestock where surgery of the penile urethra is contraindicated, urinary bladder surgery is performed. Surgical procedures involving the urinary bladder include cystotomy, tube cystostomy, and bladder marsupialization. Bladder surgery is more difficult to perform than urethral surgery under field conditions. General anesthesia is preferred; however, combinations of injectable, local, and epidural anesthesia can be used. For all procedures, the patients are placed in dorsal recumbency, so rumen tympany, excess salivation, and regurgitation are important considerations during anesthesia.

Urogenital surgery in the female

Cesarean section

Patient positioning and surgical approach for the bovine cesarean section will be influenced by multiple factors including fetal viability, patient's temperament, available facilities, and clinician experience and preference. Discussion of the benefits and drawbacks of the various approaches is beyond the scope of this text; the standing flank and ventral midline approaches are used most commonly. Both approaches are performed successfully under regional and local anesthesia. Epidural anesthesia is provided at the discretion of the surgeon. A caudal epidural anesthesia using 2% lidocaine will not provide analgesia to the surgery site but will decrease straining. In recumbent animals, this may also decrease the resultant hind limb movement and assist in restraint. In standing procedures, caution is warranted when administering epidurals as excessive anesthesia can result in recumbency. The dose of local anesthetic is 0.5 ml per 45 kg (99 lb) of body weight.

The use of sedatives or tranquilizers is optional for the bovine cesarean section and is dictated by the attitude of the patient and available facilities. When a standing approach is preferred, care must be taken not to induce recumbency. Sedation with acepromazine (0.01 mg/kg IV; 0.1 mg/kg IM) is preferred by the authors when performing standing cesarean sections on nervous or fractious patients. Xylazine is a commonly used sedative in bovine medicine and may aid in restraint of recumbent animals. However, the ecbolic activity of xylazine may hinder uterine manipulation and thus is not favored for cesarean sections. Cattle in dorsal or dorsolateral recumbency experience cardiovascular and respiratory compromise, and this must be accounted for when choosing whether to use sedation and, if so, which drug to employ. While sedation or tranquilization is acceptable, and even beneficial in select cases, local anesthesia and physical restraint are sufficient for most cesarean sections in the bovine patient.

Local blocks providing anesthesia to the paralumbar fossa include the proximal and distal paravertebral nerve blocks, inverted-L block, and line block; these are discussed in detail in Chapter 7. Selection of a particular block is influenced by the condition of the patient and surgeon's preference. For ventral midline celiotomies, local anesthesia is provided by the infusion of a field block of 2% lidocaine along the intended incision line.

An 18-gauge, 3.8-cm needle is used to infuse multiple, small injections of 10 ml of local anesthetic solution subcutaneously and into the deep layers and peritoneum. High-volume caudal epidural anesthesia (1 ml of 2% lidocaine per 5-kg (11-lb) body weight) has also been used to facilitate the procedure from the ventral midline approach [11].

Anesthetic protocols for cesarean sections in small ruminants are similar to those used in cattle and primarily depend on the surgical approach to be used. Local anesthetic techniques are performed as in the bovine. However, it must be remembered that small ruminants are much more sensitive to lidocaine than their larger counterparts with the recommended maximum dose not to exceed 6 mg/kg. Regional anesthesia using a lumbosacral epidural is a viable alternative for cesarean sections in sheep and goats; the recommended dose is 2 ml of 2% lidocaine per 10-kg (22-lb) body weight. An 18- or 20-gauge, 3.8-cm needle is sufficient in most animals. Onset of anesthesia occurs within 5–15 minutes and generally lasts 60–120 minutes. General anesthesia is also suitable for the procedure in small ruminants. Maintenance with an inhalation anesthetic, such as isoflurane, is preferred.

In swine, cesarean sections are indicated when transcervical extraction of pigs from the uterus is not feasible or electively to obtain gnotobiotic or specific pathogen-free pigs. General anesthesia is desirable for cesarean sections in swine. Anesthetics with minimal depressive effects on the piglets are favored when live births are anticipated. If the piglets will remain with the sow, it is desirable that anesthesia is chosen which allows the sow to nurse the pigs immediately after surgery. The most viable piglets are obtained when inhalation anesthetics are used to induce and maintain anesthesia of the sow. Where labeled for use, azaperone (2.2 mg/kg IM) produces a predictable and consistent sedative effect in pigs. However, the drug will cross the placental barrier and result in respiratory depression and sedation in piglets although the pigs will usually survive with appropriate postnatal care. When general anesthesia is not possible due to available facilities or the state of the patient, local anesthesia can be used in conjunction with sedation and physical restraint. A combination of ketamine and xylazine, either intravenously or intramuscularly, often yields satisfactory results when combined with a field block of 2% lidocaine. Selection of specific injectable anesthetic(s) is left to the discretion of the clinician; specific protocols are provided in Chapter 4. Alternatively, a lumbosacral epidural anesthesia (1 ml of 2% lidocaine per 4.5 kg (9.9 lb) of body weight) results in recumbency and desensitization of the ventral midline surgical site. Similar results are seen at a dose of 1 ml per 7.5 kg (16.5 lb) for pigs up to 50 kg (110 lb); for larger pigs, 1.0 ml of lidocaine is added for every additional 10 kg (22 lb) of body weight. A maximum total volume of 20 ml is suggested (Chapter 7).

Ovariectomy

In cattle, ovariectomy is most commonly performed in feedlot heifers through either a paralumbar or vaginal approach. Both approaches are done with the animal in standing restraint; sedation can be employed at the discretion of the operator but is not often necessary. When the flank approach is preferred, any of the commonly employed local or regional techniques for anesthesia of the paralumbar fossa (Chapter 7) may be satisfactorily employed. A distal paravertebral nerve block is preferred by some clinicians for its quickness and ease of administration. Original descriptions of procedures utilizing the vaginal approach did not suggest anesthesia; however, a caudal epidural can be applied easily to desensitize the pelvic and perineal regions. Occasionally, unilateral ovariectomy is indicated in mature cows with ovarian pathology. When pathology is extensive and the surgical procedure is expected to involve extensive tissue dissection, general anesthesia may be warranted. If additional local analgesia is desired in such cases, a sterile gauze soaked in 2% lidocaine can be wrapped briefly around the ovarian attachment before surgical transection. Pet animals represent the most common populations of swine and small ruminants that present to the clinician for ovariectomy. In both groups, the procedure is most commonly performed with the animal in dorsal recumbency; general anesthesia with inhalation anesthesia maintenance is preferred in both cases.

Vaginal prolapse

A variety of procedures have been described for the correction of vaginal prolapse in cattle and swine. Caudal epidural administration is indicated for the manual manipulation of the prolapse and placement of the retention sutures. In swine, local infiltration of the vestibular area provides effective analgesia when administration of a caudal epidural is difficult or ineffective. Cervicopexy by the modified Winkler method is a relatively permanent repair of cervicovaginal prolapse. Sedation is employed based on the temperament of the patient. Successful anesthesia is achieved by administration of a distal paravertebral nerve block or other technique to desensitize the paralumbar fossa. A caudal epidural is also recommended for the procedure.

Perineal laceration

Perineal lacerations are classified according to location and tissues involved; surgical repair is usually attempted after secondary healing has occurred. Standing restraint is required, and sedation can be achieved with acepromazine (0.01 mg/kg IV, 0.1 mg/kg IM) or other sedatives according to the surgeon's preference. A caudal epidural is indicated to provide anesthesia to the perineum and rectovestibular shelf. Some clinicians advocate the use of xylazine in the caudal epidural for this procedure, but this may not be advantageous in all cases. The dose for xylazine given via caudal epidural is 0.05 mg/kg diluted to 5 ml in 0.9% saline. When given by epidural, xylazine will provide approximately 2–3 hours of anesthesia beginning 20–40 minutes after administration.

Urogenital surgery in the male

Castration

Along with dehorning, castration represents one of the most common surgical procedures performed in farm animal species. The methodology and anesthesia of castration to minimize associated stress and pain is currently the focus of heavy research. The acute distress of castration is effectively eliminated by the administration of local anesthetics, which is the most commonly used anesthesia protocol for castrating food animals. However, the integrated cortisol response is less efficiently controlled with local anesthesia alone, and a multimodal approach to anesthesia should be considered, particularly when castration is performed in older animals [12]. There are currently no drugs labeled for the control of pain for farm animals in the United States other than local anesthetics. Nonsteroidal anti-inflammatory drugs (NSAIDs) in conjunction with local anesthetics effectively minimize the acute and prolonged pain response associated with castration. Labeled for the control of inflammation or as an antipyretic, flunixin meglumine (1.1–2.2 mg/kg) is the sole NSAID labeled for use for farm animals in the United States and must be given intravenously at least daily for efficacy. Longer-acting NSAIDs, such as meloxicam, may be used more effectively to control pain associated with castration when used in accordance with extralabel drug use regulations [12].

Castration in young ruminants can be done with the animal standing or in lateral recumbency; adequate physical restraint in either case is required. Infusion of 2% lidocaine in the skin and/or spermatic cord can then performed although many procedures are done with only physical restraint in order to minimize the time of the procedure and the stress of being separated from the dam. A small-gauge needle is used to infiltrate 1–3 ml of 2% lidocaine in the scrotal skin along the proposed line of the incision. An additional 1–2 ml may be injected into each spermatic cord. Vasodilation associated with lidocaine increases the risk of hemorrhage but, in the experience of the authors, has not resulted in clinically significant blood loss. Dilution of lidocaine with sterile saline to a final concentration of 0.5–1% should be considered in lambs and kids due to their sensitivity to local anesthetics. General anesthesia or heavy sedation is sometimes used in pet animals; injectable anesthesia is usually sufficient to provide ample time for the procedure. IV administration of ketamine (2–3 mg/kg) and xylazine (0.1–0.2 mg/kg) will usually provide 20–30 minutes of anesthesia. Other drugs can also be used successfully (Chapter 4), and choice of agents will depend on the surgeon's preference.

Several local blocks have been described for the castration of older, or mature, ruminants. In addition to the aforementioned techniques, anesthesia can be provided by injecting 10–15 ml of 2% lidocaine subcutaneously in a ring block of the scrotal neck, followed by the administration of 5 ml of 2% lidocaine into each spermatic cord. When castration of several patients is to be performed, the animal can be released and the block performed on other patients to allow a 10-minute period for the onset of anesthesia. Alternatively, intratesticular administration of a local anesthetic can be performed in addition to SC infiltration of the scrotal skin. In mature animals, a 3.75–7.5-cm, 16- to 18-gauge needle is used; for smaller animals, a 2.5–3.75-cm, 20-gauge is preferred. With the testicle grasped firmly, the needle is inserted just ventral to the tail of the epididymis and advanced toward the center of the testicle at approximately a 30° angle from perpendicular. Depending on the size of the animal, 2–15 ml of 2% lidocaine is deposited at the center of the testicle. Sedation is more commonly used when performing castration on older ruminants. General anesthesia using either injectable or inhalation anesthetics should be considered for mature animals or when physical restraint is inadequate.

Castration of New World camelids is best performed with some degree of sedation or general anesthesia although the procedure can be performed with adequate physical restraint and local anesthesia. Camelids are less sensitive to the effects of xylazine than small ruminants; thus, a higher dose of the drug is usually required to achieve a comparable state of sedation. Mild sedation with xylazine (0.3 mg/kg IV) with local infiltration of the skin of the surgical site is adequate. If heavier sedation is desired, xylazine can be administered in conjunction with ketamine. Xylazine (0.6 mg/kg IM) and ketamine (6 mg/kg IM) provide satisfactory sedation for castration of llamas. In alpacas, the doses are increased slightly to 0.7 mg/kg IM (xylazine) and 7 mg/kg IM (ketamine). **Llama Lullaby** produces short-term anesthesia in llamas and alpacas and for completion of short surgical procedures, including castration, when inhalation anesthesia is not employed. The solution is made by combining 1 ml (100 mg) of xylazine, 1 ml (10 mg) of butorphanol, and 10 ml (1000 mg) of ketamine. The resulting combination is administered intramuscularly at a dose of 1 ml/23 kg (50.6 lb) for llamas or 1 ml/18 kg (39.6 lb) for alpacas to provide approximately 20–30 minutes of anesthesia. General anesthesia using inhalation anesthetics is a viable option; addition of a local infiltration of 2% lidocaine to the incision site is recommended for additional pain management.

In swine, castration is ideally performed before 2 weeks of age to minimize stress and behavioral changes associated with castration. Piglets are best castrated by suspending them by the hind limbs in vertical restraint. Anesthesia is provided by injecting 0.5–1.0 ml of 2% lidocaine into the scrotal skin over each testicle and 0.5 ml into each spermatic cord in the inguinal canal. Heavy sedation or general anesthesia is preferred for the castration of older pigs. **TKX-P**, a combination of tiletamine, zolazepam, ketamine, and xylazine, is favored by many clinicians. The combination is formed by reconstituting one 500 mg vial of Telazol with 250 mg (2.5 ml) of ketamine and 250 mg of xylazine (2.5 ml). The resulting combination is dosed at 1 ml/35–75 kg (77–165 lb) in commercial pigs or 1 ml/75–140 kg (165–308 lb) in potbellied pigs. A combination of xylazine and ketamine (2 mg/kg and 11 mg/kg IM, respectively) provides deep sedation, but pigs may still respond to surgical stimulation. The same combination of drugs, albeit at lower doses (1–2 mg/kg and 3–5 mg/kg, respectively), can be administered by intratesticular injection to induce immobilization and anesthesia for castration of mature boars. Half the total dose is injected into each testicle; removal of the testicle removes unabsorbed drug residue and hastens recovery.

Penile translocation

Penile translocation surgery is performed with the patient in dorsolateral recumbency to allow access to the ventral midline and one flank. General anesthesia is preferred for the procedure, although heavy sedation and local anesthesia are also acceptable. Specific agents to be used will depend on surgeon's preference, but a combination of xylazine (0.1 mg/kg IV) and ketamine (2.0 mg/kg IV) or the use of **Bovine Triple Drip** (1 ml/kg IV induction, 2 ml/kg/hour maintenance) works well when injectable anesthesia is indicated. Local anesthesia is provided by infusing 2% lidocaine subcutaneously in a modified ring block approximately 10 cm around the periphery of the preputial orifice and prepuce to within approximately 5 cm of the scrotal neck. A second SC ring block can be performed at the translocation site in the flank.

Persistent frenulum

Correction of persistent frenula occurs with the bull in standing restraint or lateral recumbency; general anesthesia is not usually warranted. Mild sedation may be employed, but tranquilization is contraindicated as it is desirable that the bull retract the penis into the sheath postoperatively for protection against trauma and as an aid in hemostasis. Analgesia is most easily and commonly provided by local injection of the frenulum attachments with 1–2 ml of 2% lidocaine using a small-gauge needle. Local anesthesia can also be supplied by inserting a small-gauge needle through the lamina interna at the dorsal aspect of the preputial orifice. Injection of 2% lidocaine in a semicircle over the dorsal aspect of the penis will successfully desensitize the dorsal penile nerve. Alternatively, regional anesthesia can be provided by the administration of a pudendal nerve block.

Penile papilloma

Penile papillomata represent the most common penile tumor of the bovine, and anesthesia for surgical removal is adequately provided by local or regional techniques. The bull should be restrained in a standing chute or on a tilt table. Mild sedation can be used as needed for fractious animals. The dorsal penile nerve is desensitized by infusion of 2–4 ml of 2% lidocaine subcutaneously across the dorsum of the penis using a 22- or 24-gauge needle. Alternatively, local infiltration of 2% lidocaine around the base of the tumor, particularly for well-pedunculated papillomata, provides adequate analgesia. A pudendal nerve block will also successfully desensitize the surgical site but is less commonly employed due to a higher degree of technical difficulty of administration.

Epididymectomy

Epididymectomy can be performed in all farm animal species for the process of sterilization or the preparation of teaser animals, often in conjunction with other procedures. General anesthesia is indicated in mature boars and can also be used in small ruminants and camelids but is not required. The choice of injectable or inhalation anesthesia is dictated by surgical conditions, surgeon's preference, and additional procedures to be performed, if any. When local anesthetic techniques will be solely used, the choice of standing or lateral restraint is at the discretion of the surgeon. The surgical site is desensitized by local infiltration of 2% lidocaine with a small-gauge needle in the scrotal skin directly over the epididymis. Deposition of 2% lidocaine directly into the epididymis can be considered for additional analgesia but is not commonly performed.

Vasectomy

Like epididymectomies, vasectomies in ruminants are usually performed under local anesthesia; general anesthesia can be considered in small ruminants but is not often practical, and local anesthetic techniques provide adequate analgesia. After the application of standing or lateral restraint, with or without the use of sedation, 2–4 ml of 2% lidocaine is infused into the posterior scrotal skin just proximal to each testicle using a 20- or 22-gauge needle. Infusion of local anesthetic directly into each spermatic cord with a fine needle at the surgery site provides additional analgesia but is believed by some clinicians to hinder identification of the vas deferens. In swine, general anesthesia is recommended. Injectable anesthetic protocols in conjunction with local infusion of lidocaine provide adequate analgesia for the procedure. General anesthesia is also recommended when performing the procedure in New World camelids.

Musculoskeletal indications

Dehorning

Dehorning of cattle and goats is indicated to prevent tissue bruising of penmates and to enhance the safety of animal handlers; it is one of the oldest and most commonly performed surgical procedures of ruminants. It is preferable to perform the procedure in young animals to minimize pain and stress associated with the procedure. Local anesthesia effectively eliminates the acute pain and distress of dehorning but may not mitigate the prolonged stress response. Research on analgesia and pain management in cattle undergoing dehorning is abundant and has been reviewed [6, 7]. A multimodal approach is preferable for optimum alleviation of stress associated with dehorning and may include the use of NSAIDs and sedatives with analgesic properties in addition to local anesthetic techniques, particularly in older animals where the procedure is more involved. The cornual process, under the horn bud, connects to the skull at approximately 2 months of age in calves, and at 4–6 months of age, the frontal sinus becomes contiguous with the horn. The use of NSAIDs and/or sedation must be done in accordance with established regulations concerning extralabel drug use in food animal species.

In calves, a cornual nerve block is performed to provide analgesia of the horn bud and surrounding tissue. The cornual nerve, a branch of the zygomaticotemporal nerve, is desensitized by using a 20-gauge, 2.5- or 3.8-cm needle inserted under the frontal ridge midway between the lateral canthus of the eye and the base of the horn. Five to ten ml of 2% lidocaine is infiltrated subcutaneously and normally yields complete analgesia of the region in 5–10 minutes. The nerve lies superficially in young calves but may lie deeper as the animal matures. In older animals, cutaneous branches of the second cervical spinal nerve provide sensation to the caudal aspect of the horn base and are best anesthetized with an SC hemicircumferential infiltration of local anesthetic along the caudal aspect of the horn. When performing cosmetic cornuectomies in cattle, an SC ring block is performed at the horn base to anesthetize the skin.

In goats, a cornual nerve block alone is insufficient to provide adequate anesthesia for dehorning. In addition to the cornual nerve, the horn base is innervated by the cornual branches of the infratrochlear nerve. The infratrochlear branches are anesthetized by injecting 2–3 ml of local anesthetic midway between the medial canthus of the eye and the medial base of the horn as a line block due to the branching of the nerve. Alternatively, an SC ring block around the base of the horn may be performed but is likely to require a higher volume of local anesthetic and thus is less commonly used. Special care must be taken when dehorning kids and pygmy goats due to their small size and the sensitivity of the goat to lidocaine toxicity. Dilution of lidocaine to 0.5–1% using sterile saline permits injections of larger volumes without compromising anesthesia of the region. General anesthesia using a combination of ketamine (3–5 mg/kg IM) and xylazine (0.1 mg/kg IM) or an inhalation anesthetic is also popular to minimize movement and vocalization while providing analgesia of the horn base and surrounding tissues.

Claw amputation

Amputation of the claw in cattle is performed primarily as a salvage procedure for chronic infectious arthritis or other disease processes with a poor prognosis for return to function. It is important to ascertain that the contralateral claw is healthy and capable of full weight-bearing before the procedure is attempted. General anesthesia is an option although not usually necessary. IV regional perfusion is performed easily by placing a tourniquet proximal to the fetlock and injecting approximately 20 ml of 2% lidocaine intravenously. Anesthesia of the foot occurs within 5–10 minutes and lasts until removal of the tourniquet, which can be safely left in place for up to 1 hour. Sedation can be provided as needed based on the available facilities and temperament of the patient.

Excision of interdigital fibromas

IV regional perfusion (Bier block) is the preferred anesthetic technique for interdigital fibroma excision. With a tourniquet in place proximal to the fetlock, 20 ml of 2% lidocaine administered intravenously will adequately desensitize all tissue distal to the tourniquet, including the interdigital area. Local infusion of 2% lidocaine around the periphery of the fibroma will also provide anesthesia to the surgery site. The presence of lidocaine at the incision site may delay healing although this concern should not obviate the technique in cases where regional perfusion is unsuccessful. A metatarsal or metacarpal nerve block may also be used but is more technically challenging than the Bier block and is not commonly used.

Tail docking

When performed in the first 2 weeks of a lamb's life, tail docking is a relatively simple and common procedure; proper analgesia can be achieved quickly with perfusion of a local anesthetic. A caudal epidural is also effective but is time consuming and more technically challenging in small lambs. Occasionally, tail docking is requested for mature sheep that were previously overlooked or in cattle as a result of trauma. General anesthesia is recommended in sheep, though the procedure is often carried out in the field using local anesthesia. Perfusion of a local anesthetic or a caudal epidural can be performed using an 18- or 20-gauge needle at a dose of 1 ml of 2% lidocaine/50 kg (110 lb). Alternatively, a local ring block proximal to the amputation site may be employed to achieve analgesia of the surgical site.

Sacral fractures or coccygeal nerve damage in mature cows may cause a lack of tail tone and loss of function, leading to soiling of the tail and potentially, unsanitary milking conditions. For anesthesia, 5–6 ml of local anesthetic is infused into the intercoccygeal space proximal to the site of the amputation after the placement of a tourniquet farther proximal for control of hemorrhage during the procedure. A caudal epidural is recommended for additive pain management but is insufficient by itself for analgesia to more distal surgical sites. The benefit of extended duration of analgesia when including an α_2 agonist or opioid in the epidural must be weighed against the risk of associated systemic effects.

Rectal prolapse

Rectal prolapse in cattle and small ruminants can be corrected by a variety of procedures including simple replacement, submucosal resection, and rectal amputation. Adequate restraint is necessary and sedation can be employed as necessary but is often not required depending on the temperament of the patient. A caudal epidural provides effective analgesia for each of these procedures. A dose of 1 ml of 2% lidocaine per 100 kg (220 lb) is used in cattle; in small ruminants, a dose of 1 ml per 50 kg (110 lb) is preferred although dosages of up to 1 ml per 15 kg (33 lb) have been reported [13]. When caudal epidural administration is difficult or unsuccessful in small ruminants, a perianal ring block of 2% lidocaine may be substituted to adequately desensitize the perianal region.

Rectal prolapse occurs relatively commonly in swine. In sows, it is most commonly observed during, or in the first weeks following, parturition. Manual reduction of uncomplicated cases is facilitated by the use of adequate restraint and sedation as needed. The perianal region is desensitized with a lumbosacral epidural (Chapter 7) or infiltration of a local anesthetic in a ring block around the rectum. Alternative corrective procedures are indicated when the rectal mucosa has become necrotic or otherwise unviable; the most commonly performed procedure is surgical amputation. General anesthesia is indicated for such procedures, and both inhalation and injectable anesthesia have been employed satisfactorily. Inhalation anesthesia, typically isoflurane, is preferred when available.

References

1. Ames, N. (2014) *Noordsy's Food Animal Surgery*, Ames, Wiley-Blackwell.
2. Fubini, S. and Ducharme, N. (2004) *Farm Animal Surgery*, St. Louis, Elsevier.
3. Hendrickson, D. and Baird, A. (2013) *Turner and McIlwraith's Techniques in Large Animal Surgery*, Ames, Wiley-Blackwell.
4. Jorgensen, J. and Cannedy, A. (1996) Physiologic and pathophysiologic considerations for ruminants and swine anesthesia. *Veterinary Clinics of North America: Food Animal Practice*, **12**, 481–500.
5. Offinger, J., Meyer, H., Fischer, J. *et al.* (2012) Comparison of isoflurane inhalation anaesthesia, injection anaesthesia and high volume caudal epidural anaesthesia for umbilical surgery in calves; metabolic, endocrine and cardiopulmonary effects. *Veterinary Anaesthesia and Analgesia*, **39**, 123–136.
6. Stock, M., Baldridge, S., Griffin, D. and Coetzee, J.F. (2013) Bovine dehorning: assessing pain and providing analgesic management. *Veterinary Clinics of North America: Food Animal Practice*, **29**, 103–133.
7. Stafford, K. and Mellor, D. (2005) Dehorning and disbudding distress and its alleviation in calves. *Veterinary Journal*, **169**, 337–349.

8. Abrahamsen, E. (2013) Chemical restraint and injectable anesthesia of ruminants. *Veterinary Clinics of North America: Food Animal Practice*, **29**, 209–227.
9. Niahaus, A. (2008) Surgery of the abomasum. *Veterinary Clinics of North America: Food Animal Practice*, **24**, 349–358.
10. Newman, K., Harvey, D. and Roy, J. (2008) Minimally invasive field abomasopexy techniques for correction and fixation of left displacement of the abomasum in dairy cows. *Veterinary Clinics of North America: Food Animal Practice*, **24**, 359–382.
11. Anderson, D. and Edmondson, M. (2013) Prevention and management of surgical pain in cattle. *Veterinary Clinics of North America: Food Animal Practice*, **29**, 157–184.
12. Coetzee, J. (2013) Assessment and management of pain associated with castration in cattle. *Veterinary Clinics of North America: Food Animal Practice*, **29**, 75–101.
13. Plummer, P. and Schleining, J. (2013) Assessment and management of pain in small ruminants and camelids. *Veterinary Clinic of North America: Food Animal Practice*, **29**, 185–208.

CHAPTER 9

Chapter 9

Pain management for farm animals

HuiChu Lin

Department of Clinical Sciences, College of Veterinary Medicine, Auburn University, USA

Increased effort to manage pain has become standard practice in small animal medicine in recent years, but advances in pain mitigation in livestock species have been slower. Factors contributing to the slow progress are lack of analgesic drugs specifically approved for ameliorating pain of farm animals, known adverse effects including excitation and decreased gastrointestinal (GI) motility caused by opioids or GI ulcer and impairment of renal function associated with nonsteroidal anti-inflammatory drugs (NSAIDs), fear that loss of pain prompts further damage to the injured tissue, requirement of record keeping by the Drug Enforcement Administration (DEA) when using scheduled drugs, inconvenient timing to administer the drugs for effective pain relief, the need for trained personnel to administer the drug via specified route such as intravenous (IV) injection, and the increased cost to owners for analgesic drugs and their administration [1]. Untreated pain can delay wound healing and can cause significant patient discomfort, stress, depression, and inappetence. When pain is severe and prolonged, the immune system can be impaired. A goal for appropriate patient care is restoration of normal physiological functions. Judicious use of analgesic drugs should be an essential part of the treatment plan to provide adequate pain relief and ensure comfort so that normal physiological functions are not impaired or are allowed to return. It should be kept in mind that pain is easier to treat before perception of pain actually occurs (preemptive analgesia) [2].

Pain is defined by the International Association for the Study of Pain (IASP) as "an unpleasant sensory and emotional experience associated with actual or potential tissue damage, or described in term of such damage." Perception of pain involves transmission of electrical impulses in response to noxious stimuli received at the peripheral nociceptors located at the site of insult, that is, A_δ or C fibers; transduction of the impulses through the spinothalamic tract to the dorsal horn of the spinal cord; modification of these impulses by releasing central nervous system (CNS) neurotransmitters,

Farm Animal Anesthesia: Cattle, Small Ruminants, Camelids, and Pigs, First Edition.
Edited by HuiChu Lin and Paul Walz.

for example, substance P, neurokinin A, and brain-derived neurotrophic factor (glutamate); and activation of *N*-methyl-D-aspartate (NMDA) receptors. Projection of these neurotransmitters is mediated through specific pathways to the thalamus (neospinothalamic and paleospinothalamic tract neurons) and the limbic system (thalamocortical tract neurons). As a result, generation and awareness of the perception or emotion of pain occur [3, 4]. Initial response to acute pain tends to be well localized and proportional to the intensity of the insult but short-lived. This response is usually a protective mechanism with the subject moving away from the insult. Unlike acute pain, chronic pain is usually well diffused but persistent and is often associated with hypersensitivity of the neural cells in the spinal cord and brain. Chronic pain may not involve in injury to the tissue, but rather is often the result of inflammation associated with disease [4]. Hypersensitivity in the neural cells of the spinal cord and brain is reflected in the progression to central sensitization with increased sensitization of excitable nerve cells as evidenced by a disproportionally painful response to a normally mild noxious stimulation (wind-up syndrome) or greater perception of pain to a previously nonpainful stimulation (allodynia) [4, 5]. Surgery-induced pain often begins as acute pain but can progress to chronic pain as a result of prolonged inflammation.

Pain experienced by farm animal is often difficult to recognize due to their stoic temperament and the natural instinct of prey animals not to attract the attention of predators when injured. Behavioral indications of a farm animal in pain may include one or more of the following clinical signs: excessive grunting and bellowing (vocalization); lowering of the head; rigid posture; tail swishing; limping, kicking, or stomping of feet; teeth grinding; excessive licking on the affected area; reluctance to move or lay down; depression; decreased interest in surroundings; and inappetence. Physiological signs associated with pain include increased respiration, heart rate, body temperature, and pupil size. However, these signs in response to pain can be misinterpreted since vital signs are often influenced by stress or other endogenous as well as exogenous factors [6]. Therefore, close observation and monitoring of the animal by regular caretakers or a veterinarian on-site are required for objective and unbiased judgment to institute appropriate and timely administration of pain-relieving treatment. Inadequate pain management in young livestock undergoing castration surgery was evident in a survey of Canadian veterinarians in 2004 and 2005, which showed that less than 0.001% in piglets, 6.9% in beef calves, and 18.7% in dairy calves received perioperative analgesics [7]. A similar survey done in the United Kingdom showed that only 57% of adult cattle that underwent cesarean section and laparotomy received epidural anesthesia and/or postoperative analgesics [8]. A web-based survey of members of American Association of Bovine Practitioners and Academy of Veterinary Consultants of the United States (US) was conducted regarding castration methods, adverse events, and husbandry procedures. The survey results indicated that only one of five surveyed participants provided an analgesic or local anesthetic at the time of castration [9]. In 2013, a survey of Brazilian large animal veterinarians indicated that 84% of them believed their knowledge of recognition and treatment of pain to be insufficient and only 58.5% of the cattle they treated received preoperative analgesics for laparotomy as compared to the 72.9% for their equine patients [10]. Apparently, there is a need for animal caretakers, producers, and veterinarians to better recognize pain associated with disease and to promote pain management. Awareness of the need for proper pain management of farm animals has prompted several research groups worldwide, including some in the US, to promote the study of objective methods to recognize and evaluate pain and develop effective and safe analgesics.

Analgesics commonly used in veterinary practice today include local anesthetics, α_2 agonists, NSAIDs, opioids, and NMDA antagonists. These analgesics can be administered alone or in combination. The advantage of combining different classes of analgesic by their actions on different mechanisms is the potentiation of each drug's analgesic effect (synergism). Combining different classes of analgesics allows reduction of the dose requirement of each drug to produce effective analgesia which then reduces the potential for side effects of each drug. Pain perception and its signal transmission occur at different levels, that is, peripheral nociceptor site, spinal dorsal horn, and central thalamic and limbic regions. Therefore, combining analgesics acting on different mechanisms and/or receptors maximizes analgesia (multimodal analgesia). A combination of local or regional anesthesia, NSAIDs, and low doses of an opioid and/or an α_2 agonist is the most commonly practiced multimodal treatment for intra- and postoperative pain management in farm animals [11]. Pain management should be included in the context of overall case management to optimize the patient's quality of life and early return of normal physiological functions. Although analgesics may be effective in relieving pain caused by disease, they do not cure the cause of pathological tissue damages resulting from the disease. Therefore, it is imperative that the disease causing pain be appropriately treated by medication and/or surgery to remove the origin of the pain.

Currently, no medications are approved by the US Food and Drug Administration (FDA) specifically for alleviation of pain in farm animals. Flunixin meglumine is approved for use in cattle only for treatment of pyrexia and inflammation, not for alleviation of pain. Any drug administered for pain relief is considered extralabel use [12]. Under the guidelines of the Animal Medicinal Drug Use Clarification Act of 1994 (AMDUCA) [13], extralabel drug use is permitted for relief of suffering of pain in food animals as long as the following specific conditions are met: (1) extralabel drug use is allowed only by or under the supervision of a licensed veterinarian; (2) extralabel drug use is allowed only for FDA-approved animal and human drugs; (3) extralabel drug use is permitted only when the health of the animal is threatened and not for production purposes; (4) extralabel drug use in feed is prohibited; and (5) extralabel drug use is not permitted if it results in a violative drug residue in food intended for human consumption. Pain management using analgesics not approved by the FDA can be instituted to minimize suffering and pain of farm animals only as long as the aforementioned conditions are observed. Fortunately, analgesics used today with the exception of phenylbutazone are short- acting and often require repeat dosing for long-term treatment. Thus, their administrations can be terminated accordingly to avoid violative residue and to ensure protection of animal and human health [6, 14].

Local anesthetics

Local anesthetics, particularly lidocaine, can be administered locally or intravenously to produce pain relief. For local anesthetic effects, these drugs produce their effects by blocking the propagation of action potentials along nerve axons via the reversible blockade of Na^+ channels. These anesthetics can be injected into the tissue at the surgical site to produce local anesthesia, or they can be administered in the perineural area of major nerves to produce regional anesthesia. Local anesthetics block nerve fibers in the following order: β fibers (motor, touch) > nonmyelinated C fibers (pain, temperature) > A fibers (motor, proprioception) with the intensity of perception diminishing in the order of pain > cold > warmth > touch > deep pressure [15]. In domestic ruminants, many surgical procedures are performed safely and painlessly under local or regional anesthesia. All local anesthetics have similar physical properties and molecular structures. Most of these drugs are weakly basic tertiary amines, and they are generally available as acid solutions of the water-soluble salts. The acid salt is neutralized in the tissue, liberating the basic drug form, which then penetrates the cell membrane and interrupts the propagation of the action potential. Therefore, local anesthetics are less effective in inflamed tissue with lower pH because less liberation of the basic form of the drug occurs [16]. Painful, stinging sensation upon injection has been reported due to the acid nature of local anesthetics. This stinging sensation can be ameliorated by adding 5 ml of 8.5% sodium bicarbonate to 50 ml of 2% lidocaine solution (1:10 ratio) [17]. There are two types of local anesthetics: ester local anesthetics (e.g., procaine, tetracaine) and amide local anesthetics (e.g., lidocaine, bupivacaine, mepivacaine, ropivacaine). Amide local anesthetics are the most commonly used.

Administration of local anesthetics prior to castration in young calves was shown in several studies to have beneficial effects such as reduced distress and improved incisional healing, though no significant improvement on average daily gain was observed [18–21]. Lidocaine in 2% injectable solution is the only local anesthetic approved by the FDA for use in cattle. It is approved for epidural administration with a maximal volume of 15 ml or for nerve blocks for volume up to 20 ml [14]. Lidocaine is the most popular local anesthetic with onset of effect occurring within 5 minutes and a duration of 0.75–2 hours. Epinephrine induces vasoconstriction in the tissue surrounding the injected area and can be used with lidocaine to prolong the anesthetic duration of lidocaine by reducing absorption and removal of the drug by the blood circulation from the injection site. Epinephrine (1:200,000–1:50,000) at concentrations of 5–20 μg/ml can be added to lidocaine solution [22, 23]. For sheep, the maximum concentration of epinephrine that can be added to lidocaine is 12.5 μg/ml of total solution [24]. However, potential side effects associated with addition of epinephrine to lidocaine include lack of revascularization of the wound edge and tissue necrosis when injected subcutaneously, and possible spinal cord ischemia when administered intrathecally or epidurally [25, 26]. When administered at 1.5 mg/kg intravenously to adult beef cows, lidocaine has a plasma half-life ($t½$) of 1.06 ± 0.70 hours, a volume distribution of 4.6 ± 2.1 l/kg, and an elimination $t½$ of 1.52 ± 0.94 hours. When 100 ml of lidocaine was infiltrated subcutaneously for inverted-L nerve blocks to Holstein cows, maximum plasma concentration occurs at 0.52 ± 0.23 hours

CHAPTER 9

with a significant longer elimination $t½$, compared to that when the drug is administered intravenously (4.2 ± 1.7 hours) [27]. Other amide local anesthetics such as mepivacaine (5 mg/kg, 1.5–3 hours) and bupivacaine (2 mg/kg, 4–8 hours) can be used for procedures that require a longer duration of local anesthesia [28]. Bupivacaine is believed to have greater cardiotoxicity than lidocaine and mepivacaine [29]. Bupivacaine is not recommended for routine clinical use in cattle because the drug is reported to be toxic to cattle particularly in cases of accidental IV administration [17].

Administration of a large single dose or repeated small doses of local anesthetics can result in toxicity, particularly in neonates and young patients. Clinical signs of toxicity include nystagmus, muscle fasciculation, CNS stimulation progressing to opisthotonos and convulsions, hypotension, respiratory arrest, circulatory collapse, and death [16]. The maximum calculated safe dose of lidocaine was reported to be 13 mg/kg in one study [30]. In another study, accumulated IV doses of 5.8, 18, and 42 mg/kg induced signs of toxicity in adult, neonatal, and fetal sheep, respectively [31]. IV infusion of mepivacaine in sheep induced convulsions at doses of 7.5–7.9 mg/kg and cardiovascular collapse at doses as high as 52–69 mg/kg [32]. Bupivacaine is approximately four times more potent than lidocaine. Therefore, a 0.5% solution of bupivacaine produces the same degree of neuronal blockade as a 2% solution of lidocaine. Anderson and Edmondson [17] recommended a lower maximum safe lidocaine dose of 10 mg/kg for cows undergoing cesarean section since a large amount of lidocaine is required to produce effective infiltration nerve blocks. Because small ruminants appear to be more likely to experience lidocaine toxicity, a maximum safe dose of 4 mg/kg is recommended [17]. Ewing [33] suggested a maximum dose of 6 mg/kg for lidocaine and mepivacaine and 2 mg/kg for bupivacaine for small ruminants. With the maximum safe dose in mind, veterinarians should dilute lidocaine and mepivacaine solutions to 1% and 0.5%, respectively, to prevent overdosing in lambs and kids [33]. Diazepam (0.1 mg/kg IV) should be administered if seizure activity or convulsions caused by accidental overdose persist longer than 1–2 minutes [29, 34]. Ropivacaine is a newer local anesthetic with duration of effect similar to bupivacaine (6–8 hours) but has less cardiotoxicity than bupivacaine and causes less vasodilation than lidocaine [16]. Please refer to Chapter 11 for withdrawal times for lidocaine.

Systemic pain management

Opioid analgesics

Opioid analgesics such as morphine, meperidine, fentanyl, buprenorphine, and butorphanol have been used for pain management in farm animal species. These drugs bind either to μ, κ, or δ (OP3, OP1, or OP2) opioid receptors located on neuronal cell membranes. Binding of an opioid to these receptors triggers cellular changes that hyperpolarize the cell membrane and inhibit spinal pain transmission. Activation of μ receptors results in depletion of intraneuronal substance P which reduces overall inflammation and neural pain transmission. There are opioid receptors located centrally in the hypothalamus, brain stem and spinal cord; and, peripherally in the joint, and cornea. Therefore, opioid analgesics can be administered either systemically for action on the brain or they can be deposited closely to the site of action and produce their effects at all levels of pain pathways. For example, parenteral administration of an opioid provides analgesia at the central supraspinal level, intra-articular injection relieves joint pain, and epidural administration provides pain relief at the level of the spinal cord. Side effects of opioid analgesics such as respiratory depression, decreased GI motility and increased GI emptying time, increased appetite, sedation, euphoria, and nausea are also associated with activation of μ receptors [35]. Tachycardia and hyperexcitability develop occasionally when high doses of opioids are administered to farm animal species. Interestingly, hyperexcitability, though commonly observed in other species, does not occur as frequently in ruminants when administered the recommended dose [36]. Most opioids used in veterinary practice are classified as either pure μ agonists (morphine, meperidine, and fentanyl), partial μ agonist (buprenorphine), or agonist/antagonist (butorphanol). Butorphanol is classified as agonist/antagonist because it possesses agonistic effects on κ receptors but antagonistic effects on μ receptors. Thus, butorphanol should not be administered at the same time with a pure μ agonist such as morphine because these two drugs compete for binding at μ receptor sites and butorphanol can antagonize the pharmacological effects of morphine, including analgesia. Unlike in other species, opioids have not been commonly prescribed for analgesia in farm animal species due to their controlled substance status and questionable effectiveness, though they have proven to provide effective pain relief in response to thermal and pressure stimulations [37–41].

Morphine, a pure μ opioid agonist, is effective in relieving mild pain in ruminants. Good analgesia only occurred in one-third of the farm animals receiving morphine [2]. Morphine should be administered parenterally, not orally, to ruminants because the drug is inactivated by ruminal microflora. Doses of 0.05–0.5 mg/kg every 4–6 hours are recommended by IV, intramuscular (IM), or subcutaneous (SC) route [36, 42]. Superior analgesia produced by morphine was reported when administered at doses as high as 10 mg/kg to goats [36], even though 0.5 mg/kg IM is the dose recommended for use in goats [43]. Due to the slow onset of analgesic effect of morphine as a result of low lipid solubility (10 minutes IV, 20 minutes IM), an initial IV administration of the drug is recommended when significant pain is expected after surgery and maintenance of analgesia can be followed up with IM administration or constant rate infusion (CRI) of a low IV dose of morphine. Large IV doses of morphine have been reported to cause reduction of ruminoreticular contraction for up to 20 minutes [44]. However, GI side effects were not observed when morphine was administered intravenously at 0.1 mg/kg to cattle. Low-dose CRI of morphine maintains constant effective blood level but minimizes the risk of inhibition of ruminoreticular contraction [42]. Please refer to Chapter 11 for withdrawal times for morphine.

Meperidine hydrochloride is a synthetic opioid with an analgesic potency of only 10–50% that of morphine. Meperidine produces mild sedation and analgesia. Its administration has been associated with histamine release [45]. In yearling goats, meperidine (10 mg/kg IM) can be used as a preanesthetic analgesic given 10 minutes before induction of anesthesia with thiopental. After intubation, this combination provides 20 minutes of surgical anesthesia with complete recovery occurring in 90 minutes [46].

Fentanyl is a pure μ agonist similar to morphine with a potency that is approximately 75–100 times that of morphine. Fentanyl can be administered parenterally or transdermally. When administered parenterally, fentanyl induces analgesia within 5 minutes with a short duration of 20 minutes [36]. IV administration of fentanyl has been associated with abnormal behaviors and adverse effects such as pica, stall pacing, nystagmus, hyperexcitability, mania, ataxia, sedation, bradycardia, and respiratory depression [36, 47]. Transdermal patches are available at 0.025, 0.05, 0.075, and 0.1 mg/hour doses. A 0.05 mg/hour patch is an appropriate dose for a 30–50-kg (66–110-lb) goat. Onset of analgesia is observed at 18–24 hours after placement, and each patch lasts approximately 3 days. A new patch should be placed 48 hours after the first one has been applied. Variable absorption of fentanyl from the patch limits its clinical usefulness [47]. Contrary to the report in goats, transdermal fentanyl produced superior analgesia to intermittent administration of IM buprenorphine in sheep. Maximum plasma concentration was reached at 12 hours following the placement of the patch with the concentration maintained above 0.5 ng/ml for 40 hours. In addition to effective analgesia, fentanyl-treated sheep required less preanesthetic sedation to allow for tracheal intubation [48, 49]. In cattle, application of 0.05–0.1 μg/kg of fentanyl patch for pain relief was shown to be clinically beneficial [17]. Consistent skin absorption from fentanyl patch has also been reported when placed on the medial antebrachium in llamas [50]. In swine, a fentanyl 75–100-μg/hour patch can be applied to the intrascapular region to provide analgesia in 20–40-kg (44–88-lb) pigs postoperatively. Effective plasma concentrations of 0.5 and 2 ng/ml can be achieved within 24 hours following application of the transdermal patch [36]. As recommended previously, another fast-acting analgesic should be given to provide pain relief due to slow absorption of the drug from transdermal patch [2]. It is very important that the hair on the area intended for placement of the patch be clipped and skin cleaned completely to ensure secure adherence of the patch. Excessive hair, dirty skin, or insecure adherence of the patch may result in inconsistent and unreliable absorption of the drug and subsequently suboptimal analgesic effect. Keep in mind that rumenosalivary recycling may result in a bioavailability exceeding 100% and thus prolong the effects of fentanyl. This may pose a problem in establishing accurate withdrawal times [47].

Tramadol is a synthetic analog of codeine and morphine [51]. Tramadol produces analgesia by its action through central opioid, adrenergic, and serotoninergic receptors [52]. Tramadol offers advantages over other opioids. It is not a scheduled drug making its use less complicated; it causes less respiratory depression and has low potential for human abuse [51, 53]. Furthermore, tramadol is reported to produce less CNS excitation in horses [54]. Tramadol has been shown to be effective in treating moderate to more severe postoperative pain in humans and dogs [55, 56]. Tramadol has low affinity for opiate μ receptors, and its dose requirement in order to produce similar degree of analgesia for moderate pain is ten times that of morphine [57]. However, for more severe pain, tramadol administered at the same dose ratio is less effective than morphine [58]. One of the metabolites of tramadol, *O*-desmethyltramadol, is reported to be six times more potent in analgesic effect and 200 times more potent in the binding ability to the μ receptors than tramadol [59]. In calves undergoing a disbudding procedure, either IV tramadol (4 mg/kg) or rectal suppositories [200 mg/50–60 kg (110–132 lb)] provided effective analgesia to prevent head shaking, ear flicking, and head rubbing, indicators of pain from the application of caustic paste following disbudding [60]. Orally administered tramadol is well absorbed in humans, dogs, and cats with bioavailability of 70%, 65%, and 93%, respectively [61–63]. Lower absorption with a bioavailability of 23–37% and 5.9–19.1%, respectively, was reported following a single oral dose of 2 mg/kg in goats and 11 mg/kg in alpacas [64, 65]. A large volume-to-surface ratio, constantly high content of solid matter, and complex microflora and microfauna in the rumen were suggested to be the causes for the lower oral absorption of tramadol in goats and alpacas. A higher gastric pH of 6.8 in the rumen [66] as opposed to pH of 1.0–2.0 in the monogastric stomach [67] in the presence of a pK_a value of 9.41 of tramadol results in greater percentage of nonionized tramadol in plasma and enterohepatic recycling in ruminants, which increase absorption of the drug and are believed to be the primary factors responsible for the high plasma tramadol concentrations in goats (542.9 ± 219.5 ng/ml) and alpacas (1202 ± 1319 ng/ml) [64, 65]. In humans, plasma concentrations of 100–150 ng/ml are recommended as the minimum effective concentration of tramadol in relieving mild to moderate pain [55, 61]. The elimination *t*½ following oral administration was 2.67 ± 0.54 hours in goats which is shorter than that of humans [53] but longer than that of horses and alpacas [54, 65]. IV administration of tramadol at 2 mg/kg to these goats did not provide effective pain relief as the plasma concentration rapidly declined below minimum effective concentrations [64]. Adverse effects such as hyperexcitability, hyperesthesia, tremors, and ataxia occurred soon after the start of IV administration of tramadol over a period of 5 minutes, but side effects quickly dissipated 15 minutes after the termination of IV infusion to alpacas. These adverse effects were not observed following oral administration or slower IV administration over a period of 10 minutes. In alpacas, two of the metabolites, *O*-desmethyltramadol and *N*-desmethyltramadol, have slightly longer plasma *t*½, 1.53 ± 0.68 hours and 1.38 ± 0.48 hours, respectively, than tramadol itself (0.849 ± 0.463 hours) [65]. Tramadol is capable of crossing the placenta and appears in the fetal circulation, and low concentration of parent drug and its active metabolites have also been detected in human breast milk within 16 hours after administration [53]. However, no milk or meat withdrawal time for tramadol has been established at this time. In pigs anesthetized with xylazine (2.5 mg/kg IM) and ketamine (25 mg/kg IM), adding tramadol (5 mg/kg IM) to the anesthetic combination improved the quality of anesthesia and enhanced or prolonged the duration of analgesia (43.7 ± 15.5 minutes vs. 32 ± 13.3 minutes) without alteration of physiologic parameters and prolongation of recovery from anesthesia [68]. Tramadol (1.6 mg/kg IM) has also been combined with xylazine (1.2 mg/kg IM) and Telazol (3 mg/kg IM) to produce general anesthesia with excellent muscle relaxation and analgesia for approximately 80 minutes in pigs [69].

Buprenorphine is classified as partial μ agonist with an analgesic potency that is 25 times that of morphine. Buprenorphine is poorly absorbed from the GI tract. Due to its high affinity and low specificity for the μ receptors, opioid antagonists are ineffective in reversing buprenorphine's effects. Onset of analgesia occurs in 45 minutes with a duration of 240 minutes following IM administration of buprenorphine (0.005–0.01 mg/kg). Propulsive walking, rapid and frequent head movements, chewing, and hypersensitivity to auditory and visual stimuli were observed in sheep receiving buprenorphine [37]. In goats, IM buprenorphine at 0.01 mg/kg administered every 6 hours following orthopedic surgery provided satisfactory analgesia. No signs of CNS excitation as described in sheep were observed in the goats (Lin, personal observation). A 3-day meat withdrawal is suggested for buprenorphine [36]. The recommended dose of buprenorphine in pigs is 0.01–0.05 mg/kg IM or IV every 6–12 hours [70]. When compared to etorphine (0.003 mg/kg IM) and pethidine (20 mg/kg IM), buprenorphine (0.12 mg/kg IM) produced longer duration of analgesia (7–24 hours) than the other drugs in pigs. The analgesic effect of buprenorphine is deemed better than that of pethidine but not as good as etorphine's [71]. Buprenorphine has been used to provide pain relief in research pigs following thoracotomy surgery at 0.01–0.04 mg/kg administered intramuscularly (Lin, personal observation).

Butorphanol is a κ agonist and μ antagonist with an analgesic potency approximately three to five times that of morphine. Butorphanol has a unique "ceiling effect" – that is, after effective action has been attained-further increases in doses do not increase or enhance the degree of desirable pharmacologic effect [72]. Butorphanol may cause slight CNS stimulation in farm animal species, especially when administered to animals that are not in pain. Twitching of the facial muscles, lips, and head may occur. Butorphanol is the most frequently used opioids in farm animals. The recommended dose of butorphanol is 0.02–0.05 mg/kg IV or SC every 4–6 hours. Jones [2] commented that butorphanol is the best analgesic for ameliorating established pain and is capable of providing excellent visceral analgesia in 80% of the ruminant patients. Butorphanol can be given alone in sheep and goats to produce light sedation. No behavioral effects were observed when butorphanol was administered intravenously at 0.05 mg/kg in sheep, but ataxia was observed at 0.4 mg/kg while excitement occurred at 0.1–0.2 mg/kg [40, 73, 74]. In cattle, tremor and propulsive walking occurred following IV administration of butorphanol, but the signs disappeared within 30 minutes [36]. Butorphanol is frequently used in combination with a sedative or a tranquilizer to produce standing sedation and analgesia for minor surgery and diagnostic procedures. It also can be administered postoperatively for pain relief. In sheep and goats, xylazine and butorphanol can be administered simultaneously to produce deep sedation and recumbency lasting for as long as 60 minutes. In dairy cows, the $t½$ of 0.25 mg/kg IV is reported to be 82 minutes [75]. Adding xylazine (0.05 mg/kg) and ketamine (0.1 mg/kg) to butorphanol (0.025 mg/kg) did not affect the elimination $t½$ of butorphanol (71.28 ± 7.64 minutes) when the combination was administered intramuscularly to Holstein calves immediately prior to castration and dehorning [76]. This combination has been used successfully to provide analgesia for surgical procedures on very fractious cattle and also in cattle suffering extreme pain caused by disease [17]. Interestingly, when IV butorphanol (0.07 mg/kg) and xylazine (0.02 mg/kg) were administered to weanling bulls at the time of castration, the treatment did not offer significant beneficial effects in reducing distress and improving growth performance after surgery [77]. In pigs, butorphanol is recommended at 0.1–0.3 mg/kg IV or IM every 4 hours, doses slightly higher than for other farm animal species [70]. Please refer to Chapter 11 for withdrawal times for butorphanol.

Nonsteroidal anti-inflammatory drugs

NSAIDs are used for their analgesic, antipyretic, and anti-inflammatory properties through inhibition on cyclooxygenase (COX), lipoxygenase, and thromboxane enzymes. The COX acts on arachidonic acid to release prostaglandins and other mediators of inflammation, and thus, COX inhibitors like NSAIDs prevent the production of these mediators. There is evidence indicating NSAIDs may produce analgesia by central inhibition of pain response involving α_2 and μ receptors. There are two COX isoforms, COX-1 and COX-2. The COX-1 isoform presents in normal peripheral tissues and CNS. Its expression is enhanced by pain and inflammatory mediators. The COX-2 isoform is expressed in CNS but only becomes the major enzyme for prostaglandin synthesis after induction by factors released from cell damage and death. Maximal COX-2 mRNA expression occurs in peripheral tissues 2–8 hours after induction [78]. NSAIDs appear to have differential activity according to their affinity for the two COX isoforms. For example, flunixin meglumine, ketoprofen, and phenylbutazone are nonspecific COX inhibitors, whereas etodolac and carprofen are selective COX-2 inhibitors. Flunixin meglumine is an excellent visceral analgesic, and phenylbutazone is very effective in relieving musculoskeletal pain. Clinical observation suggests specific COX-2 inhibitors are not effective analgesics in ruminants [2, 79]. All NSAIDs have good oral bioavailability, making oral administration an easy and effective route to provide pain relief. However, there are significant differences in clearance of these drugs between animal species and age groups. Also, some of the NSAIDs have narrow margin of safety in that therapeutic indexes are relatively close to their toxic indexes. Therefore, extrapolation of the NSAID dosing regimens from one species to another is extremely dangerous and not recommended [80].

Aspirin (acetylsalicylic acid) and sodium salicylate are both salicylic acid derivatives and were the first NSAIDs used for their analgesic, antipyretic, and anti-inflammatory effects. Though neither drug has been approved for use in food animals by the FDA, aspirin is frequently administered at 100 mg/kg, twice daily orally, for treatment of fever and minor joint and muscle pain. Aspirin ionized extensively in the rumen pH with an ionized-to-nonionized ratio of 1000:1, indicating a low oral bioavailability and slow absorption of the drug following oral administration in ruminants [81, 82]. It is believed that the rumen serves as a slow-release reservoir for oral aspirin absorption reflecting in the longer elimination $t½$ of 3.70 ± 0.44 hours following oral administration of salicylic acid as compared to 0.54 ± 0.04 hours following IV administration of sodium salicylate to adult dairy cows [81, 83]. In humans, minimum effective serum concentration of salicylic acid to relieve mild pain resulting from headaches, aches, and pain is 30 μg/ml, but 100 μg/ml is required to relive pain caused by arthritis. In cattle, only oral administration of 100 mg/kg of aspirin resulted in a serum concentration above 30 μg/ml while 50 mg/kg did not. Therefore, 100 mg/kg of sodium salicylate is recommended to maintain serum concentration above 30 μg/ml. However, conflicting reports showed that sodium salicylate relieved pain caused by nonsuppurative tarsitis in two cows but did relieve pain in a bull suffering suppurative tarsitis [81]. There is no report on salicylic acid-induced clotting deficit in cattle [84]. For pigs, aspirin is recommended at a dose range of 10–20 mg/kg administered orally every 4–6 hours [70]. Please refer to Chapter 11 for withdrawal times for aspirin.

Flunixin meglumine (Banamine) is a COX-1 inhibitor. It is the only NSAID approved by the FDA for use in beef and lactating dairy cattle for fever and inflammation associated with respiratory diseases, endotoxemia, and acute bovine mastitis [12]. Flunixin meglumine is approved for IV administration at the dose of 1.1 mg/kg BID or 2.2 mg/kg SID, and this dosing regimen may produce analgesia for 6–12 hours. This dose can be repeated for up to three days. In calves undergoing castration with a Burdizzo clamp or surgical removal, effective pain relief was produced by flunixin meglumine administered IV along with epidural lidocaine. The report showed a significant decrease (50%) in plasma cortisol concentration and better steps and stride 6–8 hours in the postoperative period compared to the nontreated calves [85, 86]. Flunixin meglumine alone (2.2 mg/kg IV) administrated 20 minutes before castration resulted in a mild decrease (20%) in plasma cortisol concentration. Several studies showed that concurrent administration of epidural lidocaine or xylazine enhanced the analgesic effect of flunixin meglumine [85–88]. Nonetheless, significantly better appetite, defecation, and milk production have been observed in cows receiving flunixin meglumine 24 hours before and after surgical correction of left displaced abomasum [89]. In cattle, significant myonecrosis and tissue residues have been reported when flunixin meglumine is administered intramuscularly [12]. Thus, the drug should only be administered intravenously in cattle. However, this route of administration not only causes stress to the animal but also requires special training for personnel performing the task. Flunixin meglumine has become the second most common residue violation (the first being penicillin) in cull dairy calves. Veterinarians should address and emphasize the importance of following label instruction of the drug to farm personnel [90]. Doses of 2–4 mg/kg IV or SC once daily for flunixin meglumine are recommended for use in pigs [70]. However, 1–4 mg/kg IV, IM, or SC every 12 hours is recommended for pet pigs [91]. Please refer to Chapter 11 for withdrawal times for flunixin meglumine.

Phenylbutazone is clinically more effective in relieving pain associated with musculoskeletal injuries and chronic osteoarthritis than is flunixin meglumine. Phenylbutazone is a drug with high level of regulatory concern due to lack of predictable withdrawal time. The drug is highly protein bound with a very long elimination *t*½ in cattle (30–80 hours) and sheep and goats (15–20 hours) when compared to that of other large animal species. When administered to cattle at a loading dose of 24 mg/kg followed by a single daily dose of 12 mg/kg, the drug was still detectable in milk 82 hours after administration. At this time, the use of phenylbutazone in female dairy cattle older than 20 months of age is strictly prohibited, and its use in other milk- and meat-producing animals is strongly discouraged due to the concern over human consumption [92]. Phenylbutazone is capable of crossing the blood–placenta barrier, and concentration of the drug can be detected in calves born to treated cows. Continued exposure through the milk may lead to detectable plasma concentration in newborn calves with an elimination *t*½ as long as 4 days [93]. In addition, the elimination *t*½ of phenylbutazone has been reported to be age dependent, and it is twice as long in 1-month-old calves compared to those of 3-month-old calves [94]. Thus, the administration of phenylbutazone in very young calves is also discouraged. Phenylbutazone is believed to be a carcinogen and has been reported to cause blood dyscrasias (e.g., aplastic anemia, leukopenia, agranulocytosis, and thrombocytopenia) and the death rate in humans that develop aplastic anemia can be as high as 94% [95]. There are reports indicating that an idiosyncratic serum sickness, a type III hypersensitivity reaction, results from exposure to food residue of phenylbutazone; however, no threshold concentration of phenylbutazone has been established [96]. Extralabel use of phenylbutazone is not justifiable under the AMDUCA guidelines because another NSAID (flunixin meglumine) is available and approved for use in food animals. It is recommended that phenylbutazone be reserved for valuable beef breeding stock with severe chronic disease when slaughter is not an option but temporary relief of pain is necessary for embryo or semen collection followed by euthanasia. Meat withdrawal time of a minimum of 45 days for the first dose of phenylbutazone with another 5 days added to each additional day of therapy beyond the first is recommended with a duration of up to 6–8 months if needed [2, 12, 80]. Although there are no NSAIDs approved for use in small ruminants, flunixin meglumine is labeled for use in food animals and should be used preferentially over phenylbutazone.

Ketoprofen is not approved by the FDA for use in food-producing animals. In Canada and European countries, ketoprofen is approved for use in alleviation of inflammation and pain associated with arthritis and traumatic musculoskeletal injuries and also as adjunctive treatment for pain, fever, and inflammation associated with acute mastitis [97]. Compared to other NSAIDs, ketoprofen has a short plasma $t½$ (30 minutes) and a small volume of distribution (0.2 l/kg) with 80% of the parent drugs eliminated in urine within 24 hours [97, 98]. Ketoprofen comes as a racemic combination of 50:50 ratio of R(–) and S(+) enantiomeric forms in the commercial formulation. It is reported that S(+) isoform is approximately 250 times more potent than R(–) isoform in its ability to inhibit prostaglandin E_2 (PGE_2). Approximately 31% of R(–) isoform is converted to S(+) isoform following IV administration in calves [99]. In sheep, the inhibition of PGE_2 of S(+) isoform lasts four times longer than that of R(–) isoform [100]. The concentration of ketoprofen in milk, even at peak plasma concentration, was below the sensitivity level of the analytical test, suggesting that the drug can be used safely in milk-producing ruminants with a short and predictable milk withdrawal time. The FARAD recommends a 24-hour and 7-day milk and meat withdrawal time, respectively [101]. Some clinicians believe that ketoprofen does not have any advantage over flunixin meglumine for treatment of inflammatory diseases in ruminants [80]. However, if the criteria for extralabel use can be met, ketoprofen can be administered at 3.3 mg/kg SID for up to 3 days. In 4- to 8-week-old calves, ketoprofen (3 mg/kg PO) has been shown to reduce pain-related behaviors when administered prior to and at 2 and 7 hours post hot iron dehorning procedure [102]. Combining ketoprofen and cornual nerve block with or without xylazine greatly reduced the distress associated with dehorning and disbudding in calves as indicated by the reduction of the cortisol response to the surgery [103, 104]. Comparing intratesticular lidocaine alone to the combined technique of ketoprofen with intratesticular lidocaine for castration in calves less than 4 months old, the combined technique completely inhibited cortisol response to the surgery, while lidocaine alone did not inhibit cortisol response [105]. In pigs, 1–3 mg/kg IV, IM, or PO of ketoprofen every 12 hours is recommended [70, 91].

Carprofen has greater potency and lower ulcerogenicity than phenylbutazone or aspirin [106]. Carprofen is approved in European countries for use as an adjunct treatment to antimicrobial therapy to reduce clinical signs in acute infectious respiratory disease and acute mastitis in cattle [107]. Similar to ketoprofen, carprofen has two enantiomer isoforms with S(+) isoform approximately 100 times more potent than R(–) isoform on inhibiting COX-2 enzyme in a canine study [108]. However, the effect of carprofen on both COX-1 and COX-2 enzyme activities is considered as poor [106]. In sheep, the elimination *t*½ of carprofen were 26.1 and 33.7 hours when administered intravenously at 0.7 and 4 mg/kg. Plasma concentration greater than 1.5 μg/ml corresponded to the effective analgesic effect of carprofen. When administered at 4 mg/kg IV, carprofen maintained therapeutic plasma concentrations for longer than 72 hours [109, 110]. Measurable amount of carprofen was detected in the milk of cattle with mastitis following a single IV dose of 0.7 mg/kg [111]. In another study, no measurable milk concentration of greater than 25 μg/ml was detected when carprofen was administered at 1.4 mg/kg IV to healthy cows. No milk withdrawal time for carprofen is needed in European countries. Based on a maximum residue level of carprofen of 500 μg/kg in muscle and 1000 μg/kg in liver and kidney, a meat withdrawal time of 21 days is recommended following a single injection of 1.4 mg/kg IV in European countries [112]. In calves, carprofen (1.4 mg/kg IV) alone administered 20 minutes before castration using a Burdizzo clamp technique decreased plasma cortisol concentration by 19% [113], but a 59% reduction was observed when carprofen was combined with epidural lidocaine [85]. Similar to ketoprofen, carprofen is believed not to have any advantage over flunixin meglumine, and its use in food-producing animals is not recommended due to its prolonged clearance time and detectable milk distribution. Doses of 2–4 mg/kg IV or SC once daily are recommended for administration of carprofen in pigs [70]. Wolff [91] suggested that administration of carprofen at 2–3 mg/kg IM, SC, or PO every 12 hours is appropriate for treatment of pigs. Carprofen administered orally at 2 mg/kg every 12 hours for three days provided effective analgesia in a pig suffering severe joint pain (Lin, personal communication).

Meloxicam preferentially, though not specifically, inhibits COX-2 enzymes. Meloxicam (0.5 mg/kg IM or SC) is approved as adjunct treatment of cattle with acute respiratory diseases, acute mastitis, or diarrhea in several European countries and the United Kingdom [114]. A small animal formulation is approved and marketed in the US. Meloxicam has been proven to effectively relieve pain in calves resulting from castration, dehorning, and diarrhea [115–117]. Good oral bioavailability with maximum plasma concentration occurred at 10–12 hours with an elimination *t*½ of 27.5 hours after oral administration of meloxicam at 1 mg/kg to 3-month-old Holstein calves [118]. Other evidences supporting the effectiveness of meloxicam (0.5 mg/kg IV) in ameliorating pain include reduced heart rate and respiratory rate and improved weigh gain in treated calves when compared to untreated calves following dehorning and castration procedures [119–121]. It is believed that meloxicam may be useful for sustained pain relief of greater than 3 days at 0.5–1 mg/kg orally every 24–48 hours [17]. A possible fatal anaphylactoid reaction of an Ayrshire cow to IV meloxicam has been reported [122]. The cow appeared agitated and had profuse lacrimation, bilateral periocular edema, and chemosis within 10 minutes after IV administration. She became markedly ataxic and assumed recumbent position. Hyperventilation rapidly progressed to blood-tinted foaming at the mouth, tachypnea, and then dyspnea with cyanotic oral, nasal, and vulvar mucous membrane. The cow was euthanized when she began to gasp for air. Though manufacturers reported that the anaphylactoid reaction to NSAIDs is extremely rare with possibility incidence of less than 1 per 30,000 administrations, veterinarians should be aware of this possible reaction and be prepared to institute emergency treatment when an incident occurs [122]. Preemptive administration of meloxicam (0.4 mg/kg IM) to pigs not only reduces stress prior to castration but also provides analgesia following surgery [123]. Similar analgesic effect evaluated by vocal characteristics and cortisol response to castration was reported in piglets when meloxicam (0.4 mg/kg IM) with or without lidocaine local anesthesia was administered 15 minutes prior to surgery [124]. Meloxicam appeared to have wide margin of safety as evidenced by administration of 5 times the recommended dose (2 mg/kg) for 6 consecutive days to 5–6-month-old pigs with no lasting adverse effects observed [125]. Please refer to Chapter 11 for withdrawal times for meloxicam.

Diclofenac, a newly introduced NSAID, is an effective analgesic for posttraumatic pain, postoperative wound hyperalgesia, pain associated with movement and swelling, and joint pain resulting from lameness in horses [126–129]. Diclofenac was reported to be an effective analgesic for treatment of acute aseptic arthritis and myositis in cattle and buffalos [129, 130] and in relieving pain caused by castration in lambs [131, 132]. In sheep, diclofenac is proven to be effective against *Brucella* species and schistosomiasis when used in combination with streptomycin, rifampicin, or tetracycline [131, 133]. The elimination *t*½ of diclofenac following 1 mg/kg IV and IM administration to sheep was 2.84 ± 1.94 hours and 2.12 ± 1.60 hours, respectively. Therefore, twice or three times daily doses will be ideal to maintain an effective plasma concentration of the drug [134].

Tolfenamic acid is an anthranilic acid class of NSAIDs. The drug is approved in European countries and Canada for use in cattle for treatment of acute mastitis and respiratory tract diseases. Though there is no proven data indicating any advantage of tolfenamic acid over flunixin meglumine, it has been occasionally used extralabelly. The pharmacokinetic study in cattle showed that tolfenamic acid has a large volume of distribution (1 l/kg) and a long elimination *t*½ (8–10 hours). Prolonged, sustained therapeutic plasma concentration of tolfenamic acid following a single injection has been attributed to the unique enterohepatic recirculation in this species. Tolfenamic acid when administered at the recommended dose of 4 mg/kg IV has milk withdrawal time of 24 hours [14]. The maximum residue level of the drug in milk and muscle, kidneys, and liver has been set at 50, 100, and 400 μg/kg, respectively. Therefore, a meat withdrawal time of 7 days for a single IV injection of 2 mg/kg in beef cattle is recommended where the drug is approved [14, 135].

Alpha-2 agonists

Alpha-2 agonists such as xylazine, detomidine, and medetomidine, have been shown to produce good visceral analgesia. These drugs produce analgesic effects via their actions on the peripheral and central α_2 receptors. There are α_2 receptors located in the dorsal horn of the spinal cord, whereas stimulation of the α_2 receptors located at the periaqueductal gray area of the midbrain (site of origin of the descending inhibitory pain pathways) is responsible for the release of norepinephrine and modulation of pain at the spinal level. In sheep, it has been shown that approximately 60% of analgesia produced by IV xylazine is mediated via spinal α_2 receptors which is supported by the evidence of prior intrathecal administration of α_2 antagonists, idazoxan or RX811059A, results in a reduction of IV xylazine-induced analgesia [136].

Therefore, α_2 agonists can be administered parenterally, epidurally, or intrathecally to produce analgesia. Xylazine or detomidine is often the first choice for treatment of severe abdominal pain in colicky horses. In ruminants, IV or IM administration of sedative doses of xylazine produces dose-dependent analgesic effect, which may last up to 60–90 minutes. Alpha-2 agonists and opioids are often used in combination to provide good analgesia. The effects of these two classes of drugs are synergistic; thus, greater analgesia can be achieved at lower doses of both drugs. The analgesic effects of the α_2 agonists have been described in detail in Chapter 2.

Ketamine

Ketamine, at subanesthetic doses, is effective in preventing or minimizing pain resulting from windup syndrome, which is mediated through the blockade of the NMDA receptors. In addition, ketamine and its active metabolite, norketamine, have been demonstrated to bind to opioid μ and κ receptors which may be in part responsible for the analgesic effect of the drugs [137]. Result of a study in rats indicated that norketamine has one-third of the analgesic potency of ketamine [138]. Coetzee *et al.* [139] showed a correlation between plasma norketamine and substance P concentration in that lower substance P concentration is correlated to higher plasma norketamine concentration in calves receiving low doses of xylazine (0.05 mg/kg IV) and ketamine (0.1 mg/kg IV) for sedation and analgesia during surgical castration. Ketamine has been administered at 0.1–1 mg/kg IV to alleviate acute postoperative pain in humans [140]. Furthermore, a plasma ketamine concentration of 1000 ng/ml is considered minimum effective concentration for the anesthetic effect, whereas plasma concentration of 275 ng/ml or 1/10th–1/5th of the anesthetic concentration is correlated to the drug's analgesic effect [141]. Nonetheless, Grant *et al.* [142] suggested that analgesia occurred at the plasma ketamine concentration of 40–150 ng/ml. In cattle receiving xylazine (0.05 mg/kg IV) and ketamine (0.1 mg/kg IV), plasma ketamine and norketamine concentrations fell below 40 and 10 ng/ml within 30 and 60 minutes, respectively, after the administration of ketamine [143]. Ketamine can be administered alone intermittently at subanesthetic doses to produce analgesia. It can also be administered in combination with another class of analgesics such as an α_2 agonist or an NSAID or as CRI to maintain long-term analgesia. For example, ketamine has been used in combination with opioids or NSAIDs at 0.25–0.5 mg/kg IM every 6–8 hours to provide pain relief for goats suffering severe pain due to burn injury, polyarthritis, or osteomyelitis [144]. Ketamine is classified as a controlled schedule III drug, and record keeping of its use is closely monitored by the DEA, which may be viewed as a disadvantage over α_2 agonists and NSAIDs. Please refer to Chapter 11 for withdrawal times for ketamine.

Gabapentin

Gabapentin has become a popular antihyperalgesic drug for treatment of animals suffering chronic neuropathic pain or as treatment of windup syndrome in humans, dogs, and cats. Gabapentin has a chemical structure similar to the inhibitory neurotransmitter γ-amino-butyric acid (GABA) in the CNS. The drug was developed originally for use as an anticonvulsant drug [145]. Interestingly, gabapentin does not produce its pharmacologic effects through actions on the GABA receptors. There is evidence that gabapentin produces its analgesic effect by the inhibitory action on α2δ-subunits of voltage-dependent calcium-channel complexes. A decrease in calcium influx in presynaptic nerve terminal and inhibition of the release of the excitatory amino acid are the results of gabapentin binding with α2δ-subunit. These inhibitory effects of gabapentin were only observed in patients with hyperalgesia but not in normal patients [146]. Gabapentin has been used frequently in small animal patients suffering from chronic pain, but its use in larger animals is still limited. Doses of 3–5 mg/kg PO every 8 hours have been recommended to produce satisfactory analgesia in goats. The dose can be titrated up or down depending on the patient's response to the initial dose or dosing interval (Lin, personal communication). The oral bioavailability of gabapentin in goats is believed to be better than in horses. The only reported side effects of gabapentin in humans are sedation and dizziness [147] and in dogs are sedation and ataxia [148, 149]. However, sedation appears to be insignificant following IV administration of 20 mg/kg to horses [150]. Synergism of pharmacological effects has been observed when an NSAID is administered with gabapentin [145, 151]. In 6–8-month-old beef calves, oral gabapentin (15 mg/kg) has been administered concurrently with meloxicam (0.5 mg/kg) with maximum plasma concentration and elimination $t½$ occurring at 11.67 ± 3.44 hours and 20.47 ± 9.22 hours [152]. Comparable pharmacokinetics has been reported with oral meloxicam (1 mg/kg) and gabapentin (10 or 20 mg/kg) to lactating Holstein cows. Gabapentin at 10 mg/kg requires similar time to reach maximum plasma (8 hours) and milk (12 ± 6.69 hours) concentrations as meloxicam (11.33 ± 4.12 hours). Increasing the dose of gabapentin to 20 mg/kg doubles the maximum plasma concentration of gabapentin [153]. In cattle, orally administered gabapentin is useful in relieving pain caused by deep digital sepsis and septic arthritis at 10 mg/kg every 12 hours [17]. The residual milk concentration was detected for as long as 48 hours in cows receiving 10 mg/kg and 64 hours in those receiving 20 mg/kg. In lactating Holstein cows receiving gabapentin (10 or 20 mg/kg PO) with meloxicam (1 mg/kg PO), only 0.1% and 1% of administered gabapentin and meloxicam, respectively, were excreted in the milk. The concentration of either drug in the milk fell below detectable level by 3 days. Therefore, it is reasonable to predict a milk withdrawal time of 72 hours for oral meloxicam administered at 1 mg/kg and gabapentin up to 20 mg/kg [154]. If gabapentin is prescribed for long-term treatment of chronic pain, a meat withdrawal time of 21 days can be assumed until further pharmacokinetic data for repeat dosing become available [6, 153].

Drug combinations for pain management

Similar to the technique of using different classes of anesthetics to produced balanced anesthesia (i.e., unconsciousness, analgesia, and muscle relaxation), multimodal analgesia is used to produce effective analgesia using different classes of analgesics to prevent pain transmission at multiple levels and, at the same time, minimize the side effects of each drug by reducing the dose of each drug required when used alone. For example, xylazine (0.02 mg/kg IV) and butorphanol (0.05 mg/kg IV) or detomidine (0.01 mg/kg IV) and butorphanol (0.05 mg/kg) have been used to provide standing sedation in cows [155]. IM xylazine (0.02–0.05 mg/kg), butorphanol (0.01–0.025 mg/kg), and ketamine (0.04–0.1 mg/kg) is another combination commonly used to produce good standing sedation in farm animal species. For procedures that likely produce intense pain such as castration, a higher recommended dose of each drug of the combination can be administered intravenously to induce appropriate analgesia [2]. In calves, 2.2 mg/kg of flunixin meglumine IV once daily and 0.01 mg/kg of buprenorphine IV every 8–12 hours have been used to provide pain relief after thoracotomy surgery. Bupivacaine line block on the thoracotomy can be added to enhance analgesia produced by IV flunixin meglumine and buprenorphine (Lin, personal communication). Combinations of meloxicam at 0.2 mg/kg PO with buprenorphine (0.01 mg/kg IM) twice daily or carprofen (2 mg/kg PO) with buprenorphine at 0.005–0.02 mg/kg IM have been used in pigs to relieve pain due to thoracotomy or joint disease (Lin, personal communication).

Constant rate infusion

Advantages of administering CRI of an analgesic or analgesic combination is the ability to use low dose of analgesic(s) to maintain steady-state plasma concentration, avoid peak and trough fluctuation of the drug effect, and, most importantly, provide continuous pain relief to the patient suffering severe chronic pain.

Systemic administration of lidocaine for treatment of postoperative ileus following colic surgery in horses has increased dramatically in recent years. In these cases, lidocaine is believed to provide beneficial effects including analgesia via its local anesthetic effect, prevention of intestinal adhesions and ileus by promoting GI movement (prokinetic effect), and minimizing reperfusion injury of ischemic areas by its anti-inflammatory effect. In cattle, lidocaine CRI can be administered to provide long-term analgesia following laparotomy at a loading dose of 1.3 mg/kg IV followed by an infusion of 3 mg/kg/hour [2]. Concomitant CRI administration of low doses of lidocaine (3 mg/kg/hour) with intermittent administration of detomidine (0.1 mg/kg IV) every 4 hours has also been recommended to alleviate abdominal and peritoneal pain in food animals [36]. A combination of ceftiofur (10 ml), 2% lidocaine (10 ml), and saline (40 ml) administered at an infusion rate of 2 ml/hour has been used to provide pain relief in Holstein cows with chronic septic arthritis of the flexor tendon sheath, although intravenous use of ceftiofur is no longer permitted in cattle. Morphine, ketamine, and lidocaine combination CRI was administered to a Holstein heifer with severe burns over 40% of her body surface. The heifer became more comfortable and was able to lie down and stand more easily with improved appetite during infusion [156]. In calves anesthetized for umbilical surgery, lidocaine with initial bolus dose of 2 mg/kg IV followed by CRI of 3 mg/kg/hour enhanced isoflurane anesthetic effect and reduced its dose requirement for surgical anesthesia by 16.6% as compared to that of control calves [157]. Similar reduction for isoflurane requirement with CRI of lidocaine (0.12 mg/kg/hour) and ketamine (0.6 mg/kg/hour) combination has also been demonstrated in sheep undergoing orthopedic surgery [158].

Grant *et al.* [159] reported that in sheep (B.W. 45–60 kg (99–132 lb)) sedated with a bolus dose of xylazine (5 mg IM) and a continuous IV infusion of xylazine (2 mg/hour) for 90 minutes, steady-state analgesic effect tested by leg lifting in response to electrical stimulus was obtained 10 minutes after the start of the infusion until the end of the study. Ketamine produces intense analgesia by blocking NMDA receptors and stimulating μ receptors. In addition, potent anti-inflammatory effect by suppressing cytokines and neutrophil chemotaxis may also be associated with ketamine-induced analgesia. Ketamine is an effective analgesic for relieving established pain; it provides analgesia at microdose at 0.4–1.2-mg/kg/hour CRI for long-term pain relief [2].

Butorphanol is proven to be an excellent visceral analgesic in ruminants. In adult cattle, long-term analgesia can be maintained with low doses of butorphanol CRI. The solution for infusion is made up by adding 10–20 mg of butorphanol to 5 L of balanced electrolyte solution, and CRI is administered at 1–2 L/hour [2]. There is no report on the use of butorphanol CRI in sheep and goats. However, considering the concentration of butorphanol is only 0.002–0.004 mg/ml (10–20 mg in 5 L of solution) with an infusion rate of 1–2 L/hour for sheep and goats weighing 60 kg (132 lb), the total dose of butorphanol administered in an hour is only 2–4 mg (0.03–0.06 mg/kg). This dose would still be within the recommended dosage range for small ruminants [42].

A combination of an opioid, lidocaine, and ketamine (**Trifusion**) has been administered as CRI for long-term pain relief in ruminants. Either butorphanol or morphine can be used in the combination. Prior to infusion of the **Trifusion**, a loading dose of butorphanol (0.05–0.1 mg/kg IV or IM in small ruminants, 0.02–0.05 mg/kg IV or IM in large ruminants) is administered for instant increase in plasma concentration of the drug. Loading dose for lidocaine is 1 mg/kg IV, and it is administered slowly to prevent lidocaine-induced cardiovascular and CNS effects. In preparing **Trifusion** solution for a 450-kg (990-lb) animal using 3 mg/kg/hour of lidocaine as base solution, add 4000 mg of ketamine (0.6 mg/kg/hour) and 170 mg of morphine (0.025 mg/kg/hour) or 148 mg of butorphanol (0.022 mg/kg/hour) into 1 L of 2% lidocaine solution. Infusion rate of the mixture is set at 67 ml/hour. The infusion rate can be adjusted to patient size using the formula 67 ml/kg × new animal kg/450 kg (990 lb) to calculate the desired infusion rate. For example, for a 300-kg (660-lb) animal, the infusion rate is 45 ml/hour (67 ml/hour × 300 kg (660 lb)/450 kg (990 lb) = 45 ml/hour) [42]. Detomidine (0.004 mg/kg/hour) and acepromazine (0.0022 mg/kg/hour) have been added to **Trifusion**, making it a five-drug combination, and this combination is termed **Pentafusion** [42]. **Pentafusion** is used effectively to relieve extreme pain of laminitic horses. This combination has not been investigated in ruminants. Dose adjustments of the drugs will be required if **Pentafusion** be used in ruminants because of the difference in sensitivity of ruminants to the drugs included in this combination [42].

Table 9.1 and Table 9.2 summarize the doses of drugs and drug combinations that can be used for systemic pain management in cattle, small ruminants, camelids, and pigs. Many options are available to relieve pain and to ensure patient comfort. The choice of an appropriate analgesic or analgesic combination used for a patient depends on the type of pain, the patient's condition, and the experience of the veterinarian in order to maximize the beneficial effects of an analgesic or analgesic combination for patient comfort.

Table 9.1 Doses of drugs used for systemic pain management in cattle, sheep, and goats.

Drug	Dosage for cattle (mg/kg)	Dosage for sheep and goats (mg/kg)	Duration (hours)
Local anesthetics			
Lidocaine	—	1–2, SC	—
Lidocaine	—	2.5, IV	1
Lidocaine	200 mg in 40-ml saline, 2 ml/hour	Loading dose: 2–5, IV CRI: 3–6 mg/kg/hour	— —
Lidocaine	Loading dose: 1.3–2, IV, over 5 minutes CRI: 1.2–3 mg/kg/hour	Loading dose: 2.5, IV CRI during isoflurane anesthesia: 6 mg/kg/hour	—
Trifusion			
Butorphanol	Loading dose: 0.05–0.1, IV CRI: 0.02 mg/kg/hour	In sheep during isoflurane anesthesia: —	
Lidocaine	Loading dose: 1, IV CRI: 3 mg/kg/hour	CRI: 1.2 mg/kg/hour	—
Ketamine	CRI: 0.6 mg/kg/hour	CRI: 0.6 mg/kg/hour	
Or			
Morphine	0.025 mg/kg/hour		
Lidocaine	Loading dose: 1, IV CRI: 3 mg/kg/hour	In goats: CRI: 3 mg/kg/hour	—
Ketamine	0.6 mg/kg/hour		
Opioids			
Buprenorphine	—	0.0015–0.006, IV, IM	0.75–3.5
Buprenorphine	—	0.005–0.01, SC	6
Buprenorphine	—	0.005–0.1, IV or IM	4, 8–12
Buprenorphine	—	0.005, IM	12
Butorphanol	—	0.05–0.5, IV or IM	2–4
Butorphanol	0.05, SC	0.05, SC	6
Butorphanol	—	0.05–0.5, IM, sedation	—
Butorphanol	—	0.4, IV, sedation and ataxia	—
Butorphanol	—	0.5, IM, IV	2–3

Table 9.1 (*Continued*)

Drug	Dosage for cattle (mg/kg)	Dosage for sheep and goats (mg/kg)	Duration (hours)
Butorphanol	—	0.005, IM	—
Butorphanol	—	0.05–0.2, IM, IV	1–3
Butorphanol	0.005, IM	—	—
Acepromazine/ Butorphanol	0.03, IV 0.01, IV	—	—
Acepromazine/ Butorphanol	0.022, IV 0.044, IV	—	—
Diazepam/ Butorphanol	—	0.1–0.5, IM or IV 0.01, IM	—
Midazolam/ Butorphanol	—	0.05–0.025, IM or IV 0.01, IM	—
Fentanyl patch	—	0.2, transdermal	—
Fentanyl injectable	—	5 mg or 10 mg/70 kg, transdermal	72–96
Fentanyl injectable	—	0.001–0.006 μg/kg, IV; 0.001–0.005 μg/kg/hour, IV	1–2
Fentanyl injectable	—	0.01, IV in sheep	—
Meperidine	2, IM	2, IV, IM	2–4
Meperidine	3.3–4.4, IM, SC	3.3–4.4, IM, SC	—
Meperidine	—	10, IM in goats	0.25–0.5
Meperidine	5, IM	5, IM in sheep	0.25–0.5
Morphine	0.05–0.1, IM, IV	0.05–0.1, IV, SC	4–6
Morphine	0.4, IM, or 0.25–0.05, IM	0.1–0.5, IM	4
Morphine	0.05–0.5, IV, IM	0.5, IM, IV	4–6
Morphine	—	0.5–1, IV	12
Acepromazine/ Morphine	0.02–0.04, IV 0.1–0.5	—	—
Oxymorphone	0.005, IM	0.005, IM	—
α2 agonists			
Xylazine	0.05–0.2, IM, IV	0.05–0.2, IM, IV	2–4
Xylazine	0.1, IM	0.05–0.1, IM	—
Xylazine/ Butorphanol	0.01–0.02, IV 0.01–0.02, IV	0.1–0.2, IV 0.01–0.02, IV	—
Xylazine/ Butorphanol	0.05–0.1, IV 0.01–0.02, IV	0.02, IM 0.05–0.07, IM	—
Detomidine	0.003–0.01, IM, IV	0.003–0.01, IM, IV	2–4
Medetomidine	0.005–0.01, IM, IV	0.005–0.01, IM, IV	2–4
Romifidine	0.003–0.02, IM, IV	0.003–0.02, IM, IV	2–4

(*Continued*)

Table 9.1 (*Continued*)

Drug	Dosage for cattle (mg/kg)	Dosage for sheep and goats (mg/kg)	Duration (hours)
NSAIDs			
Aspirin	100, PO	50–100, PO	6–12
Aspirin	—	100, PO	12–24
Carprofen	—	2–4, IV, SC	24
Carprofen	—	1–2, IV, PO, SC	24
Carprofen	—	4, SC	24–48
Carprofen	—	0.7, IV, in sheep	—
Diclofenac	—	1, IV, IM	—
Flunixin meglumine	1–2, PO, IV	1–2.2, IV, PO, SC	12–24
Flunixin meglumine	1, IM	1, IV; 1–2, IV, PO	12
Flunixin meglumine	—	1, IM	—
Ketoprofen	2–3, IV	2, IV	12
Ketoprofen	—	3, IV, IM	24
Ketoprofen	2–3, IV, PO	2–3, IV, PO	12–24
Meloxicam	—	0.5, IV, SC, 1st day; PO, once daily for 5 days	12
Meloxicam	—	0.5, IV	8
Meloxicam	—	0.5, IM, PO	24
Meloxicam	—	2, PO, 1st day; 1 mg/kg, PO, SID	24
Phenylbutazone	2–6, PO, IV	—	24
Phenylbutazone	5, PO	5, PO	24
	10, PO	10, PO	8
Phenylbutazone	Prohibited in dairy cattle >20 months		
	Lame bull: 17–25, IV	—	24
Others			
Ketamine	CRI: 0.4–1.2 mg/kg/hour	CRI: 2.4 mg/kg/hour	—
Ketamine	CRI: 2.4 mg/kg/hour	CRI: 3 mg/kg/hour	—
Gabapentin	—	3–5, PO	8
Gabapentin	10, PO	—	12
Gabapentin/ Meloxicam	15, PO 0.5, PO	—	6–12
Gabapentin/ Meloxicam	10–20, PO 1, PO	—	—

CHAPTER 9

Table 9.2 Doses of drugs used for systemic pain management in camelids and pigs.

Drug	Dosage for camelids (mg/kg)	Dosage for pigs (mg/kg)	Duration (hours)
Local anesthetics			
Lidocaine	Loading dose: 1.3, IV CRI: 3 mg/kg/hour	—	—
	Loading dose: 1–2, IV CRI: 1.2–3 mg/kg/hour	—	—
Trifusion			
Butorphanol	Loading dose: 0.05–0.1, IV CRI: 0.02 mg/kg/hour	—	—
Lidocaine	Loading dose: 1, IV CRI: 3 mg/kg/hour		
Ketamine	CRI: 0.6 mg/kg/hour		
Or			
Morphine	CRI: 0.025 mg/kg/hour	—	—
Lidocaine	Loading dose: 1, IV CRI: 3 mg/kg/hour		
Ketamine	CRI: 0.6 mg/kg/hour		
Opioids			
Buprenorphine	—	0.01–0.05, IV, IM	6–12
Buprenorphine	—	0.005–0.01, IM	12
Buprenorphine	—	0.12, IM	7–24
Buprenorphine	—	0.02–0.03, SC	8–10
Buprenorphine	—	0.01–0.1, IM, IV	12
Buprenorphine	—	0.05–0.1, IM	—
Butorphanol	0.05–0.1, IV, IM	0.1–0.3, IM, IV	4–6
Butorphanol	0.1–0.5, IV, IM	0.1, IM	4–6
Butorphanol	—	0.1–0.4, IM, IV	—
Butorphanol	Loading dose: 0.05–0.1, IV CRI: 0.022 mg/kg/hour	—	—
Fentanyl patch	Transdermal 50 µg/hour for 30–50 kg (66–110 lb)	Transdermal 50–100 µg/hour	48–72
	4 of 75 µg/hour/ 150 kg (330 lb)	—	—
Fentanyl	—	0.05, IV, IM	4
Fentanyl	—	Loading dose: 0.05, IV CRI: 0.03–0.1 mg/kg/hour	—
Sufentanil	—	0.005–0.01, IV, IM	4
Sufentanil	—	Loading dose: 0.007, IV CRI: 0.015–0.03 mg/kg/hour	—

(*Continued*)

Table 9.2 (*Continued*)

Drug	Dosage for camelids (mg/kg)	Dosage for pigs (mg/kg)	Duration (hours)
Hydromorphone	—	0.05, IV	—
Meperidine	1–5, IM	0.4–1, IV	—
Meperidine	—	2, IM, IV	2–4
Meperidine	—	2–10, IM	4
Methadone	—	0.1–0.2, IV	—
Morphine	0.1, IV, IM	0.05–0.1, IV	4–6
Morphine	0.05–0.1, IV, IM	0.2–1, IM	4
Morphine	0.25, IV	—	4
Morphine	0.5–1, IM	—	3–6
Oxymorphone	—	0.02, IM	—
Oxymorphone	—	0.15, IM	4
Tramadol	2, IV, IM	1.6, IM	2–3
Tramadol	4, IM	5, IM	—
Tramadol	11, PO	1–4, PO	8
NSAIDs			
Aspirin	—	10, PO	4
Aspirin	—	10–20, PO	4–6
Carprofen	—	2–4, IV, SC	24
Carprofen	—	2–3, PO, IM, SC	12
Carprofen	—	4, PO	24
Etodolac	—	10–15, PO	24
Flunixin meglumine	1.1, IV	1, IV, IM	12–24
Flunixin meglumine	1.1, IV	—	8
Flunixin meglumine	—	1–2, IV, SC	24
Flunixin meglumine	—	1–4, IV, IM, SC	12
Ibuprofen	—	10, PO	6–8
Ketoprofen	—	1–3, IV, IM, SC, PO	12
Ketoprofen	1–2, IV	3, IM	24
Ketorolac	—	1, IM, IV	—
Meloxicam	—	0.1–0.2, PO	24
Meloxicam	—	0.4, SC	24
Meloxicam	—	—	—
Meloxicam	1, PO	—	72
Meloxicam	0.5, IV	—	—
Phenylbutazone	5, IV, PO	10–20, PO	24–48
Others			
Ketamine	CRI: 0.4–1.2 mg/kg/hour	CRI: 0.2–1 mg/kg/hour	—
Ketamine	CRI: 2.4 mg/kg/hour	—	—
Midazolam	—	0.5–1.5 mg/kg/hour	—
Ketamine	—	8–33 mg/kg/hour	—
Xylazine	0.1–0.3, IV, IM, SC	0.5, IM	1–2.5
Xylazine	—	1, IM	—
Xylazine	—	10, IM	12
Xylazine	—	0.05, IV	1
Ketamine		0.1, IV	
Tolfenamic acid	—	2, IM	24

Local or regional analgesia

Local or regional anesthetic techniques in farm animal species are described in detail in Chapter 7. In this chapter, only the techniques commonly involved in pain management such as caudal epidural analgesia, lumbosacral epidural analgesia, and intra-articular analgesia are included. Topical application of local anesthetics in cattle is often ineffective due to the characteristic thick bovine skin, particularly at the flank and dorsal areas. However, an analgesic effect of 5% lidocaine gel has been observed when applied to the skin of injured teats to facilitate palpation and cannulation of the teat. Analgesia is evident within 10 minutes after application of the gel to dry skin [17].

Caudal epidural analgesia

If properly performed, caudal epidural anesthesia desensitizes the perineum, vulva, vagina, and rectum. The injection site is usually between the first and second coccygeal vertebrae. As a general rule, 1 ml of 2% lidocaine per 45 kg (99 lb) of body weight is adequate; therefore, a total dose of 1–2 ml is effective for most sheep and goats and 5–7 ml for adult cattle. The onset of analgesia occurs within 1–5 minutes, and the duration is about 1 hour. The onset of perineal analgesia tends to be slower with epidural morphine or α_2 agonists, but the duration of analgesia is significantly longer as compared to that of lidocaine. Bupivacaine-induced caudal epidural analgesia was compared to lidocaine- and lidocaine–bupivacaine-induced analgesia in Holstein cows undergoing reproductive procedures [160]. The durations of analgesia produced by 0.05 and 0.06 mg/kg of bupivacaine were 226 ± 55 minutes and 247 ± 31 minutes, respectively, which were significantly longer than that of lidocaine (0.2 mg/kg, 127 ± 25 minutes) and lidocaine (0.1 mg/kg)–bupivacaine (0.025 mg/kg) combination (181 ± 33 minutes). One cow receiving 0.05 mg/kg of bupivacaine developed profuse salivation, nasal discharge, hiccough, urination, and defecation, and all of these side effects subsided within 15 minutes. Accidental IV injection was thought to be the cause of the adverse reaction, which was supported by the lack of perineal analgesia following epidural injection of the drug in this cow [160]. In another study, bupivacaine (0.25 mg/kg, 192 ± 8 minutes), xylazine (0.05 mg/kg, 127 ± 8 minutes), medetomidine (0.015 mg/kg, 212 ± 10 minutes), xylazine with bupivacaine (206 ± 7 minutes), and medetomidine with bupivacaine (228 ± 9 minutes) were shown to produce longer duration of caudal epidural analgesia in buffalos than did lidocaine [161]. Bupivacaine (9–13 minutes) and ropivacaine (15 minutes) both have significantly slower onset but longer duration of perineal analgesia than lidocaine (5–7 minutes) in cattle. Surprisingly, the duration of perineal analgesia produced by 0.11 mg/kg of ropivacaine (359 ± 90 minutes) was significantly longer than that produced by 0.06 mg/kg of bupivacaine (247 ± 31 minutes) [160, 162].

Caudal epidural injection produced by romifidine (0.05 mg/kg) and morphine (0.1 mg/kg) was capable of suppressing the response to noxious stimulation up to the flank area for 12 hours [163]. In sheep, epidural administration of fentanyl (0.0015 mg/kg) alone did not produce analgesia. When adding fentanyl to xylazine (0.2 mg/kg), fentanyl was able to shorten the time of onset (4.5 ± 0.5 vs. 10 ± 1.1 minutes) and prolong the duration of epidural analgesia (315 ± 6 vs. 96 ± 6 minutes) of that of xylazine alone [164].

Compared to morphine, caudal epidural administration of α_2 agonist not only produces excellent perineal analgesia, but these drugs also provide systemic analgesia and sensory blockade during surgery. The α_2 agonists, especially xylazine, have been used as the sole anesthetic to perform cesarean section in sheep. The CNS-depressing effects such as sedation, ataxia, and sometimes recumbency can occur following caudal epidural or lumbosacral administration of an α_2 agonist. These CNS effects are believed to be the result of (1) absorption of the drug from epidural space into systemic circulation, (2) cranial migration of the drug toward CNS, and/or (3) local anesthetic effect of the drug, particularly xylazine. IV administration of an α_2 antagonist, atipamezole (0.005 mg/kg), reversed the CNS effects induced by epidural xylazine but did not affect the epidural analgesia [165]. Hind limb paresis/paralysis resulting from trauma to the spinal cord has been reported in both small and large ruminants after epidural administration of xylazine or medetomidine [36, 166–169]. It is very likely that trauma to the spinal cord upon epidural injection is the cause for the hind limb paresis. However, this author (Lin) did not observe any adverse effects such as trauma to the spinal cord or hind limb paresis in adult cattle involved in a research project when 5 epidural injections of saline, lidocaine, clonidine, xylazine, or medetomidine were performed with at least a 2-week interval between each injection [170, 171]. The effects of three different doses of caudal epidural ketamine (0.5, 1, and 2 mg/kg, diluted to 5, 10, and 20 ml, respectively) have been investigated in standing cattle. Dose-dependent analgesia lasting from 17 to 62 minutes was observed. Ataxia but not sedation was observed throughout the study [2, 172].

Lumbosacral epidural anesthesia

Lumbosacral epidural anesthesia provides analgesia caudal to the diaphragm including abdominal wall caudal to the umbilicus, inguinal region, flank, and perineal areas if properly performed. A dosage of 0.3–0.5 ml of 2% lidocaine solution per 10 kg (22 lb) of body weight is adequate for most surgery. The onset of analgesia and hind limb paralysis usually occurs within 5–15 minutes and lasts 1–2 hours [173, 174]. Dose-dependent duration of lumbosacral epidural analgesia with recumbency of ropivacaine has been reported from 5–6 hours with 0.29–0.35 mg/kg to 7–8 hours with 0.63–0.75 mg/kg [175].

Lumbosacral injection of xylazine (0.05 mg/kg) with lidocaine (2 mg/kg) and buprenorphine (0.005 mg/kg) with lidocaine (2 mg/kg) has been used to produce intrathecal analgesia for pain relief following stifle surgery in goats [176]. The result of this study showed that intrathecal buprenorphine with lidocaine produced more profound and longer-lasting analgesia but with less sedation than that of xylazine with lidocaine. Both combinations produced satisfactory pain relief for goats following stifle surgery. However, the duration of analgesia for buprenorphine with lidocaine was at least 6 hours, which was approximately twice as long as that of xylazine with lidocaine [176]. In another study, lumbosacral epidural analgesia induced by morphine (0.1 mg/kg) or bupivacaine (1.5 mg/kg) was compared during abdominal surgery in goats. Morphine produced 22 hours of intrathecal analgesia but only 3 hours was observed with bupivacaine [177]. Goats that received morphine stood within 59 ± 9 minutes following surgery, while those that received bupivacaine remained recumbent for 285 ± 49 minutes.

Though prolonged recumbency generally does not result in long-term adverse effects in goats, lumbosacral epidural morphine is believed to be more ideal when faster recovery to standing with longer pain relief is desired [178]. In sheep, intrathecal administration of morphine (0.1 mg/kg) resulted in hind limb ataxia and licking and chewing of the flanks and the hind limbs. The higher than recommended dose of intrathecal morphine was believed to be the cause of this adverse reaction [179]. Lumbosacral administration of morphine (0.1 mg/kg), bupivacaine (0.5 mg/kg), or morphine (0.05 mg/kg) with bupivacaine (0.25 mg/kg) following thoracic surgery produced analgesia duration of 40, 70, and 140 minutes, respectively. Lumbosacral bupivacaine alone or combined with morphine resulted in hind limb paralysis during the period of analgesia. No adverse reaction to morphine was observed in this study [180]. In goats, subarachnoid administration of buprenorphine (0.005 mg/kg) combined with lidocaine (0.1 ml/kg) resulted in more profound and longer-lasting analgesia but with less sedation and ataxia than a combination of intrathecal xylazine (0.05 mg/kg) and lidocaine (0.1 ml/kg) [176]. Analgesic effects of lumbosacral administration of lidocaine (2.86 mg/kg), tramadol (1 mg/kg), and tramadol (1 mg/kg)–lidocaine (2.46 mg/kg) combination were evaluated in goats. Tramadol alone produced long duration of analgesia (235 ± 18 minutes) with a slower onset of action (12 ± 1 minutes) as compared to lidocaine. Unlike xylazine and lidocaine combination, there was no synergistic or additive analgesic effect of lidocaine when combined with tramadol, which was reflected in the shorter duration of analgesia (140 ± 2 minutes) as compared to that of tramadol alone [181].

In goats, intrathecal administration of ketamine (2.5 mg/kg) combined with romifidine (0.05 mg/kg) and an added volume of saline to produce a total volume of 2 ml was reported to produce complete analgesia in the tail, perineum, and hind limbs for 2 hours [182]. In sheep, lumbosacral epidural ketamine alone (1 mg/kg, with saline added to produce a total volume of 7–9 ml) administered prior to recovery from orthopedic surgery delayed the time for the administration of first rescue analgesic (5 hours vs. 3.5 hours for the control). In addition, sheep receiving ketamine seemed to walk with less lameness [183]. Lumbosacral ketamine (2.5 mg/kg) alone in goats produced excellent analgesia which completely abolished the response to pinprick for 5–20 minutes. Addition of xylazine (0.05 mg/kg) to ketamine prolonged the duration of analgesia to 60 minutes. Brief period of ataxia was observed with ketamine alone, whereas sedation and ataxia occurred throughout the xylazine and ketamine analgesic period [172].

The use of a combination of detomidine, ketamine, methadone, and bupivacaine administered extradurally into lumbosacral area was described for successful pain management in a Brown Swiss resulting from a pelvic limb lameness causing complex regional pain syndrome. Epidural morphine (0.1 mg/kg) was originally administered to provide pain relief but discontinued due to the development of pruritus. Initial doses of detomidine, ketamine, methadone, and bupivacaine were 7, 1640.6, 85.9, and 4.7 µg/kg/day, respectively. Each drug was diluted with saline into 10-ml solution, and the total volume of 40 ml of the mixture was infused over 24 hours. Due to significant sedation, detomidine was discontinued on day 5. The cow was monitored closely and the dose of each drug adjusted accordingly. The treatment was continued for 17 days and the cow was discharged only mildly lame with much improved physical condition [184].

Intra-articular analgesia

In sheep, pain relief was obtained after stifle arthrotomy by intra-articular injection of lidocaine (40 mg, 2 ml) prior to incision, and bupivacaine (10 mg, 2 ml) post closure. Additionally, phenylbutazone (1 g orally, once daily for 5 days) and transdermal fentanyl (15 mg) were initiated 24 hours prior to surgery. Though this study did not evaluate the total duration of analgesia induced by the combination, a similar study in dogs suggested analgesia duration of approximately 24 hours [185]. However, short duration of analgesia was observed in goats receiving intra-articular bupivacaine alone after stifle arthrotomy surgery [186]. Intra-articular injection of morphine has not been studied in adult cattle. However, the technique is proven to be an effective pain relief in dogs and horses. A dose of 0.05–0.1 mg/kg diluted with saline into 5–15 ml, according to the size of the joint, is recommended [187].

In recent *in vitro* studies, 0.5% bupivacaine has been shown to cause cytotoxicity to bovine, equine, and human chondrocytes [188–191]. Approximately 90–99% chondrocyte deaths were reported in these studies after direct in vitro exposure to 0.5% bupivacaine for 30–60 minutes. Dilution of bupivacaine to 0.25% increased both human and bovine chondrocyte viability and reduced cell death to 41% as compared with saline control group. Further dilution of bupivacaine to 0.125% resulted in similar chondrocyte viability as that of saline control group [190]. When equine chondrocytes were exposed to 0.5% bupivacaine, 2% lidocaine, and 2% mepivacaine for 30 or 60 minutes, the cell viability was reported to be $28.73 \pm 8.44\%$, $66.85 \pm 6.03\%$, and $86.27 \pm 2.00\%$, respectively, whereas the cell viability was $95.95 \pm 2.75\%$ after exposure to saline solution of a similar duration. Hence, intra-articular administration of mepivacaine, with its low cytotoxicity, could be a better choice to relieve joint pain [191]. Ropivacaine has also been shown to have less chondrocyte toxicity to *in vitro* human intact articular cartilage and cultured chondrocyte, as chondrocyte viability was reported to be $94.4 \pm 9.0\%$ for intact articular cartilage and $63.9 \pm 19\%$ for cultured chondrocyte, respectively following exposure to 0.5% ropivacaine, whereas chondrocyte viability was $78 \pm 12.6\%$ for intact articular cartilage and $37.4 \pm 12\%$ for cultured chondrocyte respectively, when exposed to 0.5% bupivacaine [188]. There are no clinical reports that support the findings of these *in vitro* studies, and intact articular cartilage apparently offers some chondrocyte-protective effects. However, the detrimental effects of bupivacaine and lidocaine on chondrocytes should be kept in mind, especially in patients with cartilage disorders, and mepivacaine and ropivacaine may be considered for intra-articular administration when indicated.

Table 9.3 and Table 9.4 summarize the doses of drugs and drug combinations that can be used to produce local and regional analgesia for pain management in cattle, small ruminants, camelids, and pigs. Similar to the options available for parenteral administration of an analgesic or analgesic combinations, there are also different options of local or regional analgesic techniques available to relieve pain and ensure patient comfort. Careful selection of an appropriate local or regional analgesic or analgesic combination best suited the type of pain and the condition of the patient.

Table 9.3 Doses of drugs used to produce local and regional analgesia for pain management in cattle, sheep, and goats.

Drugs	Dosages for cattle (mg/kg)	Dosages for sheep and goats (mg/kg)	Duration (hours)
Local anesthetics			
Bupivacaine	0.05	0.05, infiltration	2–3 in cattle
Bupivacaine	—	0.05, epidural	—
Bupivacaine	—	1, intrathecal	—
Bupivacaine	—	1.5–1.8 in goats	2–3 in goats
Bupivacaine	—	1.8, lumbosacral	11 in goats
Bupivacaine	—	10 mg, intra-articular, after surgery	—
Bupivacaine	—	1–2, SC	—
Lidocaine (2%)	0.2–0.4, epidural	0.05, infiltration	1–2 in cattle
Lidocaine (2%)	5–7 ml/450 kg (990 lb)	1–2 ml/50 kg (110 lb), epidural	1.2 in sheep and goats
Lidocaine (2%)	—	0.22, epidural	—
Lidocaine (2%)	—	1 ml/10 kg, lumbosacral	—
Lidocaine (2%)	—	1, intrapleural	—
Lidocaine (2%) Ethyl alcohol (95%)	1:1 ratio in 2–3-ml mixture, caudal epidural	—	—
Lidocaine	—	40 mg, intra-articular, presurgery	3–7 in goats
Lidocaine	20 ml/vein, intravenous regional anesthesia (IVRA)	3–4 ml/vein, IVRA	—
Lidocaine	20 ml/vein, IVRA	—	—
Morphine	40–100 mg IVRA		
α2 agonists			
Detomidine	0.04 in 5-ml saline, epidural	0.01, intrathecal in sheep, 2-ml saline	3 in cattle 1 in sheep
Medetomidine	—	0.001–0.002, lumbosacral	—
Medetomidine	0.015 in 5-ml saline, epidural	0.02 or 0.01–0.03 in 5-ml saline, epidural	7 in cattle <3 in goats
Medetomidine	0.015	—	—
Mepivacaine	0.5–1 ml/50 kg (110 lb)		
Oxymorphone	0.005, IM	0.005, IM	—
Romifidine	0.05, epidural	0.05 in 4-ml saline, intrathecal	12 in cattle 2 in goats
Romifidine	0.05	—	12 in cattle

(*Continued*)

Table 9.3 (*Continued*)

Drugs	Dosages for cattle (mg/kg)	Dosages for sheep and goats (mg/kg)	Duration (hours)
Morphine	0.1 in 30-ml saline, epidural		
Romifidine Ketamine	—	0.05 2.5 in 2-ml saline, intrathecal	2 in goats
Xylazine	0.05 in 5-ml saline, epidural	0.03, epidural	2–3 in cattle
Xylazine	0.07 in 5-ml saline, epidural	0.07–0.4 in 2.5-ml saline, epidural	1–2 in sheep
Xylazine	1 in 5-ml saline	0.15 in 5-ml saline, epidural	3 in goats
Xylazine	—	0.05 in 0.75-ml saline, intrathecal	2 in goats
Xylazine	—	0.07–0.4 in 2.5-ml saline, epidural	1–2 in sheep
Xylazine	—	0.1 in 2-ml saline, intrathecal	1.5 in sheep
Xylazine Ketamine	—	0.05 2.5 in 1.5-ml saline, epidural	0.5–1 in goats
Xylazine Ketamine	—	0.05 2.5 in 1.5-ml saline, intrathecal	2 in goats
Xylazine Lidocaine (2%)	—	0.05 1.25 in 4-ml saline, intrathecal	3 in goats
Xylazine Lidocaine (2%)	—	0.25 ml of 20 mg/ml 2 ml Mix in 73-kg (161-lb) ewe, epidural	—
Xylazine Morphine	12 mg 0.1 For 500–600-kg (1100–1320-lb) cows, caudal epidural	—	—
Opioids			
Morphine	0.1 in 0.02–0.05-ml/kg saline, epidural	0.1 in 0.2-ml/kg saline, epidural	6–12
Morphine	—	0.05–0.1, epidural	24
Morphine	—	0.1–0.2, epidural	—
Morphine	—	0.1, epidural	—
Morphine Bupivacaine	—	0.1, epidural 1.5, epidural	—

Table 9.3 (*Continued*)

Drugs	Dosages for cattle (mg/kg)	Dosages for sheep and goats (mg/kg)	Duration (hours)
Tramadol	—	1, lumbosacral	Slow onset No ataxia
Others			
Ketamine	0.5–2 in 5–20-ml saline, epidural	—	1 in cattle
Ketamine	—	1 in 7–9-ml saline, epidural	5 in sheep
Ketamine	—	2.5 in 0.75-ml saline, epidural	0.25 in goats
Ketamine	250 mg	—	0.28
Ketamine	500 mg	—	0.57
Ketamine	1000 mg	—	1.03

Table 9.4 Doses of drugs used to produce local and regional analgesia for pain management in camelids and pigs.

Drug	Dosage for camelids (mg/kg)	Dosage for pigs (mg/kg)	Duration (hours)
Local anesthetics			
Lidocaine (2%)	<4.4, IVRA	10 ml/vein, IVRA	—
Lidocaine (2%)	<1 ml/5 kg, IVRA	—	—
Lidocaine (2%)	1 ml/23 kg (51 lb), caudal epidural	0.5–1 ml/5 kg (11 lb), epidural	1–1.5
Lidocaine (2%)	1–2 ml/50 kg (110 lb), caudal epidural	—	—
Lidocaine (2%)	2–3 ml/adult llama	—	—
Lidocaine	3 mg/kg, lumbosacral	—	—
α2 agonists			
Xylazine	0.1, caudal epidural	2 in 5-ml saline, epidural	2
Xylazine	0.17 in 2-ml saline, caudal epidural	1 in 10 ml, >180 kg (396 lb) 2 in 10 ml <50 kg (110 lb)	—
Xylazine	0.17	1 in 2% lidocaine to a total of 10 ml, lumbosacral	5–8
Lidocaine	0.22 Total 1.7 ml, caudal epidural		
Detomidine	—	0.5 in 5-ml saline, epidural	—
Medetomidine	—	0.5 in 5-ml saline	<0.5
Opioids			
Morphine	0.1, caudal epidural	—	12

References

1. Coetzee, J. (2011) A review of pain assessment techniques and pharmacological approaches to pain relief after bovine castration: practical implications for cattle production within the United States. *Applied Animal Behaviour Science*, **135**, 192–213.
2. Jones, M. (2008) Clinical application in pain management. *CanWest Veterinary Conference*.
3. Muir, W. and Woolf, C. (2001) Mechanism of pain and their therapeutic implications. *Journal of the American Veterinary Medical Association*, **219**, 1346–1356.
4. Gottschalk, A. and Smith, D. (2001) New concepts in acute pain therapy: preemptive analgesia. *American Family Physician*, **63**, 1979–1984.
5. Ochroch, E., Mardini, I. and Gottschalk, G. (2003) What is the role of NSAIDs in pre-emptive analgesia? *Drugs*, **63**, 2709–2723.
6. Smith, E. and Modric, S. (2013) Regulatory considerations for the approval of analgesic drugs for cattle in the United States. *Veterinary Clinics of North America. Food Animal Practice*, **29**, 1–10.
7. Hewson, C., Dohoo, I., Lemke, K. and Barkema, H. (2007) Canadian veterinarians' use of analgesics in cattle, pigs, and horses in 2004 and 2005. *The Canadian Veterinary Journal*, **48**, 155–164.
8. Watts, S. and Clarke, K. (2000) A survey of bovine practitioners attitudes to pain and analgesia in cattle. *Cattle Practice*, **8**, 361.
9. Coetzee, J. (2012) Pain assessment and timing and method of castration. *North American Veterinary Community Conference*, pp. 14–20.
10. Lorena, S., Luna, S., Lascelles, B. and Corrente, J. (2013) Attitude of Brazilian veterinarians in the recognition and treatment of pain in horses and cattle. *Veterinary Anaesthesia and Analgesia*, **40**, 410–418.
11. Lerche, P. and Muir, W. (2009) Pain management in horses and cattle, in *Handbook of Veterinary Pain Management*, 2nd edn (eds J. Gaynor and W. Muir), Mosby-Elsevier, St. Louis, pp. 437–463.
12. Smith, G., Davis, J., Tell, L. *et al.* (2008) Extralabel use of nonsteroidal anti-inflammatory drugs in cattle. *Journal of the American Veterinary Medical Association*, **232**, 697–701.
13. Animal Medicinal Drug Use Clarification Act of 1994 (AMDUCA), US Food and Drug Administration. (1994) http://www.fda.gov/RegulatoryInformation/Legistration/FederalFoodDrugandCosmeticActFDCAct/SignificantAmendamentstotheFDCAct/AnimalMedicinalDrugUseClarificationActAMDUCAof1994/default.htm (accessed January 6, 2014).
14. Smith, G. (2013) Extralabel use of anesthetic and analgesic compounds in cattle. *Veterinary Clinics of North America. Food Animal Practice*, **29**, 29–45.
15. Muir, W., Hubbell, J., Bednarski, R. and Lerche, P. (eds) (2007) Local anesthesia in ruminants and pigs, in *Handbook of Veterinary Anesthesia*, 4th edn, Mosby-Elsevier, St. Louis, pp. 72–99.
16. Stoelting, R. (2006) Local anesthetics, in *Pharmacology and Physiology in Anesthetic Practice*, 4th edn (eds R. Stoelting and S. Hillier), Lippincott Williams & Wilkins, Philadelphia, pp. 180–207.
17. Anderson, D. and Edmondson, M. (2013) Prevention and management of surgical pain in cattle. *Veterinary Clinics of North America. Food Animal Practice*, **29**, 157–184.
18. Stafford, K., Mellor, D. and McMeekan, C. (2000) A survey of the methods used by farmers to castrate calves in New Zealand. *New Zealand Veterinary Journal*, **48**, 16–19.

19. Kent, J., Thrusfield, M., Robertson, I. and Malony, V. (1996) Castration of calves: a study of methods used by farmers in the United Kingdom. *The Veterinary Record*, **138**, 384–387.
20. Coetzee, J., Nutsch, A., Barbur, L. and Bradburn, R. (2010) A survey of castration methods and associated livestock management practices performed by bovine veterinarians in the United States. *BMC Veterinary Research*, **6**, 12–30.
21. Fisher, A., Crowe, M., Alonso, M. and Enright, W. (1996) Effect of castration method and the provision of local anesthesia on plasma cortisol, scrotal circumference, growth, and feed intake of bull calves. *Journal of Animal Science*, **74**, 2336–2343.
22. Skarda, R. (1986) Techniques in local analgesia in ruminants and swine. *Veterinary Clinics of North America. Food Animal Practice*, **2**, 621–663.
23. Muir W, Hubbell J, Bednarski R, Lerche P (eds). Local anesthetic drugs and techniques In *Handbook of Veterinary Anesthesia*. 4th ed. Mosby-Elsevier: St. Louis, 2007;51-71.
24. Vesal, N., Jahromi, A. and Oryan, A. (2012) Lidocaine containing high concentrations of a vasoconstrictor: is it safe for infiltration anesthesia? *Comparative Clinical Pathology*, **21**, 1703–1706.
25. Nelson, S. (2011) Skin lesions in cattle after use of lidokel-adrena. *Norsk Veterinaertidsskrift (NVT)*, **123**, 357–364.
26. Craig, A. (2003) Pain mechanism: labeled lines versus convergence in central processing. *Annual Review of Neuroscience*, **26**, 1–30.
27. Sellers, G., Lin, H., Riddell, M. *et al.* (2009) Pharmacokinetics of lidocaine in serum and milk of mature Holstein cows. *Journal of Veterinary Pharmacology and Therapeutics*, **32**, 446–450.
28. Rostami, M. and Vesal, N. (2011) Comparison of lidocaine, lidocaine/epinephrine or buprenorphine for thoracolumbar paravertebral anaesthesia in fat-tailed sheep. *Veterinary Anaesthesia and Analgesia*, **38**, 598–602.
29. Hall, L. and Clarke, K. (eds) (1991) General principles of local analgesia, in *Veterinary Anaesthesia*, 9th edn, Bailliere Tindall, London, pp. 173–188.
30. Scarratt, W. and Trout, H. (1986) Iatrogenic lidocaine toxicosis in ewes. *Journal of the American Veterinary Medical Association*, **188**, 184–185.
31. Morishima, H., Pedersen, H., Finster, M. *et al.* (1981) Toxicity of lidocaine in adult, newborn, and fetal sheep. *Anesthesiology*, **55**, 57–61.
32. Santos, A., Pedersen, H., Harmon, T. *et al.* (1989) Does pregnancy alter the systemic toxicity of local anesthetics? *Anesthesiology*, **70**, 991–995.
33. Ewing, K. (1990) Anesthesia techniques in sheep and goats. *Veterinary Clinics of North America. Food Animal Practice*, **6**, 759–778.
34. Alon, E., Ball, R., Gillie, M. *et al.* (1993) Effects of propofol and thiopental on maternal and fetal cardiovascular and acid-base variables in the pregnant ewe. *Anesthesiology*, **78**, 562–576.
35. KuKanich, B. and Papich, M. (2009) Opioid analgesics, in *Veterinary Pharmacology and Therapeutics*, 9th edn (eds J. Riviere and M. Papich), Wiley-Blackwell, Ames, pp. 301–335.
36. George, L. (2003) Pain control in food animals, in *Recent Advances in Anesthetic Management of Large Domestic Animals* (ed E. Steffey), International Veterinary Information Service, Ithaca,www.ivis.org (accessed January 6, 2014).
37. Nolan, A., Livingston, A. and Waterman, A. (1987) Investigation of the antinociceptive activity of buprenorphine in sheep. *British Journal of Pharmacology*, **92**, 527–533.
38. Nolan, A., Waterman, A. and Livingston, A. (1988) The correlation of the thermal and mechanical antinociceptive activity of the pethidine hydrochloride with plasma concentrations of the drug in sheep. *Journal of Veterinary Pharmacology and Therapeutics*, **11**, 94–102.

39. Waterman, A., Livingston, A. and Amin, A. (1990) Analgesic and respiratory effects of fentanyl in sheep. *Journal of the American Veterinary Medical Association*, **17**, 20.
40. Waterman, A., Linvingston, A. and Amin, A. (1991) Analgesic activity and respiratory effects of butorphanol in sheep. *Research in Veterinary Science*, **51**, 19–23.
41. Waterman, A., Livingston, A. and Amin, A. (1991) Further studies on the antinociceptive activity and respiratory effects of buprenorphine in sheep. *Journal of Veterinary Pharmacology and Therapeutics*, **14**, 230–234.
42. Abrahamsen, E. (2009) Managing severe pain in ruminants, in *Current Veterinary Therapy: Food Animal Medicine*, 5th edn (eds D. Anderson and D. Rings), Saunders/Elsevier, St. Louis, pp. 570–574.
43. Valverde, A. and Doherty, T. (2009) Pain management in cattle and small ruminants, in *Current Veterinary Therapy: Food Animal Medicine*, 5th edn (eds D. Anderson and D. Rings), Saunders/Elsevier, St. Louis, pp. 534–542.
44. Ruckebusch, Y. (1983) Pharmacology of reticulo-ruminal motor function. *Journal of Veterinary Pharmacology and Therapeutics*, **6**, 245–272.
45. Flacke, J., Flacke, W., Bloor, B. *et al.* (1987) Histamine release by four narcotics: a double blind study in humans. *Anesthesia and Analgesia*, **66**, 723.
46. Singh, B. and Kumar, A. (1988) Meperidine as preanesthetic to thiopentone anesthesia in goats. *The Indian Journal of Animal Science*, **58**, 1279.
47. Carroll, G., Hooper, R., Boothe, D. *et al.* (1999) Pharmacokinetics of fentanyl after intravenous and transdermal administration in goats. *American Journal of Veterinary Research*, **60**, 986–991.
48. Ahern, B., Soma, L., Boston, R. and Schaer, T. (2009) Comparison of the analgesic properties of transdermally administered fentanyl and intramuscularly administered buprenorphine during and following experimental orthopedic surgery in sheep. *American Journal of Veterinary Research*, **70**, 418–422.
49. Ahern, B., Soma, L., Rudy, J. *et al.* (2010) Pharmacokinetics of fentanyl administered transdermally and intravenously in sheep. *American Journal of Veterinary Research*, **71**, 1127–1132.
50. Grubb, T., Gold, J., Schlipf, J. *et al.* (2005) Assessment of serum concentrations and sedative effects of fentanyl after transdermal administration at three dosages in healthy llamas. *American Journal of Veterinary Research*, **66**, 907–909.
51. Shipton, E. (2000) Tramadol – present and future. *Anaesthesia and Intensive Care*, **28**, 363–374.
52. Raffa, R., Friserichs, E., Reimann, W. *et al.* (1992) Opioid and nonopioid components independently contribute to the mechanism of action of tramadol, an 'atypical' opioid analgesic. *The Journal of Pharmacology and Experimental Therapeutics*, **260**, 275–285.
53. Scott, L. and Perry, C. (2000) Tramadol: a review of its use in perioperative pain. *Drugs*, **60**, 139–176.
54. Shilo, Y., Britzi, M., Eytan, B. *et al.* (2008) Pharmacokinetics of tramadol in horses after intravenous, intramuscular and oral administration. *Journal of Veterinary Pharmacology and Therapeutics*, **31**, 60–65.
55. Lehmann, K., Kratzenberg, U., Schroeder-Bark, B. and Horrichs-Haermeyer, G. (1990) Postoperative patient-controlled analgesia with tramadol: analgesic efficacy and minimum effective concentrations. *The Clinical Journal of Pain*, **6**, 212–220.
56. Mastrocinque, S. and Fantoni, D. (2003) A comparison of preoperative tramadol and morphine for the control of early postoperative pain in canine ovariohysterectomy. *Veterinary Anaesthesia and Analgesia*, **30**, 220–228.

57. Hopkins, D., Shipton, E., Potgieter, D. *et al.* (1998) Comparison of tramadol and morphine via subcutaneous PCA following major orthopaedic surgery. *Canadian Journal of Anaesthesia*, **45**, 435–442.
58. Houmes, R., Voets, M., Verkaaik, A. *et al.* (1992) Efficacy and safety of tramadol versus morphine for moderate and severe postoperative pain with special regard to respiratory depression. *Anesthesia and Analgesia*, **74**, 510–514.
59. Grond, S. and Sablotzki, A. (2004) Clinical pharmacology of tramadol. *Clinical Pharmacokinetics*, **43**, 879–923.
60. Braz, M., Carreira, M., Carolino, N. *et al.* (2012) Effect of rectal or intravenous tramadol on the incidence of pain-related behavior after disbudding calves with caustic paste. *Applied Animal Behaviour Science*, **136**, 20–25.
61. Malonne, H., Sonet, B., Streel, B. *et al.* (2004) Pharmacokinetic evaluation of a new oral sustained release dosage form of tramadol. *British Journal of Clinical Pharmacology*, **57**, 270–278.
62. KuKanich, B. and Papich, M. (2004) Pharmacokinetics of tramadol and the metabolite o-desmethyltramadol in dogs. *Journal of Veterinary Pharmacology and Therapeutics*, **27**, 239–246.
63. Pypendop, B. and Ilkiew, J. (2007) Pharmacokinetics of tramadol, and its metabolite o-desmethyltramadol, in cats. *Journal of Veterinary Pharmacology and Therapeutics*, **31**, 52–59.
64. deSousa, A., Santos, A., Schramm, S. *et al.* (2007) Pharmacokinetics of tramadol and o-desmethyltramadol in goats after intravenous and oral administration. *Journal of Veterinary Pharmacology and Therapeutics*, **31**, 45–51.
65. Edmondson, M., Duran, S., Boothe, D. *et al.* (2012) Pharmacokinetics of tramadol and its major metabolites in alpacas following intravenous and oral administration. *Journal of Veterinary Pharmacology and Therapeutics*, **35**, 389–396.
66. Hinchcliff, K., Jernigan, A., Upson, D. and Constable, P.D. (1991) Ruminant pharmacology. *Veterinary Clinics of North America. Food Animal Practice*, **7**, 633–649.
67. DeRouchey, J., Goodband, B., Tokach, M., *et al.* (2009) Digestive system of the pig-anatomy and function. *North American Veterinary Community Conference*, pp. 375–376.
68. Ajadi, A., Olusa, T., Smith, O. *et al.* (2009) Tramadol improved the efficacy of ketamine-xylazine anaesthesia in young pigs. *Veterinary Anaesthesia and Analgesia*, **36**, 562–566.
69. Lu, D., Fan, H., Kun, M. *et al.* (2011) Antagonistic effect of atipamezole, flumazenil, and naloxone following anaesthesia with xylazine, tramadol, and tiletamine-zolazepam combinations in pigs. *Veterinary Anaesthesia and Analgesia*, **38**, 301–309.
70. Flecknell, P. (ed) (2009) Analgesia and post-operative care, in *Laboratory Animal Anesthesia*, 3rd edn, Academic Press, an imprint of Elsevier, London, pp. 139–179.
71. Hermansen, K., Pedersen, L. and Olesen, H. (1986) The analgesic effect of buprenorphine, etorphine and pethidine in the pig: a randomized double blind cross-over study. *Acta Pharmacologica et Toxicologica*, **59**, 27–35.
72. Murphy, M. and Hugg, C. (1981) "Ceiling effect" of butorphanol (Stadol) as an anesthetic supplement. *Anesthesiology*, **55**, 261.
73. Taylor, P. (1991) Anesthesia in sheep and goats. *In Practice*, **13**, 31–36.
74. O'Hair, K., Dodd, K., Phillips, Y. and Beattie, R. (1988) Cardiopulmonary effects of nalbuphine hydrochloride and butorphanol tartrate in sheep. *Laboratory Animal Science*, **38**, 58–61.
75. Court, M., Dodman, N., Levine, H. *et al.* (1992) Pharmacokinetics and milk residues of butorphanol in dairy cows after single intravenous administration. *Journal of Veterinary Pharmacology and Therapeutics*, **15**, 28–35.

76. Baldridge, S., Coetzee, J., Dritz, S. *et al.* (2011) Pharmacokinetics and physiologic effects of intramuscularly administered xylazine hydrochloride-ketamine hydrochloride-butorphanol tartrate alone or in combination with orally administered sodium salicylate on biomarkers of pain in Holstein calves following castration and dehorning. *American Journal of Veterinary Research*, **72**, 1305–1317.
77. Faulkner, D., Eurell, T., Tranquilli, W. *et al.* (1992) Performance and health of weanling bulls after butorphanol and xylazine administration at castration. *Journal of Animal Science*, **70**, 2970–2974.
78. Smith, W. and Langenbach, R. (2001) Why there are two cyclooxygenase enzymes? *The Journal of Clinical Investigation*, **107**, 1491–1495.
79. Anderson, D. (2007) Pain management: treatment, management, and prevention. *North American Veterinary Community Conference*.
80. Navarre, C. (2006) Prudent use of pain relief in food animals. *American Association of Bovine Practitioners,* pp. 50–52.
81. Gingerich, D., Baggot, J. and Yeary, R. (1975) Pharmacokinetics and dosage of aspirin in cattle. *Journal of the American Veterinary Medical Association*, **167**, 945–948.
82. USP Veterinary Pharmaceutical Information Monographs – Anti-inflammatories (2004) ASPIRIN Veterinary-systemic. *Journal of Veterinary Pharmacology and Therapeutics*, **27** (Suppl. 1), 4–14.
83. Kotschwar, J., Coetzee, J., Anderson, D. *et al.* (2009) Analgesic efficacy of sodium salicylate in an amphotericin B-induced bovine synovitis-arthritis model. *Journal of Dairy Science*, **92**, 3731–3743.
84. Langston, V. (2003) Therapeutic management of inflammation, in *Current Veterinary Therapy: Food Animal Practice*, 4th edn (eds J. Howard and R. Smith), WB Saunders, Philadelphia, pp. 7–12.
85. Stilwell, G., Lima, M. and Broom, D. (2008) Effects of nonsteroidal anti-inflammatory drugs on long-term pain in calves castrated by use of external clamping technique following epidural anesthesia. *American Journal of Veterinary Research*, **69**, 744–750.
86. Currah, J., Hendrick, S. and Stookey, J. (2009) The behavioral assessment and alleviation of pain associated with castration in beef calves treated with flunixin meglumine and caudal lidocaine epidural anesthesia with epinephrine. *The Canadian Veterinary Journal*, **50**, 375–382.
87. Gonzalez, L., Schwartzkopf-Genswein, K., Caulkett, N., *et al.* (2010) Pain mitigation after band castration of beef calves and its effects on performance, behavior, *Escherichia coli*, and salivary cortisol. *Journal of Animal Science*, **88**, 802–810.
88. Webster, H., Morin, D., Brown, L., *et al.* (2010) Effects of flunixin meglumine and local anesthetic on serum cortisol concentration and performance in dairy calves castrated at 2 to 3 months of age *Annual Convention of the American Association of Bovine Practitioners*, pp. 1005–1012.
89. Whittek, T., Tischer, K., Gieseler, T., Furll, M. and Constable, P. (2008) Effect of preoperative administration of erythromycin or flunixin meglumine on postoperative abomasal emptying rate in dairy cows undergoing surgical correction of left displacement of the abomasum. *Journal American Veterinary Medical Association*, **232**, 418–432.
90. United States Department of Agriculture (USDA) – Food Safety Inspection Service (2005–2010) *Red Book 2005–2010*, http://www.fsis.usda.gov/Sciences/2005_Red_Book/index.asp (accessed January 6, 2014)
91. Wolff, P. (2009) Pet pig problems. *North American Veterinary Community Conference*, pp. 416–419.
92. Davis, J., Smith, G., Baynes, R. *et al.* (2009) Update on drug prohibited for extralabel use in food animals. *Journal of the American Veterinary Medical Association*, **235**, 528–534.
93. Chamberlain, P., Fowler, B., Sexton, M. *et al.* (2003) Preliminary studies of offspring exposure to phenylbutazone and ivermectin during the perinatal period in a Holstein cow-calf model. *Toxicology and Applied Pharmacology*, **187**, 198–208.

94. Volner, Z., Nouws, J., Kozjek, F. *et al.* (1990) Age-dependent pharmacokinetics of phenylbutazone in calves. *The Veterinary Quarterly*, **12**, 98–102.
95. Inman, W. (1977) Study of fatal bone marrow depression with special reference to phenylbutazone and oxyphenbutazone. *BMJ*, **1**, 1500–1505.
96. Phenylbutazone (2003) New animal drugs; phenylbutazone; extralabel animal drug use; order of prohibition. *Federal Register*, **68**, 9528–9530.
97. USP (2004) USP veterinary pharmaceutical information monograph – anti-inflammatories. Ketoprofen. *Journal of Veterinary Pharmacology and Therapeutics*, **27** (Suppl. 1), 75–85.
98. Landoni, M., Cunningham, F. and Lees, P. (1995) Pharmacokinetics and pharmacodynamics of ketoprofen in calves applying PK/PD modeling. *Journal of Veterinary Pharmacology and Therapeutics*, **18**, 315–324.
99. Aberg, G., Ciofalo, V., Penddleton, R. *et al.* (1995) Inversion of R- to S-ketoprofen in eight animal species. *Chirality*, **7**, 383–387.
100. Landoni, M., Comas, W., Mucci, N. *et al.* (1999) Enantiospecific pharmacokinetics and pharmacodynamics of ketoprofen in sheep. *Journal of Veterinary Pharmacology and Therapeutics*, **22**, 349–359.
101. Coetzee, H. (2012) Update on pain management in cattle. *North American Veterinary Community Conference*, pp. 5–11.
102. Faulkner, P. and Weary, D. (2000) Reducing pain after dehorning in dairy calves. *Journal of Dairy Science*, **83**, 2037–2041.
103. Stafford, K. and Mellor, D. (2005) Dehorning and disbudding distress and its alleviation in calves. *Veterinary Journal*, **169**, 337–349.
104. Milligan, B., Duffield, T. and Lissemore, K. (2004) The utility of ketoprofen for alleviating pain following dehorning in young dairy calves. *The Canadian Veterinary Journal*, **45**, 140–143.
105. Stafford, K., Mellor, D., Todd, S. *et al.* (2002) Effects of local anaesthesia or local anaesthesia plus a non-steroidal anti-inflammatory drug on the acute cortisol response of calves to five different methods of castration. *Research in Veterinary Science*, **73**, 61–70.
106. Delatour, P., Foot, R., Foster, A. *et al.* (1996) Pharmacodynamics and chiral pharmacokinetics of carprofen in calves. *British Veterinary Journal*, **152**, 183–198.
107. Coetzee, J. (2013) A review of analgesic compounds used in food animals in the United States. *Veterinary Clinics of North America. Food Animal Practice*, **29**, 11–28.
108. Ricketts, A., Lundy, K. and Seibel, S. (1998) Evaluation of selective inhibition of canine cyclooxygenase 1 and 2 by carprofen and other nonsteroidal anti-inflammatory drugs. *American Journal of Veterinary Research*, **59**, 1441–1446.
109. Welsh, E., Baxter, P. and Nolan, A. (1992) Pharmacokinetics of carprofen administered intravenously to sheep. *Research in Veterinary Science*, **53**, 264–266.
110. Lees, P., Delatour, P., Foster, A. *et al.* (1996) Evaluation of carprofen in calves using a tissue cage model of inflammation. *British Veterinary Journal*, **152**, 199–211.
111. Lohuis, J., vanWerven, T., Brand, A. *et al* (1991) Pharmacodynamics and pharmacokinetics of carprofen, a non-steroidal anti-inflammatory drug, in healthy cows and cows with *Escherichia coli* endotoxin-induced mastitis. *Journal of Veterinary Pharmacology and Therapeutics*, **14**, 219–229.
112. EMEA-Carprofen (2004) European Agency for the Evaluation of Medicinal Products – Committee for Veterinary Medicinal Products: Carprofen, http//:www.emea.europa.eu/pdfs/vet/mrls/091404en.pdf (accessed January 6, 2014).
113. Pang, W., Earley, B., Sweeney, T. and Crowe, M.A. (2006) Effects of carprofen administration during banding or burdizzo castration of bulls on plasma cortisol, in vitro interferon-gamma production, acute-phase proteins, feed intake, and growth. *Journal of Animal Science*, **84**, 351–359.

114. EMEA-Meloxicam (2009) Committee for Veterinary Medicinal Products, Meloxicam, Maximum Residue Limit (MRL) Summary Report (2). *European Agency for the Evaluation of Medicinal Products (EMEA)*, http://www.emea.europa.eu/pdfs/vet/057199en.pdf (accessed January 6, 2014).
115. Theurer, M., White, B., Coetzee, J. *et al.* (2012) Assessment of behavioral changes associated with oral meloxicam administration at time of dehorning in calves using a remote triangulation device and accelerometers. *BMC Veterinary Research*, **8**, 48.
116. Heinrich, A., Duffield, T., Lissemore, K. and Millman, S. (2010) The effect of meloxicam on behavior and pain sensitivity of dairy calves following cautery dehorning with a local anesthetic. *Journal of Dairy Science*, **93**, 2450–2457.
117. Todd, C., Millman, S., McKnight, D. *et al.* (2010) Nonsteroidal anti-inflammatory drug therapy for neonatal calf diarrhea complex: effects on calf performance. *Journal of Animal Science*, **88**, 2019–2028.
118. Coetzee, J., KuKanich, B., Mosher, R. and Allen, P. (2009) Pharmacokinetics of intravenous and oral meloxicam in ruminant calves. *Veterinary Therapeutics*, **10**, E1–E8.
119. Stewart, M., Stookey, J., Stafford, K. *et al.* (2009) Effects of local anesthetic and nonsteroidal anti-inflammatory drug on pain responses of dairy calves to hot-iron dehorning. *Journal of Dairy Science*, **92**, 1512–1519.
120. Coetzee, J., Mosher, R., KuKanich, B. *et al.* (2012) Pharmacokinetics and effect of intravenous meloxicam in weaned Holstein calves following scoop dehorning without local anesthesia. *BMC Veterinary Research*, **8**, 153–167.
121. Coetzee, J., Edwards, L., Mosher, R. *et al.* (2012) Effect of oral meloxicam on health and performance of beef steers relative to bulls castrated on arrival at the feedlot. *Journal of Animal Science*, **90**, 1026–1039.
122. Okushima, S., Chesnel, M. and Clutton, R. (2013) A possible anaphylactoid reaction in a cow after intravenous meloxicam. *Veterinary Anaesthesia and Analgesia*, **40**, 333–334.
123. Keita, A., Pagot, E., Prunier, A. and Guidarini, C. (2010) Pre-emptive meloxicam for postoperative analgesia in piglets undergoing surgical castration. *Veterinary Anaesthesia and Analgesia*, **37**, 367–374.
124. Kluivers-Poodt, M., Houx, B., Robben, S. *et al.* (2012) Effects of a local anesthetic and NSAID in castration of piglets, on the acute pain responses, growth and mortality. *Animal*, **6**, 1469–1475.
125. EMEA-Meloxicam. EPARs for authorized medicinal products for veterinary use: European Public Assessment Report for Metacam. http://www.emea.europa.eu/vetdocs/vets/Epar/metacam/metacam (accessed January 6, 2014) 2001.
126. Caldwell, F., Mueller, P., Lynn, R. and Budsberg, S. (2004) Effect of topical application of diclofenac liposomal suspension on experimentally induced subcutaneous inflammation in horses. *American Journal Veterinary Research*, **65**, 271–276.
127. Bertone, J., Lynn, R. and Vatistas, N. (2002) Clinical field trial to evaluate the efficacy of topically applied diclofenac liposomal cream for the relief of joint lameness in horses. *American Association of the Equine Practitioners*, 190–193.
128. Singh, N., Kinjavdekar, P., Amarpal, S. and Pratap, K. (2001) Evaluation of epidural xylazine and ketamine for the management of posttraumatic pain in goats. *Indian Journal of Veterinary Surgery*, **22**, 73–78.
129. Mahajan, D., Ali, M. and Singh, B. (2001) Therapeutic efficacy of diclofenac sodium in clinical and experimental cases of arthritis and myositis in cattle and buffaloes. *Indian Journal of Veterinary Surgery*, **22**, 73–78.
130. EMEA-Diclofenac. Committee for Veterinary Medicinal Products (2003) *Diclofenac*. http://www.ema.europa.eu/docs/en_GB/document_library/Maximum_Residue_Limits_-_Report/2009/11/wc500013751 (accessed January 22, 2014).

131. Graham, M., Kent, J. and Molony, V. (1997) Effects of four analgesic treatments on the behavioural and cortisol responses of 3-week-old lambs to tail docking. *Veterinary Journal*, **153**, 87–97.
132. Molony, V., Kent, J., Hosie, B. and Graham, M. (1997) Reduction in pain suffered by lambs at castration. *Veterinary Journal*, **153**, 205–213.
133. Munoz-Criado, S., Munoz-Bellido, J. and Garcia-Rodriguez, J. (1996) In vivo activity of nonsteroidal anti-inflammatory agents, phenothiazines, and antidepressants against *Brucella* species. *European Journal of Clinical Microbiology & Infectious Diseases*, **15**, 418–420.
134. Altaher, A., Alkharfy, K., Al-Hadiya, B. and Khan, R. (2006) Pharmacokinetics of diclofenac in sheep following intravenous and intramuscular administration. *Veterinary Anaesthesia and Analgesia*, **33**, 241–245.
135. EMEA-Tolfenamic acid. (1997) *European Agency for the Evaluation of Medicinal Products – Committee for Veterinary Medicinal Products: Tolfenamic Acid*, http://www.emea.europa. eu/pdfs/vet/mrls/018397en.pdf (accessed January 6, 2014).
136. Waterman, A., Kyles, A. and Livingston, A. (1996) Spinal activity of analgesics in sheep. *International Congress of Veterinary Anaesthesia*, 139–141.
137. Annetta, M., Iemma, D., Garisto, C. *et al.* (2005) Ketamine: new indication for an old drug. *Current Drug Targets*, **6**, 789–794.
138. Leung, L. and Baillie, T. (1986) Comparative pharmacology in the rat of ketamine and its two principle metabolites, norketamine and (Z)-6-hydroxynorketamine. *Journal of Medicinal Chemistry*, **29**, 2396–2399.
139. Coetzee, J., Gehring, R., Tarus-Sang, J. and Anderson, D. (2010) Effect of sub-anaesthetic xylazine and ketamine ("ketamine stun") administered to calves immediately prior to castration. *Veterinary Anaesthesia and Analgesia*, **37**, 566–578.
140. Schmid, R., Sandler, A. and Katz, J. (1999) Use and efficacy of low-dose ketamine in the management of acute postoperative pain: a review of current techniques and outcome. *Pain*, **82**, 111–125.
141. Eide, P. (2000) Wind-up and the NMDA receptor complex from a clinical perspective. *European Journal of Pain*, **4**, 5–15.
142. Grant, I., Nimmo, W. and Clements, J. (1981) Pharmacokinetics and analgesic effects of IM and oral ketamine. *British Journal of Pharmacology*, **53**, 805–810.
143. Gehring, R., Coetzee, J., Tarus-Sang, J. and Apley, M. (2009) Pharmacokinetics of ketamine and its metabolite norketamine administered at a sub-anesthetic dose together with xylazine to calves prior to castration. *Journal of Veterinary Pharmacology and Therapeutics*, **32**, 124–128.
144. Wegner, K. (2008) Anesthesia and analgesia, in *Blackwell's Five-minute Veterinary Consult: Ruminant* (ed S. Hankell), Wiley-Blackwell, Ames, pp. 66–69.
145. Hurley, R., Chatterjea, D., Rose-Feng, M. *et al.* (2002) Gabapentin and pregabalin can interact synergistically with naproxen to produce antihyperalgesia. *Anesthesiology*, **97**, 1263–1273.
146. Taylor, C. (2009) Mechanisms of analgesia by gabapentin and pregabalin-calcium channel alpha2-delta [Cavalpha2-delta] ligands. *Pain*, **142**, 13–16.
147. Mao, J. and Chen, L. (2000) Gabapentin in pain management. *Anesthesia and Analgesia*, **91**, 680–687.
148. Govendir, M., Perkins, M. and Malik, R. (2005) Improving seizure control in dogs with refractory epilepsy using gabapentin as an adjunctive agent. *Australian Veterinary Journal*, **83**, 602–608.
149. Platt, S., Adams, V., Garosi, L. *et al.* (2006) Treatment with gabapentin of 11 dogs with refractory idiopathic epilepsy. *The Veterinary Record*, **159**, 881–884.
150. Terry, R., McDonnell, S., vanEps, A. *et al.* (2010) Pharmacokinetic profile and behavioral effects of gabapentin in the horse. *Journal of Veterinary Pharmacology and Therapeutics*, **33**, 485–494.

151. Picazo, A., Castañeda-Hernandez, G. and Ortiz, M. (2006) Examination of the interaction between peripheral diclofenac and gabapentin on the 5% formalin test in rats. *Life Sciences*, **79**, 2283–2287.
152. Coetzee, J., Mosher, R., Kohake, L. *et al.* (2011) Pharmacokinetics of oral gabapentin alone or co-administered with meloxicam in ruminant beef calves. *Veterinary Journal*, **190**, 98–102.
153. Malreddy, P., Coetzee, J., KuKanich, B. and Gehring, R. (2013) Pharmacokinetics and milk secretion of gabapentin and meloxicam co-administered orally with Holstein-Friesian cows. *Journal of Veterinary Pharmacology and Therapeutics*, **36**, 14–20.
154. Gehring R, Malreddy O, Coetzee J, KuKanich B. Pharmacokinetics and milk depletion of meloxicam and gabapentin in lactating Holstein. *American Association of Bovine Practitioners Annual Conference* 2011;142.
155. Lin, H. and Riddell, M. (2003) Preliminary study of the effects of xylazine or detomidine with or without butorphanol for standing sedation in dairy cattle. *Veterinary Therapeutics*, **4**, 285–291.
156. Anderson, D. and Muir, W. (2005) Pain management in cattle. *Veterinary Clinics of North America. Food Animal Practice*, **21**, 623–635.
157. Vesal, N., Spadavecchia, C., Steiner, A. *et al.* (2009) Evaluation of the isoflurane-sparing effects of lidocaine infusion during umbilical surgery in calves. *Veterinary Anaesthesia and Analgesia*, **38**, 451–460.
158. Raske, T., Pelkey, S., Wagner, A. and Turner, A. (2010) Effect of intravenous ketamine and lidocaine on isoflurane requirement in sheep undergoing orthopedic surgery. *Lab Animal*, **39**, 76–79.
159. Grant, C., Summersides, G. and Kuchel, T. (2001) A xylazine infusion regimen to provide analgesia in sheep. *Lab Animal*, **35**, 277–281.
160. Vesal, N., Ahmadi, M., Foroud, M. and Imani, H. (2013) Caudal epidural anti-nociception using lidocaine, bupivacaine or their combination in cows undergoing reproductive procedures. *Veterinary Anaesthesia and Analgesia*, **40**, 328–332.
161. Singh, V., Amarpal, K. and Aithal, H. (2009) Effects of bupivacaine on epidural analgesia produced by xylazine or medetomidine in buffalos (*Bubalus bubalis*). *Veterinary Anaesthesia and Analgesia*, **36**, 77–85.
162. Araujo, M., Albuquerque, V., Deschk, M. *et al.* (2012) Cardiopulmonary and analgesic effects of caudal epidurally administered ropivacaine in cattle. *Veterinary Anaesthesia and Analgesia*, **39**, 409–413.
163. Fiecheller, E., Caulkett, N. and Baily, J. (2004) A romifidine and morphine combination for epidural analgesia of the flank in cattle. *The Canadian Veterinary Journal*, **45**, 917.
164. Aminkov, B., Dinev, D. and Pascalev, M. (2002) The anti-nociceptive and cardiopulmonary effects of extradural fentanyl-xylazine in sheep. *Veterinary Anaesthesia and Analgesia*, **29**, 126–132.
165. Haerdi-Landerer, M., Schlegel, U. and Neiger-Aeschbacher, G. (2005) The analgesic effects of intrathecal xylazine and detomidine in sheep and their antagonism with systemic atipamezole. *Veterinary Anaesthesia and Analgesia*, **32**, 297–307.
166. Aminkov, B. and Hubenov, H. (1995) The effect of xylazine epidural anaesthesia on blood gas and acid-base parameters in rams. *British Veterinary Journal*, **151**, 579–585.
167. Aithal, H., Pratap, A and Singh, G. (1997) Clinical effects of epidurally administered ketamine and xylazine in goats. *Small Ruminant Research*, **24**, 55–64.
168. Scott, P. and Gessert, M. (1997) Evaluation of extradural xylazine injection for cesarean operation in ovine dystocia cases. *Veterinary Journal*, **154**, 63–67.

169. Mpanduji, D., Bittegeko, S., Mgasa, M. and Batamuzi, E. (2000) Analgesic, behavioural and cardiopulmonary effects of epidurally injected medetomidine (Domitor) in goats. *Journal of Veterinary Medicine. A, Physiology, Pathology, Clinical Medicine*, **47**, 65–72.
170. Lin, H., Trachte, E., DeGrave, F. *et al.* (1998) Evaluation of analgesia induced by epidural administration of medetomidine to cows. *American Journal of Veterinary Research*, **59**, 162–167.
171. Lin, H., Heath, A., Pugh, D. and Trachte, E. (2003) Comparison of the analgesic effect of clonidine and lidocaine when administered epidurally in cattle. *The Bovine Practitioner*, **37**, 83–88.
172. Lee, I., Yoshiuchi, T., Yamagishi, N. *et al.* (2003) Analgesic effect of caudal epidural ketamine in cattle. *Journal of Veterinary Science*, **4**, 261–264.
173. Purohit, R. (1999) Anesthesia, in *Large Animal Urogenital Surgery* (eds D. Wolfe and H. Moll), Williams & Wilkins, A Waverly Company, Baltimore, pp. 181–200.
174. Hooper, R. (1998) General surgical techniques for small ruminants: Part II. *Western Veterinary Conference: Small Ruminants for the Mixed Animal Practitioner*.
175. Amarpal, T., Kinjavdekar, P., Aithal, H. *et al.* (2007) Comparison of two doses of ropivacaine for lumbosacral epidural analgesia in buffalo calves (*Bubalus bubalis*). *The Veterinary Record*, **160**, 766–769.
176. Staffieri, F., Driessen, B., Lacitignolas, L. and Crovace, A. (2009) A comparison of subarachnoid buprenorphine or xylazine as an adjunct to lidocaine for analgesia in goats. *Veterinary Anaesthesia and Analgesia*, **36**, 502–511.
177. Pablo, L. (1993) Epidural morphine in goats after hindlimb orthopedic surgery. *Veterinary Surgery*, **22**, 307–310.
178. Hendrickson, D., Kruse-Elliott, K. and Broadstone, R. (1996) A comparison of epidural saline, morphine, and bupivacaine for pain relief after abdominal surgery in goats. *Veterinary Surgery*, **25**, 83–87.
179. Wegner, A., Dunlop, C. and Turner, A. (1996) Experiences with morphine injected into the subarachnoid space in sheep. *Veterinary Surgery*, **25**, 256–260.
180. DeRossi, R., Pagliosa, R., Modolo, T. *et al.* (2012) Thoracic epidural analgesia via the lumbosacral approach using multiport catheters with a low concentration of bupivacaine and morphine in sheep. *Veterinary Anaesthesia and Analgesia*, **39**, 306–314.
181. Dehkordi, S., Bigham-Sadegh, A. and Gerami, R. (2012) Evaluation of anti-nociceptive effect of epidural tramadol, tramadol-lidocaine, and lidocaine in goats. *Veterinary Anaesthesia and Analgesia*, **39**, 106–110.
182. Aithal, H., Kinjavdekar, P., Pawde, A. and Pratap, K. (2001) Analgesic and cardiopulmonary effects of intrathecally administered romifidine or romifidine and ketamine in goats (*Capra hircus*). *Journal of the South African Veterinary Association*, **72**, 84–91.
183. Guedes, A., Pluhar, G., Daubs, B. and Rudé, E. (2006) Effects of preoperative epidural administration of racemic ketamine for analgesia in sheep undergoing surgery. *American Journal of Veterinary Research*, **67**, 222–229.
184. Bergadano, A., Moens, Y. and Schatzmann, U. (2006) Continuous extradural analgesia in a cow with complex regional pain syndrome. *Veterinary Anaesthesia and Analgesia*, **33**, 189–192.
185. Sammarco, J., Conzemius, M., Perkowski, S. *et al.* (1996) Post-operative analgesia for stifle surgery: a comparison of intra-articular bupivacaine, morphine, or saline. *Veterinary Surgery*, **25**, 59–69.
186. Krohm, P., Levionnois, O., Ganster, M. *et al.* (2011) Antinociceptive activity of pre- versus post-operative intra-articular bupivacaine in goats undergoing stifle arthrotomy. *Veterinary Anaesthesia and Analgesia*, **38**, 363–373.

187. Shafford, H., Hellyer, P. and Turner, A. (2004) Intra-articular lidocaine plus bupivacaine in sheep undergoing stifle arthrotomy. *Veterinary Anaesthesia and Analgesia*, **31**, 20–26.
188. Piper, S. and Kim, H. (2008) Comparison of ropivacaine and bupivacaine toxicity in human articular chondrocytes. *The Journal of Bone and Joint Surgery*, **90**, 986–991.
189. Chu, C., Izzo, N., Papas, N. and Fu, F. (2006) In vitro exposure to 0.5% bupivacaine is cytotoxic to bovine articular chondrocytes. *Arthroscopy*, **22**, 693–699.
190. Chu, C., Izzo, N., Coyle, C. *et al.* (2008) The in vitro effects of bupivacaine on articular chondrocytes. *The Journal of Bone and Joint Surgery*, **90**, 814–820.
191. Park, J., Sutradhar, B., Hong, G. *et al.* (2011) Comparison of the cytotoxic effects of bupivacaine, lidocaine, and mepivacaine in equine articular chondrocytes. *Veterinary Anaesthesia and Analgesia*, **38**, 127–133.

Chapter 10

Fluid therapy

Paul Walz

Department of Pathobiology, College of Veterinary Medicine, Auburn University, USA

Fluid therapy prior to and during anesthesia is an important component of the anesthetic plan. Proper use of fluids can be beneficial and lifesaving, and this therapy should be viewed as a medical therapy just as important as other medications in the management of sick or debilitated livestock where anesthesia and/or surgery is required. As with other medications, inappropriate use of fluids during anesthesia can lead to detrimental or lethal outcomes. Fluid therapy can be provided during the perioperative period, which is defined as the period of time beginning when the animal is examined on the farm or clinic and completed when the animal is returned to its normal environment or discharged from the clinic. In many situations, fluid therapy provided prior to and following anesthesia is more important to the outcome of the case than the fluids administered during anesthesia and surgery.

General considerations

The physical state of the animal, especially the level of hydration, is an important consideration prior to anesthesia. Ideally, dehydration along with electrolyte and acid–base imbalances is corrected 12–24 hours prior to anesthetic induction; however, anesthesia and surgery might be necessary prior to complete fluid resuscitation. Under these circumstances, monitoring of cardiac, renal, and pulmonary function is critically important. Even when rehydration can be accomplished prior to anesthesia and surgery, another factor that impacts fluid balance is restriction of oral feed and water. Ruminants are prone to regurgitation and rumen tympany; thus, adult ruminants are often fasted for at least 12–24 hours prior to general anesthesia and restricted from oral water intake for a minimum of 8–12 hours. In very large livestock, or where greater reductions in rumen volume are preferred during abdominal surgery, longer periods of fasting of up to several

Farm Animal Anesthesia: Cattle, Small Ruminants, Camelids, and Pigs, First Edition.
Edited by HuiChu Lin and Paul Walz.

days may be preferred. This restriction of oral water intake combined with ongoing fluid losses associated with a disease process makes consideration of perioperative intravenous (IV) or other parenteral fluid therapy imperative for successful management of anesthesia and surgery. Fluid loading which is the administration of high volumes of IV fluids over a short duration prior to induction of anesthesia and surgery is one way to accomplish the goal of maintaining hydration while restricting oral intake of food and water to prevent regurgitation.

Dehydration as a result of excessive loss of body fluids or failure of fluid intake is the most common indication for fluid therapy in livestock. Examples of fluid intake failures include a lack of thirst as a result of neurologic depression or toxemia or inability to drink as would occur with esophageal obstruction. Diarrhea is the most common cause of excessive fluid loss, although vomiting and polyuria (renal disease) should also be considered, especially in small ruminants. Other indications for fluid therapy include hypovolemic shock, electrolyte abnormalities, disturbances in acid–base balance, hypoglycemia, hypothermia, diuresis following toxin exposure, malnutrition, trauma, and failure of passive transfer.

The overall goal of fluid therapy in sick livestock is to expand the vascular volume in order to improve cardiac output which will improve organ and tissue perfusion. Most drugs used for induction and maintenance of anesthesia decrease cardiac contractility and induce vasodilation which result in a relative hypovolemia. These effects lead to decreased cardiac output and decreased arterial blood pressure. Combining the effect of anesthesia with surgical manipulation, evaporative fluid loss during surgery, blood loss, and the specific disease for which surgical intervention is required, perioperative fluid therapy is an important contribution to the treatment plan in order to improve cardiac function, smooth muscle vascular tone, blood flow distribution, and correction of electrolyte and acid–base imbalances.

Physiology of body fluids

In order to administer fluids and electrolytes properly, a general understanding of fluid composition of the patient and how this fluid is altered or lost during anesthesia, surgery, and disease states is necessary. Total body water comprises between 57% and 67% of body weight for ruminants, while pigs have less total body water (40–50%) as a percentage of weight likely due to less gastrointestinal (GI) water [1]. Most estimations of total body water approximate 60% of body weight [2]. This amount can vary slightly with age, body composition, and breed. In general, neonatal ruminants have relatively more body water than adults, and total body water in neonates may approach 75–80% of body weight. The larger total body water percentage is primarily due to a large extracellular fluid volume, but by 6 months of age, the total body water and extracellular fluid space percent are similar to adult values. The larger total body water and extracellular fluid percent of neonatal ruminants does not provide a reservoir of fluid for the sick neonate [3]. Overweight animals have decreased total body water content as compared to lean animals since adipose tissue contains very little water. As an example, estimations of total body water for fattened sheep are approximately 50% of body weight [2].

Total body water is distributed within two major compartments, extracellular fluid compartment and intracellular fluid compartment. Approximately two-thirds of total body water is intracellular fluid (40% of body weight) and one-third is extracellular fluid (20% of body weight). The extracellular fluid compartment can be further subdivided into interstitial fluid (~15% of body weight), the intravascular fluid or plasma volume (~5% of body weight), and transcellular fluid (very small % of body weight). The interstitial fluid compartment consists of cerebrospinal fluid, connective tissue, and, most importantly, the contents of the reticulorumen and the rest of the GI tract. The reticulorumen is an important reservoir of fluid for adult ruminants during periods of water restriction, and the GI tract can also be a site for water deposition during disease processes such as grain overload or endotoxemia. Dehydration causes a decrease in extracellular fluid volume secondary to a decrease in total body water and is characterized by an increase in packed cell volume and total protein. Hypovolemia is generally defined as a decrease in fluid in the intravascular volume, and hypovolemia can be treated rapidly by filling the vascular compartment to improve tissue perfusion. With dehydration, all fluid compartments are affected. Initially, dehydration results in reduction of the intravascular fluid compartment followed by contraction of the interstitial and intracellular fluid compartments. For dehydration, fluid deficits should be replaced more gradually to allow for fluid equilibriums to be reestablished between the various compartments of the extracellular fluid space.

Although the intracellular and extracellular fluid compartments differ in electrolyte composition, they are in osmotic equilibrium, and water can freely diffuse between them. The movement of water and electrolytes between compartments is governed by hydrostatic and oncotic forces. Sodium is the most important cation within the extracellular fluid compartment, accounting for about 95% of the total cation pool. Potassium is the major intracellular cation. The concentrations of sodium and potassium are maintained within and outside of cells by the Na^+/K^+-ATPase pump. Chloride and bicarbonate are the major anions within the extracellular fluid space, while phosphates, proteins, and other anions maintain electroneutrality with the potassium cation in the intracellular fluid compartment. Assessment of blood electrolyte concentrations and acid–base status is performed within the extracellular fluid compartment. When fluids are administered to dehydrated animals, fluid losses are replaced within the extracellular fluid compartment, and thus, the fluids being administered should contain concentrations of ions similar to what is found in the extracellular fluid compartment. Most disease processes in ruminants result in loss of fluids and electrolytes concurrently, and this is referred to as isotonic or iso-osmolar dehydration. In these cases, providing both fluid and electrolytes (mainly sodium) is important. Hypertonic dehydration or a relative water deficit occurs when water losses exceed losses of electrolytes, and water deprivation is an example. In contrast, hypotonic dehydration or relative water excess occurs when electrolyte losses exceed water losses. Hypotonic dehydration can occur in livestock with diarrhea, where loss of electrolytes and water occurs concurrently (isotonic dehydration), but the water deficit is replaced by water consumption or administration of 5% dextrose solutions. Another example of hypotonic dehydration occurs in ruminants with obstructive urolithiasis where sodium depletion exceeds water loss as sodium moves into the peritoneal cavity. In cases of urolithiasis with urinary bladder rupture, administration of fluids containing sodium is important.

Patient assessment

Physical examination of ruminants is very important prior to anesthesia to ensure that the correct fluid type is administered at an appropriate rate, as well as for identifying underlying disease processes that could complicate anesthesia. Intercurrent disease processes, hypothermia, and perinatal asphyxia can lead to difficulty in accommodating IV fluids during anesthesia and surgery. Fluid therapy can have adverse effects such as volume overload and pulmonary edema, so particular attention should be given to the cardiovascular, pulmonary, and renal systems. Respiratory disease is common in ruminants, especially weaning-age calves, kids, and lambs. In addition, mild, chronic lung pathology can be difficult to identify on clinical examination, yet this can negatively impact anesthesia and fluid therapy. Patients with respiratory disease have difficulty with gas exchange and are at greater risk of mortality, especially when general anesthesia and dorsal or lateral recumbency are utilized and the weight of the abdominal organs is further reducing lung capacity. Careful cardiac and pulmonary auscultation is important to identify animals at risk for anesthesia and fluid overload. Cardiovascular diseases may result in an inability to cope with an acute fluid load. Oliguric renal failure results in an impaired ability to excrete excess fluid. If concern exists following physical examination, preanesthetic diagnostic evaluation becomes important. A packed cell volume and total solids should be performed prior to induction of anesthesia for all cases. For cases where disease or organ dysfunction is suspected, a complete blood count, serum chemistry profile, blood gases, and radiographs should be performed. For suspected cardiovascular disease, echocardiography and electrocardiograms should be performed. Evidence of respiratory, cardiovascular, or renal disease should delay anesthesia until the problem is resolved or characterized as to the impact on anesthesia. Life-threatening abnormalities (dehydration and hypovolemia, hyperkalemia, metabolic acidosis) should be corrected prior to anesthesia if at all possible.

Dehydration is most accurately assessed by changes in body weight before and after a disease event, but this information is not usually available to the clinician; therefore, clinical assessment is utilized to assess degree of dehydration. The packed cell volume and total plasma protein can be used as tools to assess hydration status, and the packed cell volume also provides an assessment of oxygen-carrying capacity. However, measurements of packed cell volume and total solids cannot be used solely to replace an estimation of hydration status from physical examination. For example, the reference ranges for packed cell volume in healthy ruminants can be quite large [4], which makes this measurement too variable to be useful for sole estimation of hydration status. Total plasma protein concentration is dependent on colostral intake in neonates and can be elevated in patients with chronic inflammation. In addition, sheep, goats, and camelids with anemia and hypoproteinemia in conjunction with dehydration as occurs with intestinal parasitism can have a normal packed cell volume and total plasma protein concentration. Packed cell volume and total plasma protein concentrations are most useful in monitoring the progress of fluid therapy to prevent overhydration.

Percent dehydration can be estimated by assessing heart rate, degree of eyeball recession, mucous membranes for tackiness, color and capillary refill time, and skin elasticity or turgor (Table 10.1). Degree of enophthalmos has been used to assess hydration status

Table 10.1 Estimating level of dehydration based upon physical examination findings.

Percent (%) dehydration	Physical examination findings
<5	History of fluid loss but no findings on physical examination
5	Minimal depression, normal to mildly tacky mucous membranes, minimal enophthalmos, normal heart rate, normal capillary refill time (<2 seconds)
8	Depression, mild to moderate decreased skin turgor (skin tent 2–4 seconds), obvious enophthalmos, slight tachycardia (heart rate > 90 bpm), increased capillary refill time (3–4 seconds)
≥10	Severe depression, weakness, moderate to marked degree of decreased skin turgor (skin tent > 5 seconds), dry and dark mucous membranes, tachycardia (>120 bpm), increased capillary refill time (>5 seconds), cold extremities

in calves [5] and can be used to assess hydration in young small ruminants as well. The percent dehydration can be estimated by measuring the eyeball recession (in mm) and multiplying by 2. For example, a patient with eyeball recession of 4 mm is calculated to be 8% dehydrated. However, patients exhibiting eyeball recession of 6–8 mm are 10–14% dehydrated. The duration of skin tenting can also be used to estimate hydration status. The percent dehydration is estimated by measuring the skin tent (in seconds), multiplying by 2, and then subtracting 4. For example, a calf with a skin tent of 6 seconds is estimated to be 8% dehydrated. Some caveats to this clinical assessment of dehydration exist, and it is important for the clinician to remember that emaciated ruminants have poor skin elasticity and enophthalmos which can mimic dehydration.

Acid–base and electrolyte abnormalities are more difficult to assess without the aid of laboratory testing. Serum biochemistry and blood gas analyses can provide information on serum electrolyte abnormalities (sodium, potassium, chloride, bicarbonate, calcium, magnesium, phosphorus), acid–base disorders, or glucose abnormalities that require correction. In general, most cases of diarrhea in neonates and grain engorgement in adults will be characterized by a metabolic acidosis, whereas intestinal obstructions, abomasal disease and displacements, and renal disease will have a metabolic alkalosis. A clinical scoring system has been utilized to assess the degree of acidosis in calves with diarrhea [6]; however, this scoring system has not been applied to sheep or goats with diarrhea or for other clinical conditions that result in metabolic acidosis.

Fluid and electrolyte therapy in the perioperative period

Fluid and electrolyte replacement therapy in livestock is required when fluid intake by the animal is not enough to meet their metabolic needs. Rehydration, replacement of lost electrolytes, and restoration of acid–base balance are the goals for fluid therapy. Provision of IV fluids can restore the circulatory capacity and mental status sufficiently that nutrition and replacement of ongoing losses can be provided through oral fluids. The aggressiveness of treatment is dictated by the severity of the condition as well as economic considerations. When developing the fluid and electrolyte replacement therapy plan, three basic assessments should be made: (1) quantity and rate of fluid administration, (2) fluid type, and (3) method of fluid administration.

Quantity and rate of fluid administration

All patients that are to be anesthetized should have IV access for administration of fluids and drugs. Fluid therapy is not always indicated for patients undergoing short duration of anesthesia and surgery during which no or little fluid or blood loss occurs [7]. When anesthesia and surgical time exceed 1 hour, fluid therapy is indicated to replace insensible water loss, counteract the hypotensive effects of anesthetics, and maintain tissue perfusion. Recipe-based and goal-directed fluid therapy is used to maintain vascular volume and tissue perfusion [8]. A recipe-based or liberal approach is the most often utilized method for fluid administration during anesthesia for farm animals. Fluid administration rates of 3–10 ml/kg/hour of crystalloid solutions (e.g., normal saline, lactated Ringer's solution), but not to exceed 20 ml/kg, are used when the surgical procedure does not result in significant blood loss [8]. In the majority of situations, the rate of fluid administration should not exceed 10 ml/kg/hour. If minor blood loss occurs (<20 ml/kg), patients should receive 3 ml of a balanced electrolyte solution for every 1 ml of lost blood. In surgical procedures where significant blood loss occurs (>20 ml/kg), a colloid solution or whole blood should be administered for each volume of blood lost. Attempts should be made to maintain the packed cell volume greater than 20%, since a low packed cell volume in combination with hypotension can result in poor tissue perfusion and oxygenation. In cases where the total plasma protein becomes less than 3 g/dl, plasma administration should be considered. Goal-directed fluid therapy involves administration of fluids during anesthesia and surgery based upon measurements of cardiac performance such as systolic arterial blood pressure. In this situation, combinations of crystalloids and colloids are administered to maintain mean arterial blood pressure in the normal range during surgery (90–120 mm of Hg) [8]. Colloids such as albumin, hetastarch, and dextrans are not frequently used in anesthesia or fluid therapy for farm animal patients.

For anesthesia and surgical cases that present with dehydration, the fluid therapy plan is calculated to replace deficits while supplying maintenance fluid needs and accounting for ongoing loss of fluids associated with the disease process (Table 10.2). The first priority for treating dehydration is to restore the extracellular fluid volume back to normal. Multiply the estimation of dehydration by body weight in kilograms, and this will provide the quantity of fluid in liters recommended to restore an animal to a normal hydration. IV fluid therapy is recommended in cases where the estimation of dehydration is 8% or greater because oral fluid therapy will not be effective [9]. Since the methods for precisely measuring dehydration are not available, it is important for the clinician to remember that replacing the exact fluid deficit is not of chief concern. Rather, the clinician should replace a fluid deficit to restore tissue perfusion to improve response to anesthesia and surgery. Fluid given intravenously should be warmed prior to administration because cold fluids result in energy dissipation by the patient. If rehydration can be accomplished prior to anesthesia, a general rule of thumb is to replace half of the fluid deficit over 4–6 hours with the balance given over 12–24 hours. More often, the fluid deficit is replaced more rapidly

Table 10.2 Components and formulas for perioperative fluid therapy.

Category	Amount/formula
Fluid rate during anesthesia	3–10 ml/kg/hour but not to exceed 20 ml/kg/hour
Fluid deficit	% dehydration × body weight in kg
Fluid maintenance	50 ml/kg/day (adults) 80 ml/kg/day (neonates)
Ongoing losses with disease process	Up to 5% of body weight in kg
Bicarbonate deficit	Body weight (kg) × 0.3 × base deficit (adults) Body weight (kg) × 0.6 × base deficit (neonates)
Shock rate	90 ml/kg/hour
Blood transfusion	Administer 1 ml of whole blood for every ml of blood lost during surgery when significant blood loss occurs ml of donor blood = recipient blood volume × desired PCV – actual PCV/PCV of donor blood

(6 hours); however, care should be taken in hypothermic neonates or in cases of sepsis, as generalized edema may result. Specifically, too rapid IV fluid therapy can result in pulmonary and cerebral edema. Alternatively, the rate of fluid administration can be set at 50 ml/kg/hour which is less than the shock therapy rate at 90 ml/kg/hour.

Calculation of maintenance fluids is based upon the physiologic requirements of the patient. The normal adult requires about 50 ml/kg/day to provide enough fluids for digestion and losses through urine and defecation (sensible water loss) and sweat and respiration (insensible water loss). As stated previously, neonates have higher total body water than adults and therefore have higher maintenance fluid requirements. The maintenance fluid needs for neonates can be up to 80 ml/kg/day. When developing the fluid therapy plan, replacement of the deficit is of primary importance, but including maintenance fluid requirements and accounting for ongoing fluid losses in the calculations are important if the animal is not taking in fluids on its own. The maintenance fluid needs (50 ml/kg/day) can be simply converted to 1 ml/lb/hour or 2–4 ml/kg/hour. It is also important for the clinician to remember that this maintenance fluid requirement can change with ambient temperature and feed intake as diets may vary in moisture content. Care should be taken when patients are on continuous IV fluid therapy or when large volumes of fluids are given in a short period of time, as they can become hypoproteinemic and develop edema. Monitoring packed cell volume and total plasma protein is needed to prevent overhydration.

Pathologic water losses continue to occur in livestock even while fluid therapy is initiated, especially in cases of infectious diarrhea. Losses may continue as well for third-space sequestration of fluids such as grain engorgement or ruptured urinary bladder. These losses that are expected should be included in the fluid therapy plan. While it is difficult to estimate these losses, up to 5% of the body weight per day may be estimated as extra fluid losses for animals with severe diarrhea.

Fluid type

Many different and correct fluid types are available for IV administration in veterinary patients. For all practical purposes, the decision to administer IV fluids to expand fluid volume is far more important than the specific choice of fluid type and rate. The majority of patients will respond adequately to any balanced electrolyte fluid. The type of fluid to be administered ideally should be based on the individual patient's disease process and the measured or predicted acid–base or electrolyte deficits that must be corrected. Four basic categories of fluids are utilized for IV use in farm animal practice: crystalloids, colloids, whole blood, and parenteral nutrition. Crystalloid fluids are the mainstay of fluid therapy during anesthesia and consist primarily of water with a sodium or glucose base. Crystalloid fluids can be divided into four groups based upon purpose and include replacement, maintenance, hypertonic saline, and dextrose in water. Alternatively, crystalloid fluids can be divided based on tonicity and include hypotonic, isotonic, and hypertonic. Replacement crystalloid fluids are required with deficits of either electrolytes, water, or, most commonly, both. The commonly used replacement crystalloids in farm animal medicine are isotonic solutions and include the unbalanced solutions such as normal saline (0.9% NaCl) and sodium bicarbonate (1.3% $NaHCO_3$) and the balanced electrolyte solutions such as Ringer's solution (with lactate or acetate), Normosol R® (Hospira, Inc., Lake Forest, IL), and Plasma-Lyte A® (Baxter Healthcare Corp., Deerfield, IL). Balanced solutions resemble the composition of extracellular fluid. All replacement and maintenance crystalloids have a similar osmolality to plasma and can enter all body fluid compartments. These fluids will equilibrate quickly with interstitial fluids, so only 20–25% of the infused fluid remains within the intravascular compartment 1 hour after infusion. During anesthesia, the balanced crystalloid fluids are preferred to the unbalanced crystalloids with few exceptions. Dextrose-containing solutions are indicated for treatment of primary water deficits or hypoglycemia, and normal saline can be used in cases of hyperkalemia (urolithiasis), hyponatremia, or hypochloremia.

Normal saline (0.9% NaCl) has slightly higher sodium and higher chloride than plasma. Normal saline is considered an acidifying solution because it lowers plasma bicarbonate levels through volume expansion, reduction in renal bicarbonate absorption, and increased renal tubular chloride levels, which in turn promotes bicarbonate excretion in the renal collecting ducts. For ruminants with metabolic acidosis such as occurs with grain engorgement or neonatal diarrhea, normal saline is not the fluid of choice. Normal saline is a crystalloid fluid indicated for conditions associated with metabolic alkalosis or hyponatremia as would occur with GI obstruction or stasis such as a displaced abomasum, obstructive urolithiasis, and ruptured urinary bladder.

Balanced crystalloid fluids vary in their content of electrolytes, but in general, balanced crystalloid solutions contain electrolyte concentrations similar to that of plasma. Ringer's solution is an acidifying solution and is fairly similar to normal saline except with slightly lower levels of sodium, higher levels of chloride, and additional potassium and calcium. Lactated Ringer's solution is considered an alkalinizing solution, but the lactate present requires hepatic metabolism to produce bicarbonate, and only the L-isomer of lactate is metabolized efficiently to produce bicarbonate. The balanced crystalloids Normosol R® and Plasma-Lyte A® are also considered alkalinizing fluids because they both contain sodium acetate and sodium gluconate. Acetate and gluconate are bicarbonate precursors. Unlike lactate which is metabolized by the liver, acetate is metabolized by muscle tissue. Gluconate has been shown to be ineffective as an alkalizing agent in calves when administered intravenously but is effective orally [10]. Although some of these balanced crystalloid solutions are considered alkalinizing, they are considered inferior to the alkalinizing ability of 1.3%, 5%, or 8.4% sodium bicarbonate [3].

Sodium bicarbonate is the crystalloid fluid of choice for metabolic acidosis and can be used as either isotonic sodium bicarbonate (1.3%) or hypertonic sodium bicarbonate (5% or 8.4%) or added to other crystalloid solutions. Common causes of metabolic acidosis in ruminants include absorption of D-lactate from the GI tract (grain engorgement, enterocolitis) and sodium loss due to secretory diarrhea. Sepsis or other causes of systemic shock can also result in metabolic acidosis as a result of L-lactate accumulation from poor tissue perfusion. To correct metabolic acidosis, a total carbon dioxide (CO_2) measurement from a serum biochemistry panel or blood gas analysis is needed. The base deficit is calculated by subtracting the measured total CO_2 from the normal total CO_2 (approximate normal total CO_2 is 25). The amount of bicarbonate to administer to a patient can be calculated as follows: base deficit × body weight (kg) × 0.6 for neonates and base deficit × body weight (kg) × 0.3 for adults. Neonatal animals have a larger bicarbonate space than adult animals and thus have larger bicarbonate replacement needs when losses occur [9]. None of the crystalloid fluids previously discussed can provide enough base in 500 ml to correct the acidosis in this specific example, emphasizing the need for bicarbonate therapy in cases of severe metabolic acidosis in ruminants. Acid–base disturbances should be corrected prior to induction of anesthesia. The bicarbonate needed to correct metabolic acidosis can be given as a 1.3% isotonic solution, or alternatively the deficit can be added to normal saline and administered intravenously. As a general rule of thumb, the clinician should correct half of the calculated base deficit if the metabolic acidosis results from dehydration only. The entire deficit can be corrected if the dehydration is due to neonatal diarrhea or grain engorgement. Sodium bicarbonate is available commercially as hypertonic solutions of either 5% (0.6 mEq/ml) or 8.4% (1 mEq/ml). Solutions of 5% sodium bicarbonate can be given intravenously without dilution so long as the dehydration is corrected at the same time. The administration rate for 5% sodium bicarbonate should not exceed 2 ml/kg/min [11].

Dextrose-containing IV crystalloid solutions such as 5% dextrose in water (D5W) should not be used routinely as a stand-alone therapy because once the dextrose is metabolized, the fluid contains no active solute. Infusion of 5% dextrose can lead to dilution of serum electrolytes and the development of edema. However, glucose supplementation is important for hypoglycemic, hypothermic neonates and in ewes with pregnancy toxemia. Blood glucose can easily be measured with commercially available, handheld glucometers. In cases of hypoglycemia, dextrose can be administered as a 50% solution (dose of 0.2 ml/kg) or as a 5–10% solution intravenously. Dextrose can be added to other crystalloid fluids to make a 1% or 2% solution (20 ml of 50% dextrose per liter for each 1% of dextrose needed).

Hypertonic saline solutions are a crystalloid fluid that has gained increased use in ruminants over the past two decades. Hypertonic saline solutions (7.2% NaCl) rapidly increase intravascular volume by increasing intravascular hyperosmolality, thus drawing fluid from the intracellular and interstitial fluid compartments. The effect is transient and must be supplemented by additional volume replacement. Hypertonic saline solutions should be administered at a dose of 4 ml/kg over 3–10 minutes. Indications for hypertonic saline solution administration are severe dehydration, endotoxic shock, and hemorrhagic shock.

Hypertonic saline can also be administered during anesthesia to rapidly, but transiently, expand the vascular volume while additional, longer-lasting fluids can be administered. In cases of hemorrhagic shock, blood transfusions should be performed following therapy with hypertonic saline solutions. In cases of dehydration, hypertonic saline solutions should be followed with IV isotonic solutions ideally prior to induction of anesthesia.

Colloids are high-molecular-weight compounds that, unlike crystalloids, do not readily leave the intravascular space. Examples of colloids include plasma, human serum albumin, and synthetic compounds such as hetastarch, dextrans, and modified gelatin solutions. Plasma is used primarily in cases of failure of passive transfer and hypoproteinemia and is administered at a dose rate of 20–40 ml/kg [12]. The use of plasma for colloidal effects is relatively ineffective, as 50–100 ml/kg of body weight is required to raise serum albumin concentration by 1 g/dl. Plasma for livestock species is available commercially (Midwest Animal Blood Services, Inc., Stockbridge, MI).

Whole blood transfusions are primarily indicated when the red blood cell mass is inadequate to carry oxygen to the peripheral tissues. Whole blood transfusions are recommended when clinical signs suggestive of tissue hypoxia exist, such as elevated heart and respiratory rates, weakness, and lethargy, or when the packed cell volume drops below 15–20% in acute anemia and below 10–15% in chronic kg body weight anemia. Whole blood can be administered at a dose of 10–15 ml/kg; however, this will only result in an increase in packed cell volume of the recipient by 3–4%. For hemorrhagic shock, at least half of the estimated blood loss should be replaced by whole blood [12]. Whole blood transfusions can also be used as a source of plasma and can be given at a dose of 40–80 ml/kg. Monitoring of the transfusion is important, and the whole blood transfusion should be started at a slow rate (0.1 ml/kg/hour) with vital signs evaluated every 5 minutes. Clinical signs of anaphylactic reactions to whole blood transfusions include fever, dyspnea, hiccoughing, muscle tremors, salivation, and lacrimation. If a transfusion reaction is noted, blood administration is ceased and epinephrine (1:1000) can be administered at a dose of 0.01–0.02 ml/kg intravenously.

Method of administration

Administration of fluids is performed primarily by two routes, oral and IV. Subcutaneous, intraperitoneal, and intraosseous routes can be but are not commonly used. Subcutaneous fluid therapy is limited by volume; therefore, this route cannot meet the daily fluid needs of most livestock patients. In addition, subcutaneous fluids are contraindicated in animals that are severely dehydrated as blood is shunted away from the subcutaneous vasculature leading to poor absorption of the administrated fluids. With severe dehydration (>8% dehydrated), the IV route is required. IV fluids can be given as bolus injections or as a constant rate infusion. Oral fluids have the advantage of being less costly but the disadvantage of being less effective in cases involving GI stasis or severe dehydration. In addition, oral fluids cannot be given to adult livestock within 8–12 hours of anesthesia.

Catheterization of the jugular vein is the most widely used approach for fluid therapy in livestock. A catheter should be placed prior to anesthesia in ruminant patients. In younger animals, the jugular vein is very superficial and easy to visualize. For small ruminants and camelids, the fleece or hair might need to be clipped in order to visualize the jugular vein. In patients with severe dehydration, jugular catheterization can be difficult when the vessel is collapsed and not visible, in spite of prolonged occlusion. In addition, skin elasticity is diminished in dehydrated livestock, and this can cause problems with jugular catheterization. Placement of jugular catheters is best accomplished with proper positioning and restraint. For small ruminants and calves, jugular catheterization is easiest with the patient positioned in lateral recumbency if possible. After aseptic preparation of the jugular furrow, a local block can be performed over the catheterization site with 0.5–1 ml of 2% lidocaine using a 3-ml syringe and 25-gauge, 5/8-in. needle. After the site is blocked, a small stab incision through the skin is made with a #15 scalpel blade. The skin can either be pinched up away from the jugular or slid dorsally over the neck muscles during this incision to prevent inadvertent incision of the jugular vein. The small stab skin incision is very helpful in decreasing the amount of tissue drag and collapse of the jugular vein during catheter placement. Prior to placing the catheter, maximally expand the jugular vein by holding off at the thoracic inlet and allowing time for it to distend. In severely dehydrated or hypotensive sheep and goats, this may take time. Hold the catheter horizontally and flush it out with sterile heparinized saline. Heparinized saline can be purchased commercially or made in normal saline as 10 units/ml. The catheter is held by the hub with the index finger over and occluding the end of the hub. Insert the catheter through the stab incision. If there is any skin drag, set the catheter aside and deepen or extend the skin incision with the scalpel blade. Once the catheter is through the skin, line it up with the distended jugular at an angle of 45–60° and give a quick, short, forceful insertion. Lift your finger off the hub and watch for a flash of blood. If a flash of blood is evident, advance the catheter and stylet an additional 1 cm. Check for blood flash again, and if you are still in the jugular vein, slide the catheter off the stylet into the jugular vein and remove the stylet. In patients with severe hypovolemia or hemoconcentration, a flash of blood may not be observed in the catheter. This is more common if the animal is standing or in sternal recumbency than if the animal is in lateral recumbency. In these cases, check for position of the catheter within the jugular vein by attaching a syringe filled with heparinized saline to an extension set and periodically aspirating as you are trying to perform the initial venipuncture. Once the catheter is inserted, an injection port or extension set can be attached to the catheter, and the catheter should be checked for blood withdrawal and then flushed with heparinized saline. There are several methods for securing and protecting jugular catheters. The catheter and extension set or injection port can be sutured to the skin. White, porous tape can also be attached to the catheter injection port or extension set, and this tape can be sutured to the skin. The catheter can be additionally secured to the skin using a cyanoacrylate glue (Superglue®). Glue can also be placed where the end of the hub and catheter enters the skin. Extension sets are very useful but must be secured at another site on the body to prevent the catheter from being pulled out if the extension set or fluid line gets caught or tangled. Heparinized saline can be used to keep catheters patent when IV fluids are not running, and catheters should be flushed every 6–8 hours with heparinized saline.

IV catheters are available in various lengths, diameter, and construction materials. Teflon, polypropylene, polyurethane, and silastic catheter types are available for use. Teflon catheters need to be changed every 3 days, whereas polyurethane catheters can remain in the patient for up to 2 weeks. For adult cattle, a 14-gauge, 5¼-in. Teflon catheter is often used; however, 10- and 12-gauge catheters can be placed for rapid administration of fluids. For adult sheep and goats, a 16-gauge, 3¼-in. Teflon catheter is often used. For kids and lambs, an 18-gauge, 2-in. catheter is the appropriate size and length for jugular catheterization. The rate of fluid administration is proportional to the diameter of the catheter and inversely proportional to the length of the catheter.

Oral fluid therapy can be utilized for diseases of neonatal and adult farm animal patients. In general, oral fluid therapy is preferred since it is the most physiologic, but use of oral fluids is limited in cases set to undergo anesthesia and surgery. Oral fluids can be administered by orogastric or nasogastric intubation or through a rumenostomy surgery site. Syringe barrels or syringe cases can be adapted as a speculum. Orogastric tubes can be passed all the way down the esophagus into the reticulorumen in adult ruminants. For neonates, small red rubber feeding tubes or esophageal feeders are suitable, and these are ideally passed down to the midesophageal region. Deposition of milk and bicarbonate- or sodium-enriched fluids will stimulate esophageal groove closure and diversion of the fluid to the abomasum for digestion and absorption. Oral rehydration solutions formulated for calves can be utilized for the treatment of small ruminants. These solutions all contain variable concentrations of glucose, sodium, potassium, and chloride, and many contain an alkalinizing agent (bicarbonate, acetate, propionate), while others do not. All oral rehydration solutions must be mixed according to their label directions to avoid alterations in tonicity. Oral fluids can be administered at a dose of 3.5% of body weight at any one time.

Monitoring fluid administration

Fluid administration during anesthesia and surgery is performed to expand the vascular volume in order to improve cardiac output which will improve organ and tissue perfusion. As most drugs used for induction and maintenance of anesthesia decrease cardiac contractility and induce vasodilation, hypovolemia is a common negative effect encountered during or after anesthesia. Use of monitoring equipment including electrocardiogram and arterial blood pressure analyzers is important to monitor the effects of inadequate or excessive fluid administration. Mean arterial blood pressure should be maintained at least above 60 mm of Hg, preferably 70 mm of Hg in adult cattle [7]. IV fluids in combination with judicious use of vasopressors can help to maintain adequate blood pressure. Please refer to Chapter 6 for treatment of hypotension. Close monitoring of heart rate, pulse strength, respiratory rate, and color of mucous membranes should be performed during anesthesia and recorded. Monitoring for fluid overload is also extremely important and can be evaluated by central venous pressure measurements and pulmonary auscultation. Central venous pressure or jugular venous pressure measurements are often not performed during anesthesia in farm animals, but if available and pressures are greater than 15 mm of Hg, volume overload is occurring. Pulmonary auscultation is performed to detect increased bronchovesicular lung sounds that may be associated with pulmonary edema. Packed cell volume and total protein should be maintained above 20% and 3.5 g/dl, respectively, and serum electrolytes should be maintained within the reference ranges.

References

1. Sheng, H. and Huggins, R. (1979) A review of body composition studies with emphasis on total body water and fat. *The American Journal of Clinical Nutrition*, **32**, 630–647.
2. Carlson, G. and Bruss, M. (2008) Fluid, electrolyte, and acid–base balance, in *Clinical Biochemistry of Domestic Animals*, 6th edn (eds J. Kaneko, J. Harvey and M. Bruss), Elsevier, Amsterdam, pp. 529–560.
3. Berchtold, J. (1999) Intravenous fluid therapy of calves. *The Veterinary Clinics of North America. Food Animal Practice*, **15**, 505–531.
4. Kaneko, J., Harvey, J. and Bruss, M. (1997) Blood analyte reference values in large animals (Appendix VIII), in *Clinical Biochemistry of Domestic Animals*, 4th edn (eds J. Kaneko, J. Harvey and M. Bruss), Academic Press, San Diego, pp. 890–894.
5. Constable, P., Walker, P., Morin, D. and Foreman, J. (1998) Clinical and laboratory assessment of hydration status of neonatal calves with diarrhea. *Journal of the American Veterinary Medical Association*, **212**, 991–996.
6. Naylor, J. (1989) A retrospective study of the relationship between clinical signs and severity of acidosis in diarrheic calves. *The Canadian Veterinary Journal*, **30**, 577–580.
7. Riebold, T., Geiser, D. and Goble, D. (1995) Clinical techniques for food animal anesthesia, in *Large Animal Anesthesia: Principles and Techniques*, 2nd edn, Iowa State University Press, Ames, pp. 140–173.
8. Muir, W., Hubbell, J., Bednarski, R. and Lerche. (2013) Perioperative fluid administration, in *Handbook of Veterinary Anesthesia*, 5th edn (eds W. Muir, J. Hubbell, R. Bednarski and P. Lerche), Elsevier, St. Louis, pp. 306–329.
9. Roussel, A. and Navarre, C. (2009) Fluid therapy, transfusion, and shock therapy, in *Current Veterinary Therapy: Food Animal Medicine*, 5th edn (eds D. Anderson and D. Rings), Saunders/Elsevier, St. Louis, pp. 526–533.
10. Naylor, J. and Forsyth, G. (1986) The alkalinizing effects of metabolizable bases in the healthy calves. *Canadian Journal of Veterinary Research*, **50**, 509–516.
11. Constable, P. (2003) Fluid and electrolyte therapy in ruminants. *The Veterinary Clinics of North America. Food Animal Practice*, **19**, 557–597.
12. Divers, T. (2005) Blood component transfusions. *The Veterinary Clinics of North America. Food Animal Practice*, **21**, 615–622.

Chapter 11

Regulatory and legal considerations of anesthetics and analgesics used in food-producing animals

Thomas Passler

Department of Clinical Sciences, College of Veterinary Medicine, Auburn University, USA

Veterinarians and farm animal owners involved in the production of animals for human consumption are charged with providing a healthy, wholesome, and safe product. Consumers demonstrate an increased interest in the origin of their food and demand it be produced under standards that ensure the well-being of food-producing animals and prevent contamination of food with harmful microorganisms or residues. While much misconception about the use of pharmaceuticals in food-producing animals exists in the general public, ensuring that edible animal products are free from harmful residues is the legal and moral obligation of producers and veterinarians. To aid in this goal, labels for all drugs approved for use in food-producing animals must provide a withdrawal time for meat, milk, and/or eggs, and animal products cannot be harvested until this time elapses. This requirement is the result of important amendments to the Federal Food, Drug, and Cosmetics Act of 1938 (replaced the Pure Food and Drug Act of 1906), including the Delaney Clause of 1958 and the Kefauver–Harris Drug Amendments of 1962, that impose that drugs must be safe and efficacious and must not leave unsafe residues in edible animal products [1].

To achieve approval for marketing of a new animal drug, the sponsor must file a New Animal Drug Application (NADA) with the Food and Drug Administration (FDA) of the United States (US). The sponsor then must demonstrate in studies that the new drug is safe and efficacious in the target animal species, is safe for the environment, and can be manufactured to uniform standards of purity, strength, and identity. In addition, for food-producing animals, the sponsor must demonstrate that food products derived from treated animals are safe for human consumption. The goal of human food safety studies is a risk standard of "reasonable certainty of no harm," which is assessed in toxicity and residue chemistry studies [2]. Toxicity studies are performed to assess the toxic hazard of a drug and its metabolites resulting from consumption of products from treated animals and include genetic toxicity studies, 90-day feeding studies, and a two-generation reproduction study to assess cross-generational toxicity and teratogenic potential of a new drug [2].

Farm Animal Anesthesia: Cattle, Small Ruminants, Camelids, and Pigs, First Edition.
Edited by HuiChu Lin and Paul Walz.

Residue and metabolism studies are performed to describe the fate of a drug following administration to the target species. For drugs demonstrated to require a withdrawal time, residue depletion studies are performed. The drug is administered at the largest label dose for the longest label duration to evaluate residue depletion to below a tolerated concentration (tolerance). For withdrawal time calculations, the FDA, using parametric statistical methods, determines 99% tolerance limits with 95% confidence, indicating that there is only a 5% chance that 1 of 100 animals treated in accordance with label directions has tissue residues that exceed the tolerance value [2]. While similar in approach, the European Committee for Veterinary Medicinal Products (CVMP) determines withdrawal periods using different statistical methods and suggests that 95% tolerance limits are more appropriate [3]. Support and criticism exist for these methods, and alternative statistical procedures have been proposed including nonparametric methods that do not require the satisfaction of assumptions of parametric methods to estimate withdrawal times [4–7]. Additional concerns have been expressed regarding withdrawal time calculations for injection sites, from which the depletion of residues is extremely slow and erratic [8, 9]. Various factors influence metabolism and degradation of injectable pharmaceuticals at the injection site, which can result in different residue depletion profiles as compared to other tissues [10]. In different countries, varying assessments are used by licensing authorities to evaluate human food safety implications of injection site residues, and the necessity for an internationally harmonized approach has been emphasized [10].

Veterinarians are commonly faced with the need to administer medications in a fashion or to a species that is not in accordance with label directions. When using pharmaceuticals in an extralabel fashion, the veterinarian assumes the legal responsibility of assuring that the product is safe, efficacious, and will not leave harmful residues in animal products intended for human consumption. The Animal Medicinal Drug Use Clarification Act (AMDUCA) of 1994 amended the Federal Food, Drug, and Cosmetics Act to allow veterinarians to prescribe approved animal drugs in an extralabel fashion but also defined several conditions and stipulations, including [11]:

- Extralabel drug use is permitted only by the order of a licensed veterinarian within the context of a valid veterinarian–client–patient relationship.
- No other approved animal drug is labeled and contains the same active ingredient in the required dosage and concentration, except when the veterinarian finds the approved drug to be clinically ineffective.
- The health of the animal is threatened, or suffering or death may result from failure to treat.
- Extralabel drug use is not permitted to enhance production or for feed additives.
- Extralabel use of an approved human drug is not permitted in food-producing animals if an approved animal drug can be used in extralabel fashion.
- Appropriate labeling information including withdrawal times for meat, milk, and/or eggs as specified by the veterinarian must be provided.
- Assure that the identity of the treated animal is recorded and records are maintained.
- Extralabel use that may result in residues above an established safe level or tolerance or present a risk to public health is not permitted.

The effects of antimicrobial use in food animals and resulting residues in animal products have received much attention, but human safety concerns unique to residues associated with anesthetic and analgesic drugs exist. At least four idiosyncratic or allergic responses related to anesthetic or anesthetic adjuncts can occur in humans, including malignant hyperthermia, halothane hepatitis, porphyria, and allergic reactions [1]. Violative residues of anesthetics are much less frequently detected than those of antimicrobials or anthelmintics, and adverse reactions in humans exposed to anesthetic residues are not reported. For the year of 2010, the United States Department of Agriculture Food Safety and Inspection Service (USDA FSIS) reported the greatest proportions of violative residues were antibiotics, anthelmintics, and pesticides with 0.1%, 0.43%, and 0.21% of samples above tolerance limits, respectively [12]. While sensitive detection methods exist, the infrequency of detecting anesthetic residues in food animal tissues may in part result from paucity of routine testing. Additional factors that decrease the risk of anesthetic residues include the following: (1) short-term use for single procedures reduces the risk of accumulation; (2) short half-life ($t½$) of most available anesthetics; (3) common intravenous (IV) or inhalation anesthetic administration results in more rapid absorption as compared to other routes of administration; (4) potency of current anesthetics results in low doses; and (5) unlike many other drugs, anesthetics are usually used under direct supervision of a veterinarian [13]. Following the use of an anesthetic for surgery, sufficient time for drug elimination usually elapses before slaughter; however, risk of violative residues exists when fractious animals are tranquilized for transportation to slaughter or show animals are sedated in shows preceding sale. As most anesthetic or anesthetic adjunct drugs are not approved for use in food animals, their use commonly falls under the regulations of AMDUCA. Considerable heterogeneity exists in the metabolism and excretion of pharmaceuticals within and especially between species, limiting the ability to extrapolate residue information from one species to another. Therefore, an extended withdrawal time should be considered when using a drug approved for one food animal species in another species.

The primary resource for information for veterinarians using pharmaceuticals in an extralabel fashion is the Food Animal Residue Avoidance Databank (FARAD) that was established as part of the USDA FSIS Residue Avoidance Program of 1982 [14, 15]. On its webpage, veterinarians can search the database for approved food animal drugs and find recommended withdrawal times for extralabel use of some drugs. In addition, veterinarians can contact FARAD by email or in emergencies by phone, and FARAD personnel will recommend an appropriate withdrawal interval according to individual features of each case. Recommendations are based on available pharmacokinetic studies, and members of FARAD developed an extrapolated withdrawal-interval estimator (EWE) algorithm that facilitates the calculation of extended withdrawal times in a repeatable and scientifically valid fashion [16]. The accuracy of the recommended withdrawal times depends on available pharmacokinetic data, and more conservative estimates are provided when little data is available.

When tissue residue depletion data are not available, the plasma $t½$ can be used to calculate withdrawal times, and this approach is a viable alternative for many drugs [17, 18]. For other drugs, such as those that concentrate in target tissues or that have metabolites that are excreted at a slower rate than the parent drug, plasma $t½$-derived estimates of withdrawal time may be too short. Furthermore, pharmacokinetic studies are performed in healthy animals and drug elimination in sick animals with compromised kidney or liver function may be prolonged [13]. The animal groups in which violative residues are most often reported are veal calves and culled dairy cows, in which elimination kinetics are often altered due to disease and reduced excretory function [19]. Considering the various factors that can influence drug elimination, adding a safety margin to the withdrawal time in sick and debilitated animals is prudent.

Some general rules apply when extrapolating withdrawal times in the absence of available information from FARAD [19, 20]:

1 For drugs that are eliminated in a linear fashion, doubling the dose will add an additional $t½$ to the withdrawal time, provided the same route and volume per site are administered.
2 99.9% of a drug is eliminated after $10t½$, which can be a good rule of thumb to extrapolate the withdrawal time for many drugs. However, the remaining 0.01% must be below the tolerance level for tissue residues, and tissue deposition must not occur.
3 In smaller species, $t½$ are generally shorter than in larger species, and directly extrapolating withdrawal times from cattle to small ruminants is often appropriate.

With some exceptions, most anesthetics and anesthetic adjuncts have very short elimination $t½$ and should be largely cleared from the body after 48–96 hours [13].

Alpha-2 agonists

Alpha-2 agonists include xylazine, detomidine, and medetomidine that induce sedation and analgesia. While xylazine and detomidine are commonly used in farm animals, in the US, xylazine is approved only for horses and Cervidae and detomidine is approved only for horses. Cattle and small ruminants are very sensitive to the effects of xylazine. For systemic administration of xylazine, typical doses range from 0.05 to 0.3 mg/kg in cattle and 0.05 to 0.2 mg/kg in small ruminants. The pharmacokinetic profile of xylazine is best described by a two-compartment model with a rapid distribution phase and a large volume of distribution [21]. Following IV administration, the distribution $t½$ was 1.2 minutes in cattle and 1.9 minutes in sheep [22]. The elimination $t½$ of xylazine following IV administration is 36 minutes in cattle and 23 minutes in sheep and is very similar when the drug is administered intramuscularly. Xylazine is rapidly metabolized to inactive compounds, and elimination occurs mainly by urinary excretion of these metabolites. In cattle, the primary metabolite of xylazine is 2,6-dimethylaniline, a toxic substance demonstrated to be carcinogenic in rats [21]. The toxicity of 2,6-dimethylaniline, which is used for many industrial manufacturing processes, has been studied extensively, and its genotoxic and carcinogenic properties have prevented the FDA from establishing an acceptable daily intake [21, 23]. However, there is currently no evidence that xylazine has carcinogenic potential for livestock at sedative doses and ingestion of edible tissues from xylazine-treated animals appears to pose an extremely low risk [24, 25].

In contrast to the US, xylazine is approved for use in food animals in various countries and withdrawal times vary nationally. The FARAD has updated its previous recommendations for xylazine withdrawal times, based on approval of the drug in New Zealand [26]. In that study, a single intramuscular (IM) dose of 0.35 mg/kg of xylazine followed by 4 mg/kg of IV tolazoline was administered, and concentrations of xylazine and 2,6-dimethylaniline were below the limit of detection (10 μg/kg) by 72 hours in tissues and 12 hours in milk [27]. Currently, a withdrawal time of 4 days for meat and 24 hours for milk is recommended for doses of 0.05–0.3 mg/kg by IM administration [26]. For larger doses of xylazine (0.3–2 mg/kg) administered intramuscularly, the recommended meat withdrawal time is 10 days and milk withdrawal time is 120 hours. For IV administration of 0.016–0.1 mg/kg of xylazine, recommended withdrawal times are 5 days for meat and 72 hours for milk. These recommendations pertain to single and multiple doses and are identical to those for sheep and goats [28]. For swine, a withdrawal time of 18 days is recommended for a single IM xylazine administration of up to 2.2 mg/kg (FARAD, email communication, December 2013). For Cervidae, including elk, fallow deer, mule deer, sika deer, and white-tailed deer, species-specific IM doses are provided. Xylazine should not be administered 15 days before or during the hunting season, and a minimum withdrawal time of 14 days is recommended [28]. In an emergency, xylazine is approved for use in organic livestock production, which requires a meat withdrawal time of 8 days and a milk discard period of 4 days [29].

The newer α_2 agonist detomidine has similar effects as xylazine, but in contrast to xylazine treatment, animals usually remain standing after an IV dose of detomidine [24]. When administered intramuscularly at 0.05 mg/kg to facilitate castration of rams and bucks, detomidine affected body temperature, heart and respiratory rates, and blood pressure similarly but provided superior analgesia to xylazine administered at 0.2 mg/kg [30]. Detomidine is labeled for IV or IM use in horses, but IV use has been recommended for most clinical scenarios [24]. An IV dose of 0.01 mg/kg is commonly used [24]. In goats, 0.01 mg/kg of detomidine produced sedation only when administered intravenously, and this dose did not result in observable analgesia. In contrast, doses of 0.02 or 0.04 mg/kg produced effective sedation and moderate analgesia by IV or IM administration. Ataxia and sternal recumbency were observed in all goats when detomidine was administered at 0.04 mg/kg [31]. In cattle, detomidine is characterized by rapid distribution and elimination, with elimination *t*½ of 1.32 hours after IV administration and 2.56 hours after IM administration [32]. Excretion of detomidine in milk is very low and concentrations of 0.4 ng/g were present at the first milking 11 hours after dosing, and no detectable amounts were present at 23 hours following administration [32]. Recommended withdrawal times for single or multiple IM or IV doses of up to 0.08 mg/kg are 3 days for meat and 72 hours for milk for cattle and small ruminants [28].

The pharmacologic effects of α_2 agonist are commonly reversed using the α_2 antagonist tolazoline, which is generally administered at 2–4 mg/kg by slow IV infusion. In 13 steers and 10 lactating dairy cows, tolazoline was administered 10 minutes after sedation produced by xylazine, and tissue and milk concentrations were evaluated [27]. Concentrations of tolazoline were below the limit of quantification (10 μg/kg) by 96 hours in tissues and 48 hours in milk. These data served as basis for current FARAD withdrawal time recommendations for tolazoline, which are 8 days for meat and 48 hours for milk following a single IV dose of 2–4 mg/kg [26].

Barbiturates

The short-acting barbiturate thialbarbitone and ultrashort-acting barbiturates thiamylal and thiopental are approved for use in food animals, but they are not currently available. The short duration of narcosis following single IV infusion of *N*-methyl-barbiturates and thiobarbiturates is not a result of rapid metabolism, but instead of redistribution to less vascularized muscle and fat tissues. After administration, the short-acting barbiturates almost instantly enter the brain and other organs that receive large proportions of the cardiac output. Subsequently, redistribution to larger, less vascularized muscle and fat tissues occurs, resulting in recovery and consciousness. A large proportion of short-acting and ultrashort-acting barbiturates can redistribute to adipose tissues, depending on the amount of body fat, and accumulation in adipose tissues can occur with repeated administration. The FARAD has established withdrawal times of 1 day for meat and 24 hours for milk after administration of the ultrashort-acting barbiturates, thiamylal (up to 5.5 mg/kg) and thialbarbitone (up to 9.4 mg/kg) [28]. In small ruminants, recommended withdrawal times for a single IV dose of up to 5 mg/kg of thiopental are 1 day for meat and 24 hours for milk [33]. Ultrashort-acting barbiturates are most commonly used for induction of anesthesia. Today, their uses have been replaced by other injectable anesthetics capable of producing short-term anesthesia such as ketamine and propofol.

Benzodiazepines

The minor tranquilizers, diazepam and midazolam, are used for their anxiolytic, anticonvulsant, and central muscle-relaxing effects. They are suitable for use alone to produce mild tranquilization, or for induction of anesthesia when combined with an anesthetic such as ketamine. Benzodiazepines can be especially useful for use in high-risk animals, such as geriatric or debilitated livestock, because of their minimal cardiovascular and pulmonary effects. Additionally, benzodiazepines have a short-lived appetite-stimulating effect. An injectable formulation containing brotizolam (Mederantil®) is commercially available and approved for use as appetite stimulation in cattle in some European countries.

Benzodiazepines rapidly penetrate the blood–brain barrier, and maximal brain concentrations are achieved within a minute following IV administration [34]. In sheep, diazepam reaches maximal serum concentrations in 14.6 ± 7.2 minutes following IM administration, which is much more rapid than in humans [35]. Diazepam and midazolam are metabolized by the liver, and high concentrations of active diazepam metabolites are present in the blood stream following administration. Elimination kinetics and other pharmacokinetic characteristics vary greatly between species [36], making the extrapolation of appropriate withdrawal times from other species difficult. The prevention of benzodiazepine residues in tissues of farm animals is critical because a variety of adverse effects can occur in humans [13]. Pharmacokinetic and residue studies guiding withdrawal time recommendations for benzodiazepines in food-producing animals are currently lacking. Therefore, a conservative estimate of withdrawal time of 30 days for meat should be used [13]. For IV doses of diazepam of up to 0.1 mg/kg in cattle and small ruminants, FARAD recommends a withdrawal time of 10 days (FARAD, email communication, December 2013). Benzodiazepines should not be used in lactating dairy cattle [13].

Dissociative anesthetics

Dissociative anesthesia differs from narcosis induced by other anesthetics, as in addition to the depressive components such as unconsciousness and analgesia, catalepsy and spasms are also induced. The mechanism of action is understood to be a noncompetitive blockade of glutamate at the *N*-methyl-D-aspartate (NMDA) receptor. Only two dissociative anesthetics, ketamine and tiletamine, are used in veterinary medicine. Ketamine is usually administered in combination with other anesthetics and can be used for anesthesia induction and maintenance protocols. Tiletamine is available only in combination with a benzodiazepine derivative, zolazepam, and this combination (Telazol®) is widely used for immobilization and anesthesia in various species.

While tissue residue data for ketamine are not available, the European Committee for Veterinary Medicinal Products concluded that a maximum residue limit (MRL) does not need to be established for ketamine, because "ketamine is rapidly absorbed and extensively excreted" and the drug is used only in individual animals that are not sent for slaughter during or immediately after treatment [37]. Different studies have investigated the pharmacokinetics of ketamine in food animals, demonstrating rapid elimination following administration. Ketamine is rapidly metabolized, and its major metabolite norketamine contributes to the analgesic effects of ketamine [38, 39].

In calves administered with 5 mg/kg of ketamine intravenously, the elimination $t½$ was 60.5 ± 5.4 minutes. In the same study, the administration of xylazine did not significantly alter the elimination $t½$ of ketamine in calves receiving ketamine 10 minutes after premedication with 0.2 mg/kg of xylazine. However, premedication with xylazine resulted in a significantly lower volume of distribution and clearance of ketamine and prolonged the duration of anesthesia [40]. In calves administered subanesthetic doses of xylazine (0.05 mg/kg) and ketamine (0.1 mg/kg) to provide sedation without recumbency (**Ketamine Stun**) prior to castration, similar pharmacokinetic parameters were determined [38]. In lactating dairy cows receiving IV administration of 5 mg/kg of ketamine, the plasma elimination $t½$ was 1.8 ± 0.5 hours, and ketamine was undetectable at 12 hours with the last detectable concentration present at 8 hours following administration [41]. In milk samples, ketamine was detectable until 48 hours of the study, and no residues were present at 60 hours after administration [41].

In sheep, a similar but shorter $t½$ of 40 minutes of ketamine was reported [39]. Ketamine and its metabolites were rapidly detected in the urine of intravenously injected sheep, with peak concentrations occurring at 20 minutes. At 24 hours following administration, large concentrations of ketamine metabolites are present, but only trace amounts of ketamine are present in the urine samples [39]. In swine, ketamine is highly bioavailable and rapidly absorbed following IM administration with peak plasma concentrations detected between 1 and 15 minutes [42]. Considerable individual differences of maximal plasma concentrations

(1.5–12 μg/ml) and total amount of ketamine (AUC, 14.5–42.5 μg/hour/ml) were detected between pigs. Immobilization and sternal recumbency were observed 1–5 minutes after IM injection. The duration of lateral recumbency varied from 9 to 48 minutes in young pigs, while a considerably longer duration was observed in adult sows (78–88 minutes). Elimination *t*½ varied between 1.7–2.9 hours for ketamine and 1.4–3.2 hours for norketamine. Analgesic effects of ketamine varied between individual animals, and the duration of recumbency correlated directly with plasma concentrations of ketamine [42].

Recommended withdrawal times following single and multiple IM administrations of up to 10 mg/kg of ketamine in cattle and small ruminants are 3 days for meat and 48 hours for milk. For IV doses of up to 2 mg/kg, withdrawal time recommendations are also 3 days for meat and 48 hours for milk [28]. For larger doses of intravenously administered ketamine (up to 5 mg/kg), a milk withdrawal time of 48 hours is recommended by FARAD based on a previous publication [41]. However, as discussed earlier, ketamine was still present in the milk of five of six cows in that study, and the authors recommend adherence to a longer withdrawal time (72 hours) than currently provided by FARAD [41]. For swine, a meat withdrawal time of 2 days is recommended for a ketamine dose of 10 mg/kg by IM or IV administration (FARAD, email communication, December 2013). Many anesthetic protocols use larger doses of ketamine for swine, prompting the necessity for longer withdrawal times. For IM doses of up to 20 mg/kg in swine, a meat withdrawal time of 4 days was recommended (Food Animal Residue Avoidance Databank (FARAD) (A component of the Food Animal Residue Avoidance and Depletion Program), email communication, December 2013).

While the use of Telazol is reported in various species, there was no published report on the pharmacokinetics and tissue residues in cattle or small ruminants; hence, FARAD was unable to make a recommendation for withdrawal time of the anesthetic [28]. In pigs administered with a single IM dose of Telazol of 10 mg/kg, maximal plasma concentrations were detected at 31.92 minutes (range 15–75 minutes) for tiletamine and 65.17 minutes (range 15–135 minutes) for zolazepam. The *t*½ were 3.67 ± 3.01 hours and 8.39 ± 5.67 hours for tiletamine and zolazepam, respectively [43]. A 30-day meat withdrawal time for IM Telazol up to 2 mg/kg was recommended for swine by (FARAD, email communication, December 2013).

Local anesthetics

Local anesthetics include lidocaine, mepivacaine, and bupivacaine that can be used as local analgesics for minor or standing surgeries and for epidural anesthesia in farm animals. The mechanism of action is the blockade of fast voltage-gated Na^+ channels of neuronal membranes, thus preventing signal transduction. Only lidocaine is approved for use in food animals in the US and can be used in cattle for epidural anesthesia with a total volume of up to 15 ml or nerve blocks up to 20 ml. Frequently, larger volumes must be locally infiltrated during surgeries on adult cattle, which constitutes an extralabel drug use. As for xylazine, the toxic metabolite 2,6-dimethylaniline (2,6-xylidine) is produced and can be detected in tissues and milk of animals treated with lidocaine [44]. However, a risk assessment report indicated that hazard to human health from lidocaine and 2,6-dimethylaniline was deemed unlikely due to rapid excretion and the presence of insignificant concentrations in consumed food animal products [45].

In cattle, lidocaine is rapidly metabolized and excreted following administration [46]. In adult cattle, the plasma *t*½ was 1.06±0.70 hours following IV administration [47]. Following an inverted-L block using 100 ml of 2% lidocaine subcutaneously, maximal lidocaine concentrations were detected in plasma at 0.521±0.226 hours [48]. The serum *t*½ following subcutaneous (SC) administration was 4.19±1.69 hours, which is considerably longer than after IV administration [47, 48]. Lidocaine was detectable in serum for 8.5±1.4 hours and milk for 32.5±16.2 hours following administration for inverted-L nerve block [48]. The administration of 0.22 mg/kg of 2% lidocaine (~6 ml per adult cow) for caudal epidural anesthesia did not result in detectable concentrations of lidocaine in serum and milk [48].

A study in fetal, neonatal, and adult sheep evaluated pharmacokinetic parameters after IV administration of 5 or 10 mg/kg of lidocaine and demonstrated a rapid decline of drug concentrations following administration [49]. The elimination *t*½ of lidocaine was 30.9 minutes in adult nonpregnant sheep and 51.0 minutes in neonatal sheep. In another study, similar elimination *t*½ were detected, which were 38.1±2.1 minutes in nonpregnant and 31.9±3.0 minutes in pregnant sheep [50]. Lidocaine rapidly crosses the placental barrier. IV administration of catheterized fetuses showed detectable lidocaine concentrations in maternal blood within 2 minutes, indicating rapid equilibration of lidocaine between a dam and her fetus [49]. During constant rate infusion of lidocaine, fetuses receive approximately half of the maternal dose by weight (weight-normalized fetal–maternal dose ratio, 0.45) [51]. While toxic doses of lidocaine can cause neurologic signs including convulsions, low doses of lidocaine can be used therapeutically as an anticonvulsant [52, 53]. A study evaluating pharmacokinetics and toxicity of lidocaine in neonatal pigs determined an elimination *t*½ of 2.67±1.28 hours. As in sheep, it is longer in neonatal pigs than in adult pigs in which an elimination *t*½ of 1.12 hours was described [52, 54].

While lidocaine is labeled for use in cattle, a withdrawal time is not provided. The FARAD recommendations for withdrawal times in cattle at label indications and doses are 1 day for meat and 24 hours for milk following single and multiple doses or up to 15 ml by epidural administration. For single SC infiltrations (inverted-L block) with a total volume of up to 100 ml (2 gm) of lidocaine based on a previous report in lactating dairy cows, a withdrawal time of 4 days for meat and 72 hours for milk is recommended [48]. These recommendations should also be appropriate for other farm animals that have shorter elimination *t*½ than cattle. In horses, the lidocaine clearance time is reported to be of 60 hours, which is longer than those of mepivacaine and bupivacaine [13]. There are no similar comparisons reported in food animals.

Opioids

The mechanism of action of opioids is binding of μ, κ, and δ opioid receptors, located in the central and peripheral nervous systems, as well as joints and cornea. Opioids used in veterinary medicine are either selective or partially selective μ receptor agonists, which include morphine, meperidine, fentanyl, oxymorphone, methadone, buprenorphine, and butorphanol [24]. While limited pharmacokinetic data are available in food animals, opioids exhibit rapid elimination with elimination $t½$ approximately 3–4 hours in most species [13].

In food animals, morphine has poor analgesic properties when used parentally, and frequent administration is necessary to maintain therapeutic blood concentrations [24]. Recommended analgesic doses for morphine in food animals include 0.05–0.1 mg/kg for cattle, 0.2 mg/kg intramuscularly (up to 20 mg) for swine, and doses up to 10 mg intramuscularly for small ruminants, but larger doses in goats (up to 10 mg/kg) have also been recommended [24, 55]. The elimination $t½$ of morphine in farm animals is approximately 1–2 hours, which was reported to be 87.9 minutes in horses and 86 minutes in sheep [24, 56, 57].

In addition to parenteral administration, morphine can be administered epidurally at 0.1 mg/kg to relieve pain of the perineum, posterior abdomen, or rear limb. This route of administration has two major benefits: (1) the duration of activity is prolonged and thought to be approximately 12 hours in cattle, and (2) unlike with local anesthetics such as lidocaine, epidural administration of morphine does not paralyze the motor nerves of the hind limbs [24]. Diffusion of morphine into the spinal cord is slow with peak activity observed at 210–250 minutes following administration. Epidural morphine can be administered via the lumbosacral space or caudal epidural space, and the dose should be repeated every 12 hours for management of chronic pain. In a study in horses given an IV dose of morphine of 0.1 mg/kg, a serum elimination $t½$ of 87.9 minutes was determined. Morphine was detected for 48 hours in the blood and 144 hours in the urine. The authors recommended that horses should not be treated with morphine within 1 week of a race [56]. Because of lack of information regarding tissue pharmacokinetics, FARAD currently does not recommend the use of morphine in food animals (FARAD, email communication, December 2013). From the limited data in goats, morphine has a large volume of distribution which can be taken up into cells and may persist in tissues after plasma clearance. For cattle, sheep, and goats receiving a single dose of 0.1 mg/kg by IV, IM, or epidural administration, FARAD suggests a meat withdrawal time of 14 days and milk withdrawal time of 48 hours. For repeated dosing, up to six doses, the recommended meat and milk withdrawal times are 28 days and 96 hours, respectively (FARAD, email communication, December 2013).

Butorphanol is likely the most commonly used opioid in farm animals and is administered either alone or in combination with other drug for analgesia or as part of the anesthetic protocols. Furthermore, butorphanol is used as an appetite stimulant, but this use is based on anecdotal efficacy [46]. In addition to affinity for μ receptors, butorphanol is a κ receptor agonist which provides visceral analgesia [34]. In farm animals, butorphanol is commonly used at doses between 0.02 and 0.25 mg/kg, and repeated dosing every 4 hours is necessary to maintain analgesic plasma concentrations [24]. In nonlactating dairy cows administered 0.25 mg/kg of butorphanol by single IV administration, rapid and extensive distribution followed by a slower elimination phase was observed [58]. The mean elimination $t½$ was 82 minutes (range 69–15 minutes). In the same study, three lactating dairy cows received a smaller IV dose of 0.045 mg/kg, and trace quantities of butorphanol in milk were detected for 36 hours [58]. Butorphanol is commonly used in combination with other sedatives to enhance the analgesic effect of xylazine [59]. In calves receiving IM xylazine (0.05 mg/kg), ketamine (0.1 mg/kg), and butorphanol (0.025 mg/kg), butorphanol was rapidly absorbed (T_{max} 9.5 ± 0.5 minutes) and cleared from the plasma [60]. The elimination *t*½ for butorphanol in these calves was 68.23 ± 7.13 minutes. Withdrawal times of 5 days for meat and 72 hours for milk or 4 days for meat and 72 hours for milk have been recommended following butorphanol administration in cattle [24, 46]. Butorphanol is an allowed substance for use in organic livestock production, which requires a meat withdrawal time of at least 42 days and a milk withdrawal time of at least 8 days [29].

Relatively little information is available regarding the use and the pharmacokinetics of other opioids such as fentanyl in farm animals. In sheep, IV administration of 2.5 μg/kg of fentanyl resulted in a short elimination *t*½ of 3.08 hours [61]. In the same study, transdermal fentanyl patches with a total dose of 12.8 ± 1.8 mg/kg/sheep were applied to sheep for 72 hours [61]. Adverse effects associated with opioids were not observed in these sheep. The time to maximum concentration following transdermal application was 12 hours (range 4–24 hours), and the elimination *t*½ was 15.6 hours (range 10.9–27.2 hours). An average plasma concentration of 84.6 ± 45.7 pg/ml of fentanyl was detectable in samples 12 hours after patch removal. While the optimal concentration for analgesia has not been determined in sheep, maximal plasma concentrations of fentanyl applied transdermally (C_{max} = 1302.0 pg/ml) were within the range of concentrations considered sufficient for analgesia in humans [61]. In goats, IV administration of 2.5 μg/kg of fentanyl resulted in an elimination *t*½ of 1.20 ± 0.78 hours [62]. However, transdermal application of fentanyl (50 μg/hour) in these goats resulted in large variation of peak plasma concentrations (1.12–16.69 ng/ml, mean 6.99 ± 6.03 ng/ml) and time to peak plasma concentrations (8–18 hours, mean 13 ± 4.5 hours). The elimination *t*½ following patch removal was 5.34 ± 5.34 hours [62]. Because of large variability in pharmacokinetic data and lack of tissue residue studies, conservative withdrawal time recommendations should be made following treatment with transdermal fentanyl patches.

Nonsteroidal anti-inflammatory drugs

Nonsteroidal anti-inflammatory drugs (NSAIDs) exert antipyretic, anti-inflammatory, and analgesic properties by inhibition of cyclooxygenase enzymes that synthesize proinflammatory prostaglandins. Currently, only flunixin meglumine is labeled for use in food animals in the US, but other NSAIDs including aspirin, carprofen, meloxicam, and phenylbutazone have also been used by veterinarians [46]. In this chapter, the most frequently used flunixin meglumine, aspirin, and meloxicam will be discussed in detail. The administration of phenylbutazone is discouraged in food animals, and because flunixin meglumine is approved in the US, the extralabel use of carprofen and ketoprofen would be difficult to justify under the guidelines of AMDUCA. Carprofen, ketoprofen, and phenylbutazone are reviewed in detail in other reports [46, 63] and also in Chapter 9 of this book.

In cattle, flunixin meglumine is labeled for the control of pyrexia associated with bovine respiratory disease, endotoxemia, and acute bovine mastitis at a dose of 2.2 mg/kg every 24 hours or 1.1 mg/kg every 12 hours. Use of other NSAIDs in cattle would be in an extralabel fashion and would be illegal under the guidelines of AMDUCA if used for the same indications, unless the veterinarian can justify that flunixin meglumine would not be effective for that patient. An injectable solution labeled for swine for the control of pyrexia associated with swine respiratory disease is also available. This product is labeled for IM administration at 2.2 mg/kg and is not recommended for use in breeding swine.

In cattle, flunixin meglumine is labeled only for IV use. In addition to causing significant tissue damage, SC or IM administration could prolong the elimination of flunixin meglumine from tissues and may result in violative residues [64, 65]. Multiple studies demonstrated prolonged elimination $t½$ for flunixin meglumine when administered subcutaneously or intramuscularly as compared to that following IV administration. The elimination $t½$ following a single IV dose of flunixin meglumine (1.1 mg/kg) in dairy cattle was 3.1 hours but was 5.2 hours after IM administration of the same dose [66]. In a study evaluating plasma pharmacokinetics and milk residues of flunixin meglumine and its metabolite, 5-hydroxy flunixin meglumine, in dairy cows receiving two doses of 1.1 mg/kg of the drug, significantly longer terminal $t½$ were detected following IM or SC administration (4.48 ± 1.77 and 5.39 ± 2.48 hours) as compared to that of IV administration (3.42 ± 0.98 hours) [67]. While 5-hydroxy flunixin meglumine was undetectable in milk at 36 hours after the second IV dose, violative residues were detected in one intramuscularly and one subcutaneously administered cow. Cows producing less than 20 kg (44 lb) of milk per day eliminated 5-hydroxy flunixin meglumine slower than those with greater milk production. The authors concluded that the large number of reported flunixin meglumine residues in culled dairy cows is likely related to administration of the drug via an unapproved route. In addition, lower milk production may also be a contributing factor for the occurrence of violative residues in this study [67]. The current tolerance for flunixin meglumine concentrations in milk is 2 ng/ml [two parts per billion (ppb)]. However, following IV administration of 2.2 mg/kg/day for 3 days, the concentrations of the drug in milk of the first, second, and third milking were 66, 20, and 14 ng/ml, respectively, exceeding the approved tolerance [46, 68].

In weaned dairy calves, flunixin meglumine administration at the time of dehorning improved average daily gains, reduced biomarkers of pain, and decreased circulating cortisol levels [69]. The median plasma $t½$ of flunixin meglumine in these calves was 6.0 hours (range 3.4–11 hours) following an IV dose of 2.2 mg/kg [69]. In tissues, the reported elimination $t½$ of flunixin meglumine were 9–51 hours for liver and 22–37 hours for kidney after IV administration of three daily doses of 2.2 mg/kg, which is approximately ten times longer than the plasma elimination $t½$ [46]. In sheep, plasma elimination $t½$ of flunixin meglumine were reported to be 229 minutes (3.82 hours) and 205 minutes (3.42 hours) after IV administration of 1.0 and 2.2 mg/kg, respectively [70]. Very similar plasma elimination $t½$ were reported in goats following IV (3.6 hours, range 2.0–5.1 hours) and IM administration (3.4 hours, range 2.6–7.1 hours) [71]. In swine, the elimination $t½$ of flunixin meglumine following administration of a single IV dose of 2.0 mg/kg was 7.76 hours. The authors suggested that enterohepatic recycling may occur in swine similar to that reported in other species [72]. The withdrawal time for flunixin meglumine in cattle following administration at the approved dose and route is 4 days for meat and 36 hours for milk. If flunixin meglumine is administered intramuscularly, a meat withdrawal time of 30 days is recommended, which may need to be extended to 60 days when multiple IM doses are administered [46]. In swine, a meat withdrawal time of 12 days following IM administration of 2.2 mg/kg of flunixin meglumine has been established [15].

While aspirin is believed by some veterinarians to fall under the grandfather clause of the Animal Drug Amendments of 1968, this is not the position of the FDA [65]. There are currently no approved veterinary products containing salicylic acid available in the US; the use of commercially available products in food animals is of questionable legality and discouraged by FARAD [63, 65]. Following oral administration to cattle, aspirin is slowly absorbed (absorption *t*½ of 2.91 hours) and rapidly eliminated (elimination *t*½ of 32 minutes). However, oral doses of 100 mg/kg every 12 hours maintained serum salicylate concentrations that were considered therapeutically effective (30 µg/ml) [73]. In calves treated with 50 mg/kg of oral aspirin, plasma salicylate concentrations remained below 10 µg/kg and failed to mitigate an effect on acute cortisol response [74]. But an elimination *t*½ of 0.63 hours was detected following IV administration of 50 mg/kg of sodium salicylate prior to castration. In calves treated with 2.5–5.0 mg/l of sodium salicylate in drinking water for approximately 5 days, the time to maximal plasma concentration was 41.7 hours, and the mean plasma salicylate concentration was 32.2 µg/ml. Plasma concentrations rapidly declined after removal of salicylate from drinking water and were undetectable within 24 hours [60]. Elimination *t*½ of aspirin in sheep and goats (38.2 ± 4.0 and 27.3 ± 3.6 minutes) are similar to those reported in cattle, and a dose of 20 mg/kg by IV or IM administration achieved therapeutic plasma concentrations [75]. Recommended withdrawal times for aspirin following oral administration to cattle are 1 day for meat and 24 hours for milk [65].

Meloxicam is an NSAID of the oxicam class that is approved for use in cattle in Europe for IM or SC administration. In the US, meloxicam is commercially available in oral and injectable formulations for use in small animals. Several generic tablet formulations (7.5 and 15 mg) are available for relief of signs and symptoms of osteoarthritis in people. The use of oral meloxicam as an analgesic compound in cattle could be considered under the guidelines of AMDUCA, as FDA-approved drugs for this purpose in food animals are currently unavailable [63]. In cattle, meloxicam was demonstrated to be effective in alleviating pain associated with painful procedures including castration, dehorning, and resection of the coffin joint [69, 76–78]. Furthermore, clinical efficacy was demonstrated when meloxicam was included in therapeutic protocols for medical conditions such as respiratory disease, mastitis, and calf diarrhea [79–82]. In studies evaluating the pharmacokinetics of oral meloxicam in calves, the drug had good bioavailability, and approximate mean peak plasma concentrations of 3.0–3.5 µg/ml were achieved at 10–12 hours. In these studies, the plasma *t*½ of meloxicam was approximately 25 hours [83, 84]. The bioavailability of meloxicam was significantly different in calves receiving meloxicam in milk replacer as compared to that administered by stomach tube [85]. In lactating dairy cattle, plasma pharmacokinetics of meloxicam were similar to those described for calves [86]. Meloxicam was detectable in milk for up to 80 hours, and the *t*½ in milk was 10.38 ± 1.20 hours [86]. Withdrawal times following the use of injectable formulations of meloxicam in cattle at a dose of 0.5 mg/kg range from 8 to 20 days for meat and 84 to 144 hours (6 days) for milk in countries where the drug is approved [85]. A conservative meat withdrawal time of 21 days based on ten terminal *t*½ in the plasma of calves was recently suggested [46].

Phenothiazine derivatives

The mechanism of action of phenothiazine derivatives is by antagonism of dopaminergic receptors of the ascending reticular formation and other central nervous systems [34]. Despite its common use as a tranquilizer and anesthetic adjunct, little information regarding the disposition of acepromazine in food animals is available. In horses, the elimination *t*½ was determined to be in the range of 50–150 minutes following a dose of 0.15 mg/kg in one study [87]. In another equine study, the elimination *t*½ was 184.8 minutes, and acepromazine was detectable in plasma for 8 hours after administration of 0.3 mg/kg [88]. Acepromazine is not approved for use in food animals in the US, but it is approved in Canada and Australia. The recommendation of withdrawal time provided by FARAD is primarily based on foreign approvals [28]. For cattle, FARAD recommends a withdrawal time of 7 days for meat and 48 hours for milk for doses of up to 0.44 mg/kg by IM administration or up to 0.13 mg/kg by IV administration [28]. Identical recommendations are provided for small ruminants [33]. For swine, a 7-day meat withdrawal is recommended for up to 0.055 mg/kg by IV administration or up to 0.44 mg/kg by IM administration [28].

Propofol

Propofol is an injectable, highly lipophilic, and short-acting anesthetic used for induction and maintenance of anesthesia. Propofol crosses the blood–brain barrier very rapidly, but unlike ultrashort-acting barbiturates, repeated dosing of propofol to maintain anesthesia does not result in tissue accumulation. In general, propofol has a very large volume of distribution, rapid clearance, and short terminal *t*½ [34]. In a pharmacokinetic study in calves, propofol was administered at 3 mg/kg following the administration of xylazine (0.1 mg/kg) to induce general anesthesia for umbilical hernia repair [89]. Following administration of propofol, plasma concentrations decreased rapidly in all calves. However, propofol was still detectable in plasma of three of five calves at 8 hours after administration and in one calf at 12 hours after administration. A volume of distribution of 330.7 ± 171.1 ml/kg, a clearance of 1,182.61 ± 443.24 ml/hour/kg, and an elimination *t*½ of 3.27 ± 2.34 hours were reported in these calves [89]. Because of the paucity of sufficient plasma and tissue pharmacokinetics in food animals, FARAD recommends the use of other anesthetics instead of propofol (FARAD, email communication, December 2013). A meat withdrawal time of at least 72 hours was recommended for propofol, but due to lack of data, a milk withdrawal time cannot be determined [47] (Table 11.1).

Table 11.1 Recommended withdrawal times for anesthetics and analgesics in farm animals.

		Cattle			Small ruminants			Swine	
Drug class	Drug name	Meat (days)	Milk (hours)	Dose (mg/kg)	Meat (days)	Milk (hours)	Dose (mg/kg)	Meat (days)	Dose (mg/kg)
α_2 agonists	Detomidine	3	72	≤0.08, IV, IM	3	72	≤0.08, IV, IM		
	Xylazine	5	72	0.016–0.1, IV	5	72	0.016–0.1, IV	18	2.2, IM
		10	120	0.3–2.0, IM	10	12	0.3–2.0, IM		
		4	24	0.05–0.3, IM	4	24	0.05–0.3, IM		
α_2 antagonists	Tolazoline	8	48	2–4, IV					
Barbiturates	Thiamylal	1	24	≤5.5, IV					
	Thialbarbitone	1	24	≤9.4, IV					
	Thiopental				1	24	≤5.0, IV		
Benzodiazepines	Diazepam	10		≤10, IV	10		≤10, IV		
Dissociative anesthetics	Ketamine	3	48	≤10, IM	3	48	≤10, IM	2	10, IM
		3	48	≤2	3	48	≤2	4	20
	Telazol®							30	≤2
Local anesthetics	Lidocaine	1	24	≤15 ml, epidurally					
		4	72	≤100 ml, SQ					
Opioids	Morphine	14	48	0.1, once, IV, IM, epidurally	14	48	0.1, once, IV, IM, epidurally		
	Butorphanol	5	72						
NSAIDs*	Flunixin	4	36	≤2.2, IV				12	2.2, IM
Phenothiazine derivatives	Acepromazine	7	48	≤0.13, IV	7	48	≤0.13, IV	7	≤0.055, IV
		7	48	≤0.44, IM	7	48	≤0.44, IM	7	≤0.44, IM

*NSAIDs: nonsteroidal anti-inflammatory drugs.

References

1. Heavner, J. and Teske, R. (1986) Legal implications of the extra-label use of drugs in food animals. *Veterinary Clinics of North America: Food Animal Practice*, **2**, 517–525.
2. Friedlander, L., Brynes, S. and Fernandez, AH. (1999) The human food safety evaluation of new animal drugs. *Veterinary Clinics of North America: Food Animal Practice*, 15, 1–11, vii.
3. The European Agency for the Evaluation of Medicinal Products: Veterinary Medicine Evaluation Unit: Committee for Veterinary Medicinal Products (1996) *Note for guidance: approach towards harmonisation of withdrawal periods (EMEA/CVMP/036/95)*, London.
4. Concordet, D. and Toutain, P. (1997) The withdrawal time estimation of veterinary drugs revisited. *Journal of Veterinary Pharmacology and Therapeutics*, **20**, 380–386.
5. Concordet, D. and Toutain, P. (1997) The withdrawal time estimation of veterinary drugs: a non-parametric approach. *Journal of Veterinary Pharmacology and Therapeutics*, **20**, 374–379.
6. Fisch, R. (2000) Withdrawal time estimation of veterinary drugs: extending the range of statistical methods. *Journal of Veterinary Pharmacology and Therapeutics*, **23**, 159–162.
7. Martinez, M., Friedlander, L., Condon, R. *et al.* (2000) Response to criticisms of the USFDA parametric approach for withdrawal time estimation: rebuttal and comparison to the nonparametric method proposed by Concordet and Toutain. *Journal of Veterinary Pharmacology and Therapeutics*, **23**, 21–35.
8. Nouws, J., Smulders, A. and Rappalini, M. (1990) A comparative study on irritation and residue aspects of five oxytetracycline formulations administered intramuscularly to calves, pigs and sheep. *The Veterinary Quarterly*, **12**, 129–138.
9. Sanquer, A., Wackowiez, G. and Havrileck, B. (2006) Critical review on the withdrawal period calculation for injection site residues. *Journal of Veterinary Pharmacology and Therapeutics*, **29**, 355–364.
10. Reeves, P. (2007) Residues of veterinary drugs at injection sites. *Journal of Veterinary Pharmacology and Therapeutics*, **30**, 1–17.
11. US Food and Drug Administration (1994) *Animal Medicinal Drug Use Clarification Act (AMDUCA) of 1994*, http://www.fda.gov/AnimalVeterinary/GuidanceComplianceEnforcement/ActsRulesRegulations/ucm085377.htm (accessed March 28, 2013).
12. US Department of Agriculture – Food Safety and Inspection Service (USDA FSIS) (2012) *Residue Sample Results, 2010*, http://www.fsis.us (accessed January 22, 2014).
13. Papich, M. (1996) Drug residue considerations for anesthetics and adjunctive drugs in food-producing animals. *Veterinary Clinics of North America: Food Animal Practice*, **12**, 693–706.
14. Baynes, R. (2011). Review of AMDUCA and extra-label drug use in food animals. *American Association of the Bovine Practitioners*; pp. 8–10.
15. Food Animal Residue Avoidance Databank (FARAD) *A component of the Food Animal Residue Avoidance and Depletion Program*, http://www.farad.org (accessed January 22, 2014).
16. Martin-Jimenez, T., Baynes, R., Craigmill, A. and Riviere, J. (2002) Extrapolated withdrawal-interval estimator (EWE) algorithm: a quantitative approach to establishing extralabel withdrawal times. *Regulatory Toxicology and Pharmacology*, **36**, 131–137.
17. Gehring, R., Baynes, R., Craigmill, A. and Riviere, J. (2004) Feasibility of using half-life multipliers to estimate extended withdrawal intervals following the extralabel use of drugs in food-producing animals. *Journal of Food Protection*, **67**, 555–560.
18. Gehring, R., Baynes, R., Wang, J. *et al.* (2004) A web-based decision support system to estimate extended withdrawal intervals. *Computers and Electronics in Agriculture*, **44**, 145–151.

19. Riviere, J. (1991) Pharmacologic principles of residue avoidance for veterinary practitioners. *Journal of the American Veterinary Medical Association*, **198**, 809–816.
20. Fajt, V. (2001) Label and extra label drug use in small ruminants. *Veterinary Clinics of North America: Food Animal Practice*, **17**, 403–420.
21. Chamberlain, P. and Brynes, S. (1998) The regulatory status of xylazine for use in food-producing animals in the United States. *Journal of Veterinary Pharmacology and Therapeutics*, **21**, 322–329.
22. Garcia-Villar, R., Toutain, P., Alvinerie, M. *et al.* (1981) The pharmacokinetics of xylazine hydrochloride: an interspecific study. *Journal of Veterinary Pharmacology and Therapeutics*, **4**, 87–92.
23. Chamberlain, P. (1996) Xylazine. *WHO Food Additives Series*, 38.
24. George, L. (2005) Pain control in food animals, in *Recent Advances in Anesthetic Management of Large Domestic Animals* (ed E.P. Steffey), International Veterinary Information Service, Ithaca, p. 13.
25. Yasuhara, K., Kobayashi, H., Shimamura, Y. *et al.* (2000) Toxicity and blood concentrations of xylazine and its metabolite, 2,6-dimethylaniline, in rats after single or continuous oral administrations. *The Journal of Toxicological Sciences*, **25**, 105–113.
26. Haskell, S., Gehring, R., Payne, M. *et al.* (2003) Update on FARAD food animal drug withholding recommendations. *Journal of the American Veterinary Medical Association*, **223**, 1277–1278.
27. Delehant, T., Denhart, J., Lloyd, W. and Powell, J. (2003) Pharmacokinetics of xylazine, 2,6-dimethylaniline, and tolazoline in tissues from yearling cattle and milk from mature dairy cows after sedation with xylazine hydrochloride and reversal with tolazoline hydrochloride. *Veterinary Therapeutics*, **4**, 128–134.
28. Craigmill, A., RangelLugo, M., Damian, P. and Riviere, J. (1997) Extralabel use of tranquilizers and general anesthetics. *Journal of the American Veterinary Medical Association*, **211**, 302–304.
29. US Code of Federal Regulations (2000) *7 CFR Part 205 National Organic Program. §205.603 Synthetic substances allowed for use in organic livestock production.*
30. Khan, M., Ashraf, M., Pervez, K. *et al.* (2004) Comparative effects of detomidine and xylazine as sedative and analgesic agents in small ruminants. *Pakistan Veterinary Journal*, **24**, 62–69.
31. Singh, A., Peshin, P., Singh, J. *et al.* (1991) Evaluation of detomidine as a sedative in goats. *Acta Veterinaria Hungarica*, **39**, 109–114.
32. Salonen, J., Vaha-Vahe, T., Vainio, O. and Vakkuri, O. (1989) Single-dose pharmacokinetics of detomidine in the horse and cow. *Journal of Veterinary Pharmacology and Therapeutics*, **12**, 65–72.
33. Webb, A., Baynes, R., Craigmill, A. *et al.* (2004) Drugs approved for small ruminants. *Journal of the American Veterinary Medical Association*, **224**, 520–523.
34. Ebert, U., Frey, H. and Schulz, R. (2002) Pharmakologie des zentralen nervensystems (ZNS), in *Lehrbuch der Pharmakologie und Toxikologie für die Veterinärmedizin*, 2nd edn (eds H. Frey and W. Loscher), Enke Verlag, Stuttgart, pp. 87–138.
35. Moore, D., Smallridge, R., von Bredow, J. and Lukey, B. (1991) The pharmacokinetics of atropine and diazepam in sheep: intramuscular co-administration. *Biopharmaceutics & Drug Disposition*, **12**, 525–536.
36. Klotz, U., Antonin, K. and Bieck, P. (1976) Pharmacokinetics and plasma binding of diazepam in man, dog, rabbit, guinea pig and rat. *The Journal of Pharmacology and Experimental Therapeutics*, **199**, 67–73.

37. EMEA-Ketamine (1997) *European Agency for the Evaluation of Medicinal Product-Committee for Veterinary Medicinal Products*, http://www.emea.europa.eu/pdfs/vet/mrls/315/97-Final (accessed 13 January 2014).
38. Gehring, R., Coetzee, J., Tarus-Sang, J. and Apley, M. (2009) Pharmacokinetics of ketamine and its metabolite norketamine administered at a sub-anesthetic dose together with xylazine to calves prior to castration. *Journal of Veterinary Pharmacology and Therapeutics*, **32**, 124–128.
39. Waterman, A. and Livingston, A. (1978) Studies on the distribution and metabolism of ketamine in sheep. *Journal of Veterinary Pharmacology and Therapeutics*, **1**, 141–147.
40. Waterman, A. (1984) The pharmacokinetics of ketamine administered intravenously in calves and the modifying effect of premedication with xylazine hydrochloride. *Journal of Veterinary Pharmacology and Therapeutics*, **7**, 125–130.
41. Sellers, G., Lin, H., Riddell, M. *et al.* (2010) Pharmacokinetics of ketamine in plasma and milk of mature Holstein cows. *Journal of Veterinary Pharmacology and Therapeutics*, **33**, 480–484.
42. Loscher, W., Ganter, M. and Fassbender, C. (1990) Correlation between drug and metabolite concentrations in plasma and anesthetic action of ketamine in swine. *American Journal of Veterinary Research*, **51**, 391–398.
43. Kumar, A., Mann, H. and Remmel, R. (2006) Pharmacokinetics of tiletamine and zolazepam (Telazol) in anesthetized pigs. *Journal of Veterinary Pharmacology and Therapeutics*, **29**, 587–589.
44. Puente, N. and Josephy, P. (2001) Analysis of the lidocaine metabolite 2,6-dimethylaniline in bovine and human milk. *Journal of Analytical Toxicology*, **25**, 711–715.
45. Norwegian Scientific Committee for Food Safety (2005) *Risk assessment of lidocaine residues in food products from cattle, swine, sheep and goats: withdrawal periods for meat and milk (05/508-4-final).*
46. Smith, G. (2013) Extralabel use of anesthetic and analgesic compounds in cattle. *Veterinary Clinics of North America: Food Animal Practice*, **29**, 29–45.
47. Cox, S., Wilson, J. and Doherty, T. (2012) Pharmacokinetics of lidocaine after intravenous administration to cows. *Journal of Veterinary Pharmacology and Therapeutics*, **35**, 305–308.
48. Sellers, G., Lin, H., Riddell, M. *et al.* (2009) Pharmacokinetics of lidocaine in serum and milk of mature Holstein cows. *Journal of Veterinary Pharmacology and Therapeutics*, **32**, 446–450.
49. Morishima, H., Finster, M., Pedersen, H. *et al.* (1979) Pharmacokinetics of lidocaine in fetal and neonatal lambs and adult sheep. *Anesthesiology*, **50**, 431–436.
50. Santos, A., Pedersen, H., Morishima, H. *et al.* (1988) Pharmacokinetics of lidocaine in non-pregnant and pregnant ewes. *Anesthesia and Analgesia*, **67**, 1154–1158.
51. Kennedy, R., Bell, J., Miller, R. *et al.* (1990) Uptake and distribution of lidocaine in fetal lambs. *Anesthesiology*, **72**, 483–489.
52. Satas, S., Johannessen, S., Hoem, N. *et al.* (1997) Lidocaine pharmacokinetics and toxicity in newborn pigs. *Anesthesia and Analgesia*, **85**, 306–312.
53. Scarratt, W. and Troutt, H. (1986) Iatrogenic lidocaine toxicosis in ewes. *Journal of the American Veterinary Medical Association*, **188**, 184–185.
54. Mets, B., Allin, R., van Dyke, J. and Hickman, R. (1993) Lidocaine decay and hepatic extraction in the pig. *Journal of Veterinary Pharmacology and Therapeutics*, **16**, 8–14.
55. Jenkins, W. (1987) Pharmacologic aspects of analgesic drugs in animals: an overview. *Journal of the American Veterinary Medical Association*, **191**, 1231–1240.
56. Combie, J., Nugent, T. and Tobin, T. (1983) Pharmacokinetics and protein binding of morphine in horses. *American Journal of Veterinary Research*, **44**, 870–874.

57. Sloan, P., Mather, L., McLean, C. *et al.* (1991) Physiological disposition of i.v. morphine in sheep. *British Journal of Anaesthesia*, **67**, 378–386.
58. Court, M., Dodman, N., Levine, H. *et al.* (1992) Pharmacokinetics and milk residues of butorphanol in dairy cows after single intravenous administration. *Journal of Veterinary Pharmacology and Therapeutics*, **15**, 28–35.
59. Dodman, N., Levine, H. and Court, M. (1992) Clinical assessment of analgesic effects of butorphanol in cattle, in *Animal Pain* (eds C.E. Short and A. Van Poznak), Churchill Livingstone, New York, pp. 396–401.
60. Baldridge, S., Coetzee, J., Dritz, S. *et al.* (2011) Pharmacokinetics and physiologic effects of intramuscularly administered xylazine hydrochloride-ketamine hydrochloride-butorphanol tartrate alone or in combination with orally administered sodium salicylate on biomarkers of pain in Holstein calves following castration and dehorning. *American Journal of Veterinary Research*, **72**, 1305–1317.
61. Ahern, B., Soma, L., Rudy, J. *et al.* (2010) Pharmacokinetics of fentanyl administered transdermally and intravenously in sheep. *American Journal of Veterinary Research*, **71**, 1127–1132.
62. Carroll, G., Hooper, R., Boothe, D. *et al.* (1999) Pharmacokinetics of fentanyl after intravenous and transdermal administration in goats. *American Journal of Veterinary Research*, **60**, 986–991.
63. Coetzee, J. (2013) A review of analgesic compounds used in food animals in the United States. *Veterinary Clinics of North America: Food Animal Practice*, **29**, 11–28.
64. Pyorala, S., Laurila, T., Lehtonen, S. *et al.* (1999) Local tissue damage in cows after intramuscular administration of preparations containing phenylbutazone, flunixin, ketoprofen and metamizole. *Acta Veterinaria Scandinavica*, **40**, 145–150.
65. Smith, G., Davis, J., Tell, L. *et al.* (2008) Extralabel use of nonsteroidal anti-inflammatory drugs in cattle. *Journal of the American Veterinary Medical Association*, **232**, 697–701.
66. Anderson, K., Neff-Davis, C., Davis, L. and Bass, V. (1990) Pharmacokinetics of flunixin meglumine in lactating cattle after single and multiple intramuscular and intravenous administrations. *American Journal of Veterinary Research*, **51**, 1464–1467.
67. Kissell, L., Smith, G., Leavens, T. *et al.* (2012) Plasma pharmacokinetics and milk residues of flunixin and 5-hydroxy flunixin following different routes of administration in dairy cattle. *Journal of Dairy Science*, **95**, 7151–7157.
68. Feely, W., Chester-Yansen, C., Thompson, K. *et al.* (2002) Flunixin residues in milk after intravenous treatment of dairy cattle with (14)C-flunixin. *Journal of Agricultural and Food Chemistry*, **50**, 7308–7313.
69. Glynn, H., Coetzee, J., Edwards-Callaway, L. *et al.* (2013) The pharmacokinetics and effects of meloxicam, gabapentin, and flunixin in postweaning dairy calves following dehorning with local anesthesia. *Journal of Veterinary Pharmacology and Therapeutics*, **36** (6), 550–561.
70. Welsh, E., McKellar, Q. and Nolan, A. (1993) The pharmacokinetics of flunixin meglumine in the sheep. *Journal of Veterinary Pharmacology and Therapeutics*, **16**, 181–188.
71. Konigsson, K., Torneke, K., Engeland, I. *et al.* (2003) Pharmacokinetics and pharmacodynamic effects of flunixin after intravenous, intramuscular and oral administration to dairy goats. *Acta Veterinaria Scandinavica*, **44**, 153–159.
72. Buur, J., Baynes, R., Smith, G. and Riviere, J. (2006) Pharmacokinetics of flunixin meglumine in swine after intravenous dosing. *Journal of Veterinary Pharmacology and Therapeutics*, **29**, 437–440.
73. Gingerich, D., Baggot, J. and Yeary, R. (1975) Pharmacokinetics and dosage of aspirin in cattle. *Journal of the American Veterinary Medical Association*, **167**, 945–948.

74. Coetzee, J., Gehring, R., Bettenhausen, A. *et al.* (2007) Attenuation of acute plasma cortisol response in calves following intravenous sodium salicylate administration prior to castration. *Journal of Veterinary Pharmacology and Therapeutics*, **30**, 305–313.
75. Ali, B. (2003) Comparative pharmacokinetics of salicylate in camels, sheep and goats. *European Journal of Drug Metabolism and Pharmacokinetics*, **28**, 125–128.
76. Theurer, M., White, B., Coetzee, J. *et al.* (2012) Assessment of behavioral changes associated with oral meloxicam administration at time of dehorning in calves using a remote triangulation device and accelerometers. *BMC Veterinary Research*, **8**, 48.
77. Heinrich, A., Duffield, T., Lissemore, K. *et al.* (2009) The impact of meloxicam on postsurgical stress associated with cautery dehorning. *Journal of Dairy Science*, **92**, 540–547.
78. Offinger, J., Herdtweck, S., Rizk, A. *et al.* (2013) Postoperative analgesic efficacy of meloxicam in lame dairy cows undergoing resection of the distal interphalangeal joint. *Journal of Dairy Science*, **96**, 866–876.
79. Friton, G., Cajal, C., Ramirez Romero, R. and Kleemann, R. (2004) Clinical efficacy of meloxicam (Metacam) and flunixin (Finadyne) as adjuncts to antibacterial treatment of respiratory disease in fattening cattle. *Berliner und Munchener tierarztliche Wochenschrift*, **117**, 304–309.
80. Friton, G., Cajal, C. and Ramirez-Romero, R. (2005) Long-term effects of meloxicam in the treatment of respiratory disease in fattening cattle. *The Veterinary Record*, **156**, 809–811.
81. McDougall, S., Bryan, M. and Tiddy, R. (2009) Effect of treatment with the nonsteroidal anti-inflammatory meloxicam on milk production, somatic cell count, probability of re-treatment, and culling of dairy cows with mild clinical mastitis. *Journal of Dairy Science*, **92**, 4421–4431.
82. Todd, C., Millman, S., McKnight, D. *et al.* (2010) Nonsteroidal anti-inflammatory drug therapy for neonatal calf diarrhea complex: Effects on calf performance. *Journal of Animal Science*, **88**, 2019–2028.
83. Coetzee, J., Kukanich, B., Mosher, R. and Allen, P. (2009) Pharmacokinetics of intravenous and oral meloxicam in ruminant calves. *Veterinary Therapeutics*, **10**, E1–E8.
84. Coetzee, J., Mosher, R., Kohake, L. *et al.* (2011) Pharmacokinetics of oral gabapentin alone or co-administered with meloxicam in ruminant beef calves. *Veterinary Journal*, **190**, 98–102.
85. Mosher, R., Coetzee, J., Cull, C. *et al.* (2012) Pharmacokinetics of oral meloxicam in ruminant and preruminant calves. *Journal of Veterinary Pharmacology and Therapeutics*, **35**, 373–381.
86. Malreddy, P., Coetzee, J., Kukanich, B. and Gehring, R. (2013) Pharmacokinetics and milk secretion of gabapentin and meloxicam co-administered orally in Holstein-Friesian cows. *Journal of Veterinary Pharmacology and Therapeutics*, **36**, 14–20.
87. Marroum, P., Webb, A., Aeschbacher, G. and Curry, S. (1994) Pharmacokinetics and pharmacodynamics of acepromazine in horses. *American Journal of Veterinary Research*, **55**, 1428–1433.
88. Ballard, S., Shults, T., Kownacki, A. *et al.* (1982) The pharmacokinetics, pharmacological responses and behavioral effects of acepromazine in the horse. *Journal of Veterinary Pharmacology and Therapeutics*, **5**, 21–31.
89. Cagnardi, P., Zonca, A., Gallo, M. *et al.* (2009) Pharmacokinetics of propofol in calves undergoing abdominal surgery. *Veterinary Research Communications*, **33** (Suppl 1), 177–179.

Chapter 12

Euthanasia of farm animals

Thomas Passler

Department of Clinical Sciences, College of Veterinary Medicine, Auburn University, USA

As implied by the Greek terms "eu" meaning good and "thanatos" meaning death, the process of euthanasia should end the life of an animal by procedures that eliminate or minimize pain and distress [1]. When a decision to euthanize an animal has been made, three phases of the process must be considered in an effort to achieve this ideal balance: (1) appropriate animal handling prior to euthanasia to minimize pain and distress, (2) appropriate technique of euthanasia, and (3) legal and safe disposal of the carcass. The decision to euthanize a farm animal is often not exclusively influenced by the desire to relieve animal suffering, as factors such as financial costs and practicality of continued therapy have to be considered; however, it is the veterinarians' and caregivers' responsibility to utilize a method of euthanasia that provides the ideal balance of minimal pain and distress while considering the environment in which the euthanasia is performed.

Considerations prior to euthanasia

Veterinary guidance is critical in forming the decision to euthanize a farm animal, as the prognoses for life and function as based on a veterinary examination can establish whether euthanasia is the most appropriate option or whether salvage by slaughter of a chronically ill animal is a morally and financially sound option. While euthanasia is easily recognized as the only viable option in certain condition such as fractures of the spine or severe painful trauma that cannot be relieved by treatment, the necessity for euthanasia may not be as appreciable with other disorders, especially by farm managers and caregivers. An increasing body of research has evaluated physiological and behavioral indicators of pain in farm animals [2–4]; however, accurate and objective assessment of pain and resulting physical suffering remains difficult. In surveys assessing perceptions of bovine veterinarians

Farm Animal Anesthesia: Cattle, Small Ruminants, Camelids, and Pigs, First Edition.
Edited by HuiChu Lin and Paul Walz.

on pain in cattle, significant variation existed among individuals concerning the perceived amount of pain associated with disease or veterinary procedures, and the utilized methods of pain control also differed significantly among veterinarians [5–7]. It is reasonable to infer that for animal caregivers, who have varying degrees of knowledge and experience, accurate assessment of the amount of pain in farm animals can be even more challenging. Some diseases may be more visually striking but less painful (e.g., rectal prolapse), while others are more painful but inconspicuous (e.g., chronic arthritis) [8], and misinterpretation of clinical signs could result in inappropriate administration of euthanasia procedures. In situations where immediate and direct veterinary advice is not available and the decision to euthanize is made by animal caregivers, creation of clear criteria for euthanasia in the form of standardized euthanasia protocols can help to alleviate employee stress associated with euthanasia and improve the overall welfare of a herd [8, 9].

On-farm euthanasia plans should be part of the overall herd health management program and should include specific planning for the three phases of euthanasia. A decision tree can be used to determine the approach to a sick or debilitated animal (Figure 12.1). This decision tree can be modified to include treatment modalities, duration of attempted therapy before deciding on euthanasia, and methods of euthanasia as part of a farm-specific herd management plan. Developing clear criteria for sick animals

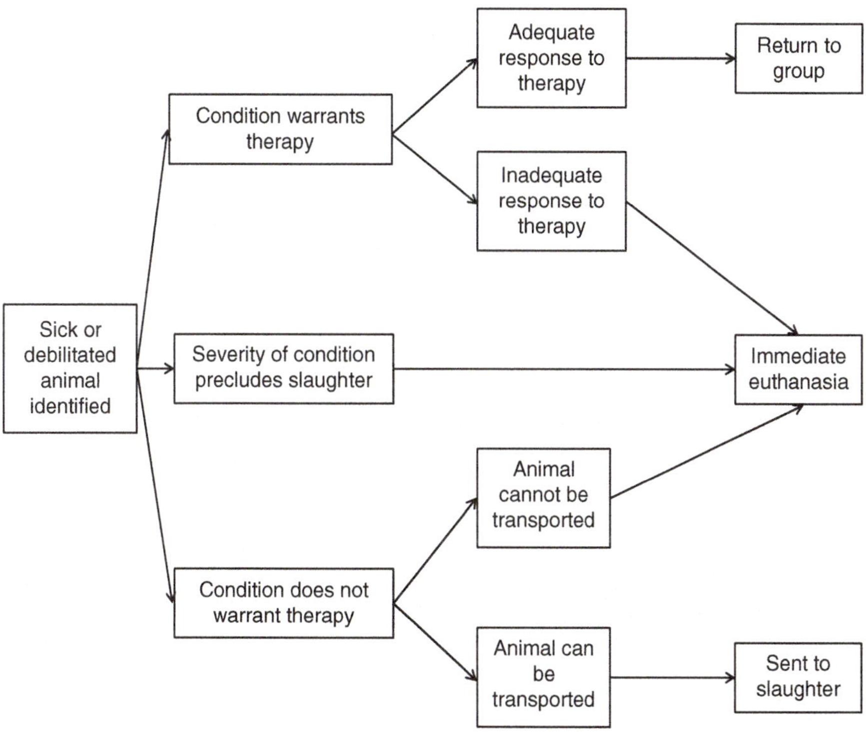

Figure 12.1 Example of a decision algorithm that can be implemented as part of an on-farm euthanasia plan to provide farm personnel with clear direction for the handling of sick and debilitated animals. Adapted from Turner PV, Doonan G. Developing on-farm euthanasia plans. *The Canadian Veterinary Journal* 2010;51:1031-1034..

can ensure consistent decisions among farm personnel and timely implementation of euthanasia procedures [10].

General guidelines have been proposed to aid in the decision-making process on whether an animal should be euthanized [10–12]. Guidelines commonly include specific end point criteria that form indications for euthanasia such as [11]:

- Fractured leg (irreparable) and severe trauma
- Loss of production and quality of life (severe mastitis, advanced systemic diseases)
- Inability to stand or walk (disabled livestock)
- Diagnostic (e.g., potential for human disease, such as rabies)
- Advanced ocular neoplasia (cancer eye)
- Debilitating or toxic conditions
- Cost of treatment prohibitive and poor prognosis
- Extended withdrawal time for sale of meat and poor prognosis

In adaption of euthanasia guidelines for small animals, generalized guidelines for use in swine operations have been proposed [8]:

- Weight loss of 20–25% of total body weight, characterized by muscle wasting
- Extreme weakness or the inability or lack of desire to eat or drink, persisting for 24 hours or more
- Suffering from any infection/disease that fails to respond to treatment

As part of an on-farm euthanasia plan, procedures for handling debilitated animals prior to euthanasia should be reviewed. The prevention of pain and distress during handling before euthanasia can often be achieved by simple environmental changes, and animal welfare recommendations for cattle transported and handled for slaughter apply [13, 14]. Separation of the animal to be euthanized from healthy conspecifics is generally advisable to prevent distress and safety concerns, such as from a missed or ricocheting gunshot. Stress responses including vocalization, fearful behavior, and olfactory stress signals can communicate anxiety and apprehension among animals [15–17], and it is often easiest to remove all healthy animals from the area in which euthanasia will be performed. While ambulatory animals may be moved for short distances to a location where euthanasia procedures and carcass removal can be more effectively performed, fractious or recumbent animals may best be euthanized at their present location. Ensuring the prevention of pain and distress, animals that tolerate human contact can be moved using appropriate carts or sleds. As most methods of euthanasia require close contact to the animal, animals must be restrained by a halter or chute. The required restraint should be chosen based on the disposition of the animal and the method of euthanasia. Restraint by a halter can be adequate for small and large farm animals accustomed to human handling, and allows for intravenous (IV) administration of barbiturates or accurate placement of a penetrating captive bolt. Premedication with sedatives or tranquilizers should be considered to ensure safety of personnel and reduce distress when euthanizing fractious animals. Premedication can be administered in a chute if possible with minimal pain and distress, or it can be administered by blow dart or dart gun. For some animals, gunshot may be the most appropriate form of euthanasia, as it requires the least amount of human contact.

The process of euthanasia

Any appropriate method of euthanasia is aimed at inducing unconsciousness as rapidly as possible. Unconsciousness is defined as the loss of individual awareness and occurs when the brain's ability to integrate information is blocked or disrupted [1]. The underlying mechanisms that achieve unconsciousness in anesthetized individuals are still not completely understood, but most anesthetic drugs appear to induce an unconscious state by deactivation and disintegration of the posterior corticothalamic complex [18]. In animals under general anesthesia, movement due to continued spinal cord activity, can be observed despite the presence of a state of unconsciousness and amnesia, as memory and awareness are abolished at anesthetic concentrations which are less than half of those needed to abolish movement [19]. While much more pronounced deactivation of cortical function and rapid loss of consciousness are expected with methods of euthanasia, it is important to ensure that all activities observed in an animal to which a method of physical or chemical euthanasia has been administered occur subsequent to unconsciousness. In animals, the loss of unconsciousness is defined as loss of the righting reflex [1]. By means of electroencephalography (EEG), various studies have evaluated brain function in animals at slaughter, and although data obtained from EEG are limited in their ability to precisely determine the onset of unconsciousness [20–23], indicators of successful stunning in slaughtered animals also apply to euthanasia. While weakly present in rare cases, the corneal reflex is expected to be absent after successful stunning by captive bolt [20, 24]. After stunning, immediate collapse, followed by a period of tetanic spasticity and then clonic slow hind limb movements with increasing frequency, occurs [1]. In cattle and small ruminants, loss of righting reflex, loss of rhythmic breathing, protrusion of tongue, absence of corneal reflex, and absence of nystagmus indicate successful stunning by captive bolt [25, 26]. During euthanasia, loss of residual muscle movement and cardiac and respiratory arrest follow closely after loss of unconsciousness. Before movement and disposal of the carcass, death must be confirmed. A combination of criteria is most reliable to confirm death, which include absence of pulse and corneal reflex, failure to respond to strong pinches to the nose or interdigital space, inability to auscultate respiratory and heart sound by stethoscope, graying of mucous membranes, and rigor mortis. Only the presence of rigor mortis can, by itself, serve as confirmation of death, and other criteria must be verified in combination [1].

Methods of euthanasia

The American Veterinary Medical Association (AVMA) Panel on Euthanasia categorizes methods of euthanasia as being acceptable, conditionally acceptable, or unacceptable. Additionally, the panel provides species-specific adjunctive methods that can be used in conjunction with other methods to produce a humane death and ensure death in an unconscious animal. An acceptable method of euthanasia is one that consistently produces a humane death when used as the only means of euthanasia. For all farm animals, euthanasia by injection of barbiturates and barbituric acid derivatives is categorized as an acceptable method. Methods that are considered conditionally acceptable vary by species and age, but for all farm animals including cattle, small ruminants, and swine, physical methods such as gunshot and penetrating captive bolt are conditionally accepted. Properly administered, conditionally accepted methods ensure a humane death, but because of the greater potential for operator error or safety hazards, they might not do so as consistently as acceptable methods. Additionally, conditionally acceptable methods include those not well documented in the literature [1].

Injectable euthanasia drugs

In addition to barbiturates and barbituric acid derivatives, the AVMA Guidelines on Euthanasia discuss other injectable euthanizing drugs, including tributame, T-61, and ultrapotent opioids. Unavailable in the United States (US), T-61 was recently evaluated in German cattle, which induced death less rapidly and with more excitatory events than a sodium pentobarbital-containing euthanasia solution [27]. Availability and practicality make barbiturate-containing solutions the most commonly used injectable method of euthanasia in farm animals. Barbiturates rapidly induce unconsciousness by depressing the function of the cerebral cortex and result in collapse of the animal. In a stepwise fashion, other central nervous system (CNS) functions are subsequently depressed, with reduction in blood pressure, depression of the medullary respiratory center and apnea, cerebral death, and subsequently, cardiac arrest.

Various manufacturers currently provide commercially available euthanasia solutions containing sodium pentobarbital at similar concentrations, often in combination with local anesthetics and other CNS depressants such as phenytoin sodium. Additionally, euthanasia solutions contain a dye to ensure ease of identification. Unlike sodium pentobarbital, which is a Drug Enforcement Administration (DEA) schedule II drug, many commercially available euthanasia solutions are categorized as schedule III drugs, enabling less strict regulations concerning their availability and storage.

Most euthanasia solutions are labeled only for dogs or dogs and other small animals, and dosing information for farm animals is extrapolated. Product information from a euthanasia solution labeled for large animals recommends a dose of 1 ml per 4.5 kg (9.9 lb) of body weight, to a maximum of 100 ml, in accordance with its small animal dosage and label information for other products (40 mg of sodium pentobarbital per kg of body weight) [27, 28]. Barbiturate solutions should always be administered by IV route, which ensures rapid distribution to the CNS. However, IV injection can be complicated in fractious or aggressive animals. In these cases, tranquilization or identification of alternative methods of restraint prior to euthanasia should be considered. Alternatively, intraperitoneal administration of sodium pentobarbital may be a substitute to IV injection and is considered acceptable by the AVMA Panel on Euthanasia; however, it is not practical for many large farm animals [1]. For euthanasia by intraperitoneal route, larger quantities of barbiturate solution should be administered, which can be cost prohibitive. Intraperitoneal injection of euthanasia solutions results in significantly increased duration until loss of consciousness as compared to IV administration [29]. While some solutions that do not contain a local anesthetic are labeled for intraperitoneal injection, this route of administration may result in pain, and this nociception can be reduced when lidocaine is included [30]. Failure of injecting the peritoneal cavity was reported in 6.7% and 58% of intraperitoneally injected piglets and adult cats, respectively, and subsequent necropsies demonstrated that the euthanasia solution was delivered into the urinary bladder, gastrointestinal tract, or spleen [29, 31]. While nonvascular administration of injectable euthanasia agents including subcutaneous, intramuscular, or intrathoracic is not acceptable, injection into organs such as intracardiac injection is considered conditionally acceptable in unconscious animals.

Unacceptable as the sole method of euthanasia, saturated solutions of potassium chloride, magnesium chloride, or magnesium sulfate are categorized as adjunctive methods of euthanasia for large and small ruminants [1]. These can be used in anesthetized or unconscious animals and induce cardiac or respiratory arrest following IV or intracardiac administration. Prior to administration, the surgical plane of anesthesia must be confirmed [1]. While injectable anesthetic protocols such as ketamine/xylazine are able to induce unconsciousness, sole use of α_2 agonists such as xylazine prior to potassium chloride or magnesium sulfate administration comprises an unacceptable method of euthanasia [1, 32].

Physical methods

The AVMA Panel on Euthanasia categorizes euthanasia by gunshot and penetrating captive bolt as conditionally accepted methods for cattle, small ruminants, and all age groups of swine, except suckling pigs [1]. Firearms are widely available and gunshot is often the most practical method of euthanasia, especially when veterinary assistance is unavailable. On dairy farms, on-farm euthanasia is most commonly performed by gunshot (85–90%), and only a minority of farms utilized barbiturates or captive bolt for euthanasia [33, 34]. On dairy farms, decisions regarding euthanasia were made in absence of veterinary consultation in 67.7% of surveyed farms, and larger farms were less likely to seek veterinary assistance for euthanasia [34]. The absence of veterinary supervision, safety concerns for personnel that perform euthanasia, and the emotional effects of the procedure on farm personnel are challenges of on-farm euthanasia by physical methods [8]. These challenges should be addressed by providing adequate training by veterinarians and farm managers because physical methods of euthanasia may be best suited to ensure rapid relief of pain and suffering in different situations [8, 35].

The goal of euthanasia by gunshot or captive bolt is the immediate loss of consciousness by inducing massive brain damage. To reliably achieve this goal, accurate placement of the shot or captive bolt on the animal's head is critical and has been reviewed [1, 36]. For cattle, the appropriate point of entry is the intersection of two imaginary lines drawn from the top of the eye or lateral canthus to the opposite horn (Figure 12.2a and b). This placement differs from previous recommendations which suggested that the imaginary lines be drawn from the medial canthus to the horn base, which can result in improper stunning due to penetration of the frontal sinus. While breed variations exist, using the lateral canthus to determine the point of entry results in greater frequencies of brain stem disruption and proper stunning [37, 38]. The shot should be placed perpendicular to the skull, aiming at the foramen magnum to reduce the risk of ricochet and increase brain damage [35]. Due to smaller brain size, accurate placement of a gunshot or penetrating bolt is more difficult in calves. Placement at the intersection of an imaginary line from the lateral canthus to the site of horn formation on the contralateral site also applies to calves,

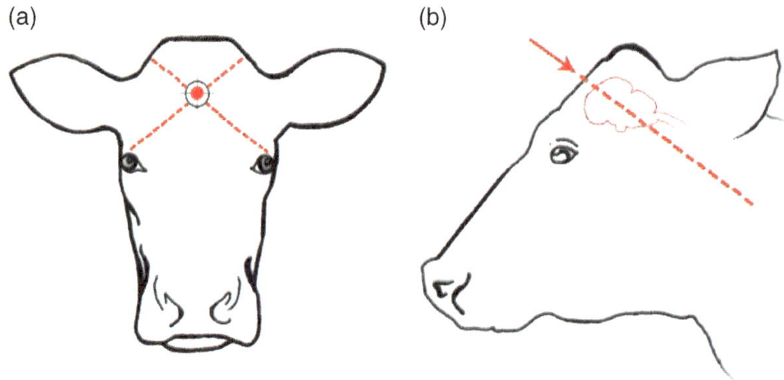

Figure 12.2 (a) Frontal view of the accurate site and angle for placement of a gunshot or captive bolt in cattle. (b) Lateral view of the accurate site and angle for placement of a gunshot or captive bolt in cattle. (Illustration by Katlyn King). With permission from Shearer JK and Ramirez A (2014). *Procedures for the Humane Euthanasia of Sick, Injured and/or Debilitated Livestock*, University Extension, Iowa State University.).

and aiming the shot at the foramen magnum is critical [1]. Alternate stunning locations such as the poll position are less effective in cattle and can result in misdirection of the shot into the spinal cord and prolong the presence of consciousness [22, 39]. The frontal placement of a gunshot or penetrating bolt is effective in most groups of cattle, but reduced effectiveness of stunning has been observed in animals with thick frontal bones such as adult bulls or water buffalo [40]. For these animals, selection of firearms with greater muzzle energy or the use of penetrating captive bolts with larger bolt velocities is necessary.

In sheep and goats, the point of entry for gunshot or penetrating captive bolt varies depending on whether the animal is horned. In hornless small ruminants, the ideal position is the midline of the top of the head or slightly behind the poll, and the frontal position is an alternative site (Figure 12.3) [12, 36]. In horned small ruminants, the thickness of the skull precludes the top of the head as an effective stunning site and the preferred position at the poll with the shot aimed at the mandible (Figure 12.4) [12, 36]. In sheep stunned in the poll position, return to sensibility was observed, and a second kill step such as exsanguination or administration of saturated potassium chloride solution should be promptly applied. Preparedness for an adjunctive method of euthanasia is recommended when using physical methods in small ruminants but is especially important when a captive bolt rather than a firearm is used [1, 12].

For pigs, three points of entry for a gunshot or penetrating captive bolt can be used. The frontal position is preferred and can be used for gunshot or captive bolt methods. On the midline of the forehead, the shot is placed approximately one-half of an inch (1.25 cm) above eye level, aiming at the tail or spinal cord (Figure 12.5a and b). Alternatively, a gunshot can be placed in the temporal region, or from behind the ear, aiming at the opposite eye [1, 12, 36].

While widely available, 0.22-caliber handguns or rifles are not sufficient to euthanize most farm animals as they lack the muzzle energy necessary to penetrate the skull and

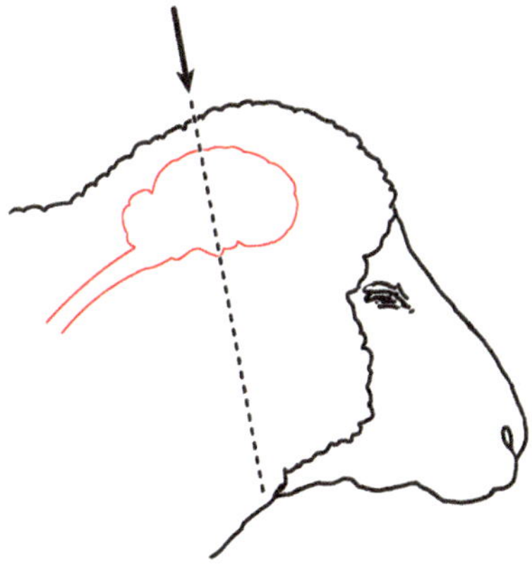

Figure 12.3 Lateral view of the proper placement of a gunshot or captive bolt for euthanasia of hornless small ruminants. (Illustration by Katlyn King). With permission from Shearer JK and Ramirez A (2014). *Procedures for the Humane Euthanasia of Sick, Injured and/or Debilitated Livestock*, University Extension, Iowa State University.)

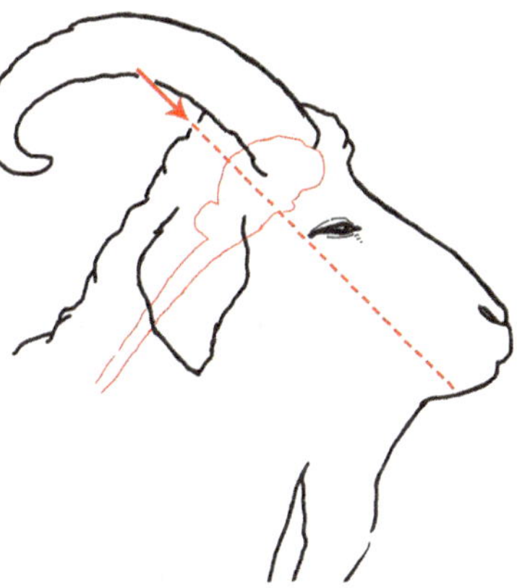

Figure 12.4 Lateral view of the proper placement of a gunshot or captive bolt for euthanasia of horned small ruminants. (Illustration by Katlyn King). With permission from Shearer JK and Ramirez A (2014). *Procedures for the Humane Euthanasia of Sick, Injured and/or Debilitated Livestock*, University Extension, Iowa State University.)

induce severe brain damage reliably [1]. Muzzle energy is a function of bullet weight and velocity and can be calculated as E (in ft-lb) = bullet weight (in grains) × bullet velocity^2 (in ft/s)/450,450 [1]. While 0.22-caliber firearms provide approximately 150 ft-lb of muzzle energy, a minimum of 300-ft-lb energy is recommended for animals weighing up to 181.8 kg (400 lb), which should be available from various handgun cartridges such as 0.38 special, 9 mm, or 0.45 ACP (automatic colt pistol). For animals larger than 181.8 kg (400 lb), firearms providing muzzle energies greater than 1000 ft-lbs are recommended [1, 41]. Solid-point bullets should be used, especially when euthanizing adult cattle and other animals with thick frontal bones. In contrast to hollow-point

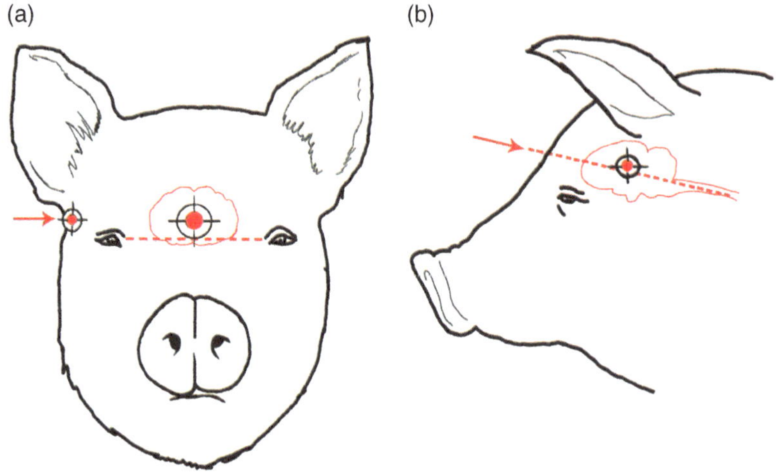

Figure 12.5 (a) Frontal view of the proper placement of a gunshot or captive bolt for euthanasia of swine. (b) Lateral view of the proper placement of a gunshot or captive bolt for euthanasia of swine. (Illustration by Katlyn King). With permission from Shearer JK and Ramirez A (2014). *Procedures for the Humane Euthanasia of Sick, Injured and/or Debilitated Livestock*, University Extension, Iowa State University.).

bullets that fragment on contact with the skull, solid-point bullets are more reliable to penetrate the frontal bones [1]. As an alternative to handguns and rifles, shotguns can be ideal for effective euthanasia of animals at close ranges. Unlike for captive bolts, a secondary kill step is usually not necessary for shotguns or other appropriate firearms. Shotguns are safer than handguns or rifles, as the shot disperses in the cranium and is less likely to exit reducing the risk for the shooter and bystanders. For small farm animals such as calves, lambs, or kids, smaller bore shotguns (0.410 or 28 gauge) are sufficient; however, for adult cattle and other large livestock, larger gauges should be used (20 gauge or larger) [42, 43].

When using physical methods of euthanasia, sufficient training, comfort with the technique, and awareness of safety hazards are critical. While penetrating captive bolts must be placed firmly against the restrained animal's head, firearms must be held off the animals head to prevent buildup of pressure and catastrophic barrel failure. To reduce the risk of ricochet, firearms should not be used in enclosed spaces or on hard surfaces, and bystanders should always be behind the shooter or removed from the area. While less restraint is necessary and animals can be euthanized at greater distances with firearms, patience is critical for accurate placement of the shot. Means of a secondary kill step such as a second cartridge or shell, knife for exsanguination, or potassium chloride solution should be available regardless of whether a firearm or captive bolt is used.

Although massive brain damage sufficient to cause death can be inflicted using penetrating captive bolts, they are considered stunning devices, and secondary kill steps need to be implemented immediately following stunning and determining unconsciousness. Stunning effectiveness is determined by accuracy of placement, bolt velocity, and depth of bolt penetration. Ineffective stunning and misfires are most commonly caused by poor maintenance [35]. Captive bolt guns require regular maintenance, and guns and powder charges must be stored in a dry location to ensure proper function [44].

Use of nonpenetrating captive bolt combined with adjunctive methods of euthanasia is a conditionally acceptable method for euthanasia in calves, kids, lambs, and young pigs. Species-specific purpose-built and general nonpenetrating captive bolts are available and deliver a controlled blunt force trauma to the head [1]. Immediate loss of consciousness results from concussive forces to the brain with greatest efficacy in young animals, which have not developed thick frontal bones. Adjunctive methods of euthanasia are applied immediately after unconsciousness has been confirmed to prevent return to sensibility and eliminate pain or distress.

Adjunctive and other methods of euthanasia

Adjunctive methods of euthanasia include IV administration of potassium chloride or magnesium sulfate solution, second shot, exsanguination, and pithing and are administered to unconscious animals to ensure a humane death [1]. Adjunctive methods must be prepared prior to inducing unconsciousness and administered immediately after loss of consciousness is confirmed. During administration, violent involuntary movements can occur and pose safety concerns to personnel. The safest location for personnel is at the dorsum, close to the head of the recumbent animal and away from the extremities [12].

Saturated solutions of potassium chloride or magnesium sulfate are prepared using hot water, and frequent agitation enhances the solubility of the salt. Both salts are readily available as water softener (potassium chloride) or Epsom salt (magnesium sulfate). Potassium chloride solutions can be made by adding 30 gm of potassium chloride to 100 ml of water. For adult dairy cattle, 120 ml of saturated potassium chloride given rapidly by IV administration should be sufficient to cause death [35]; however, salt solutions are administered to effect. When magnesium sulfate is used, larger volumes may be required and death may not occur as rapidly.

Exsanguination is performed by severing the common carotid artery, jugular vein, and trachea using a very sharp pointed knife. The knife is inserted into the neck just behind the jaw and ventral to the neck bones. A deep incision is then made away from the neck which allows rapid loss of large blood volumes and death. Bleeding may continue for several minutes, but increased blood flow can be achieved by dissecting the vessels closer to the thoracic inlet where they are larger in diameters [1]. Alternatively, exsanguination can be performed by severing the brachial vasculature by deeply incising the axillary area until the limb can be reflected dorsally [12]. The large amount of accumulating blood can be challenging and aesthetically displeasing; therefore, internal exsanguination can be achieved by severing the aorta via the transrectal route.

Pithing using commercially available, disposable pithing rods can be performed following the use of a firearm or penetrating captive bolt. The pithing rod is inserted into the entry site and manipulated to maximize destruction of the brain and spinal cord and ensure death. Pithing prevents the necessity to exsanguinate stunned animals during euthanasia or is used to reduce involuntary movement during exsanguination [12].

In addition to the injectable and physical methods discussed earlier, swine can be euthanized by inhalation agents including carbon dioxide, nitrous oxide, and argon, as well as by electrocution. These methods are commonly used to stun pigs at slaughter and are considered conditionally accepted methods of euthanasia by the AVMA Panel on Euthanasia [1]. Specialized equipment, which is generally unavailable to most veterinarians and farm managers, is required for both methods, precluding their discussion in this chapter. For suckling pigs, manually applied blunt force trauma meets the definition of euthanasia and is classified as a conditionally accepted method. As uncertainty of success and fatigue during repeated application can lead to inconsistency in the success of this method, the AVMA encourages the identification of alternatives to manually applied blunt force trauma to ensure that criteria for euthanasia are reliably met [1].

Considerations subsequent to euthanasia

After confirmation of death, appropriate means of carcass handling and disposal in accordance with local, state, and federal laws have to be taken. Disposal of farm animal carcasses may be regulated by a state's solid waste, medical waste, agriculture, or emergency management regulations. In many states, carcasses have to be disposed of within 24 hours of death [45]. Depending on the size of the animal, method of euthanasia, and environmental conditions, disposal in an approved landfill or by rendering, burial, burning, or composting may be appropriate. Important concerns when disposing euthanized animals include protection of ground and surface water, containing the spread of infectious diseases, and protection of domestic and wild animals from pharmaceutical residues.

While little information is available on the effects of most pharmaceuticals and other residues such as heavy metals from carcasses on environmental parameters and health of scavengers, increased residues are detected in apex predators such as bald eagles and are cause for concern [46, 47]. Of most immediate concern is the presence of pentobarbital in euthanized animals, and label information for all commercially available euthanasia solutions must contain environmental warnings [48]. Barbiturates are characterized by high stability to biotic and abiotic degradation and are highly stable in aquatic environments [49]. Barbiturates remain toxic in carcasses of euthanized animals for extended periods following death. The carcass of a horse remained lethally toxic for domestic dogs more than 2 years following euthanasia, emphasizing the necessity for proper disposal of euthanized animals [50]. Multiple reports on secondary pentobarbital intoxication exist in the literature, affecting domestic, zoo, and free-ranging animals [50–56]. Owners have been held responsible for the death of raptors killed by the presence of sodium pentobarbital in euthanized animals and are legally responsible for proper carcass disposal [45, 46].

Presence of barbiturates in pet food from rendered animal products has also raised concerns. While barbiturates are stable through the rendering process and are distributed approximately equally between meat, bone, and tallow fractions, combination with other raw materials results in low concentrations that are unlikely to cause adverse health effects [57, 58]. Renderers have become reluctant to accept carcasses from euthanized animals, and alternatives for carcass disposal should be considered [1].

Disposal in approved landfills is accepted by many authorities but can also expose scavengers to residues of pentobarbital when carcasses are not covered [59]. If not prevented by close vicinity to water or high-ground water tables, deep burial can be used for carcass disposal. Carcasses should be buried at least 2 ft below ground level. For carcasses of diseased animals that could be potentially contagious, incineration in licensed facilities is preferred and also abolishes concerns of barbiturate residues.

References

1. Euthanasia APo (2013) AVMA Guidelines for the Euthanasia of Animals: 2013 Edition. *AVMA Panel on Euthanasia*. https://www.avma.org/KB/Policies/Documents/euthanasia.pdf (accessed January 8, 2014).
2. Coetzee, J., Lubbers, B., Toerber, S. *et al.* (2008) Plasma concentrations of substance P and cortisol in beef calves after castration or simulated castration. *American Journal of Veterinary Research*, **69**, 751–762.
3. Theurer, M., White, B., Coetzee, J. *et al.* (2012) Assessment of behavioral changes associated with oral meloxicam administration at time of dehorning in calves using a remote triangulation device and accelerometers. *BMC Veterinary Research*, **8**, 48.
4. Gibson, T., Johnson, C., Stafford, K. *et al.* (2007) Validation of the acute electroencephalographic responses of calves to noxious stimulus with scoop dehorning. *New Zealand Veterinary Journal*, **55**, 152–157.
5. Huxley, J. and Whay, H. (2006) Current attitudes of cattle practitioners to pain and the use of analgesics in cattle. *The Veterinary Record*, **159**, 662–668.
6. Laven, R., Huxley, J., Whay, H. and Stafford, K. (2009) Results of a survey of attitudes of dairy veterinarians in New Zealand regarding painful procedures and conditions in cattle. *New Zealand Veterinary Journal*, **57**, 215–220.
7. Fajt, V., Wagner, S. and Norby, B. (2011) Analgesic drug administration and attitudes about analgesia in cattle among bovine practitioners in the United States. *Journal of the American Veterinary Medical Association*, **238**, 755–767.
8. Meyer, R. and Morrow, W. (2004) Euthanasia, in *The Well-Being of Farm Animals Challenges and Solutions* (eds G. John Benson and B. Rollin), Blackwell Publishing, Ames, pp. 351–362.
9. Morrow, W., Meyer, R., Roberts, J. and Lascelles, D. (2006) Financial and welfare implications of immediately euthanizing compromised nursery pigs. *Journal of Swine Health and Production*, **14**, 25–34.
10. Turner, P. and Doonan, G. (2010) Developing on-farm euthanasia plans. *The Canadian Veterinary Journal*, **51**, 1031–1034.
11. Animal Welfare Committee of the American Association of Bovine Practitioners (2013) *Practical Euthanasia of Cattle*, http://aabp.org/resources/AABP_Guidelines/Practical_Euthanasia_of_Cattle-September_2013_pdf (accessed January 22, 2014).
12. Shearer, J. and Ramirez, A. (2013) Human Euthanasia of Sick, Injured and/or Debilitated Livestock. *Procedures for Human Euthanasia*. January 28, 2013 Edition. University Extension, Iowa State University; 1–13. http://vetmed.iastate.edu/HumaneEuthanasia (accessed January 8, 2014).
13. Grandin, T. (2001) Welfare of cattle during slaughter and the prevention of nonambulatory (downer) cattle. *Journal of the American Veterinary Medical Association*, **219**, 1377–1382.
14. Grandin, T. (1994) Farm animal welfare during handling, transport, and slaughter. *Journal of the American Veterinary Medical Association*, **204**, 372–377.
15. Boissy, A., Terlouw, C. and Le Neindre, P. (1998) Presence of cues from stressed conspecifics increases reactivity to aversive events in cattle: evidence for the existence of alarm substances in urine. *Physiology & Behavior*, **63**, 489–495.

16. Grandin, T. (1994) Euthanasia and slaughter of livestock. *Journal of the American Veterinary Medical Association*, **204**, 1354–1360.
17. Vieuille-Thomas, C. and Signoret, J. (1992) Pheromonal transmission of an aversive experience in domestic pig. *Journal of Chemical Ecology*, **18**, 1551–1557.
18. Alkire, M., Hudetz, A. and Tononi, G. (2008) Consciousness and anesthesia. *Science*, **322**, 876–880.
19. Antognini, J., Barter, L. and Carstens, E. (2005) Overview movement as an index of anesthetic depth in humans and experimental animals. *Comparative Medicine*, **55**, 413–418.
20. Anil, M. and McKinstry, J. (1991) Reflexes and loss of sensibility following head-to-back electrical stunning in sheep. *The Veterinary Record*, **128**, 106–107.
21. Blackmore, D. and Delany, M. (1988) *Slaughter of Stock. A Practical Guide and Review*, Massey University, Veterinary Continuing Education, Palmerston North.
22. Lambooy, E. and Spanjaard, W. (1981) Effect of the shooting position on the stunning of calves by captive bolt. *The Veterinary Record*, **109**, 359–361.
23. Wotton, S. and Gregory, N. (1986) Pig slaughtering procedures: time to loss of brain responsiveness after exsanguination of cardiac arrest. *Research in Veterinary Science*, **40**, 148–151.
24. Gregory, N., Lee, C. and Widdicombe, J. (2007) Depth of concussion in cattle shot by penetrating captive bolt. *Meat Science*, **77**, 499–503.
25. Gregory, N., Lee, C. and Widdicombe, J. (2007) Depth of concussion in cattle shot by penetrating captive bolt. *Meat Science*, **77**, 499–503.
26. Grandin T (2012) *How to Determine Insensibility in Cattle, Pigs, and Sheep in Slaughter Plants, 2012*. 2012 Edition. http://www.grandin.com/humane/insensibility.html (accessed January 8, 2014).
27. Blank, C., Metzner, M., Lorch, A. and Klee, W. (2010) Euthanasia of cattle: a clinical comparison of T 61 and pentobarbital (Eutha 77). *Berliner und Munchener tierarztliche Wochenschrift*, **123**, 96–102.
28. Anonymous (2013) Socumb™ – 6 GR (Butler ScheinTM Animal Health, Dublin, OH). http://butler.naccvp.com/product/view/1082163Butler.naccp.com (accessed January 8, 2014).
29. Grier, R. and Schaffer, C. (1990) Evaluation of intraperitoneal and intrahepatic administration of a euthanasia agent in animal shelter cats. *Journal of the American Veterinary Medical Association*, **197**, 1611–1615.
30. Svendsen, O., Kok, L. and Lauritzen, B. (2007) Nociception after intraperitoneal injection of a sodium pentobarbitone formulation with and without lidocaine in rats quantified by expression of neuronal c-fos in the spinal cord – a preliminary study. *Laboratory Animals*, **41**, 197–203.
31. Whiting, T., Steele, G., Wamnes, S. and Green, C. (2011) Evaluation of methods of rapid mass killing of segregated early weaned piglets. *The Canadian Veterinary Journal*, **52**, 753–758.
32. Evers, A., Crowder, C. and Balser, J. (2006) General anesthetics, in: *Goodman and Gilman's the Pharmacological Basis of Therapeutics*, 11th edn (Bruton L, Lazo J, Parker K, eds.), Mc Graw-Hill Medical Publishing Division, New York, p. 362.
33. Fulwider, W., Grandin, T., Rollin, B. *et al.* (2008) Survey of dairy management practices on one hundred thirteen north central and northeastern United States dairies. *Journal of Dairy Science*, **91**, 1686–1692.
34. Hoe, F. and Ruegg, P. (2006) Opinions and practices of Wisconsin dairy producers about biosecurity and animal well-being. *Journal of Dairy Science*, **89**, 2297–2308.
35. Shearer, J. and Reynolds, J. (2011) Euthanasia techniques for dairy cattle, in *Dairy Production Medicine* (eds C. Risco and P. Melendez Retamal), Wiley-Blackwell, Ames, pp. 331–344.

36. Health OWOfA (2012) *Slaughter of Animals*. OiE World Organization for Animal Health, Paris. http://www.oie.int/index.php?id=169&L=0&htmfile=chapitre_1.7.5.htm (accessed January 8, 2014).
37. Gilliam, J., Shearer, J., Woods, J. *et al.* (2012) Captive-bolt euthanasia of cattle: determination of optimal-shot placement and evaluation of the Cash Special Euthanizer Kit (R) for euthanasia of cattle. *Animal Welfare*, **21**, 99–102.
38. Shearer, J. (2010) Observations on stunning placement in cattle. *AMI Foundation Animal Care and Handling Conference*, Kansas City.
39. Gregory, N. (2008) Animal welfare at markets and during transport and slaughter. *Meat Science*, **80**, 2–11.
40. Gregory, N., Spence, J., Mason, C. *et al.* (2009) Effectiveness of poll stunning water buffalo with captive bolt guns. *Meat Science*, **81**, 178–182.
41. Woods, J., Shearer, J. and Hill, J. (2010) Recommended on-farm euthanasia practices, in: *Improving Animal Welfare: A Practical Approach* (ed. T. Grandin) CABI, Wallingford Oxfordshire, pp. 186–213.
42. Humane-Slaughter, C. (2007) *Humane dispatch and disposal of infant calves*. Humane Slaughter Association, Hertfordshire. http://www.hsa.org.uk/downloads/technical-notes/TN2-calves-human-dispatch-disposal-HSA.pdf (accessed January 22, 2014).
43. Humane Slaughter Association-Kids L. 2008 *Humane dispatch and disposal of kids and lambs*. http://www.hsa.org.uk/downloads/technical-notes/TN7-kids-and-lambs-humane-dispatch.pdf (accessed January 22, 2014).
44. Grandin, T. (2012) *Recommended Captive Bolt Stunning Techniques for Cattle*, January 4, 2012 Edition. http://www.grandin.com/humane/cap.bolt.tips.html (accessed January 8, 2014).
45. O'Rourke, K. (2002) Euthanatized animals can poison wildlife: veterinarians receive fines. *Journal of the American Veterinary Medical Association*, **220**, 146–147.
46. Mierzykowski, S., Smith, J., Todd, C. *et al.* (2011) Liver contaminants in bald eagle carcasses from Maine, in: *Spec Proj Rep FY09-MEFO-6-EC*. (ed. USFWS), Maine Field Office, Orono, p. 53.
47. Scheuhammer, A., Basu, N., Burgess, N. *et al.* (2008) Relationships among mercury, selenium, and neurochemical parameters in common loons (Gavia immer) and bald eagles (Haliaeetus leucocephalus). *Ecotoxicology*, **17**, 93–101.
48. Food, U.S. and Administration, D. (2003) 21 CFR Part 522 injectable or implantable dosage form new animal drugs. Euthanasia solution. Technical amendment. *Federal Register*, **68**, 42968–42969.
49. Peschka, M., Eubeler, J. and Knepper, T. (2006) Occurrence and fate of barbiturates in the aquatic environment. *Environmental Science & Technology*, **40**, 7200–7206.
50. Kaiser, A., McFarland, W., Siemion, R. and Raisbeck, M. (2010) Secondary pentobarbital poisoning in two dogs: a cautionary tale. *Journal of Veterinary Diagnostic Investigation*, **22**, 632–634.
51. Anderson, J., Filkins, D., Stowe, C. and Arendt, T. (1979) Accidental relay toxicosis caused by pentobarbital euthanasia solution. *Journal of the American Veterinary Medical Association*, **175**, 583–584.
52. Fucci, V., Monroe, W., Riedesel, D. and Jackson, L. (1986) Oral pentobarbital intoxication in a bitch. *Journal of the American Veterinary Medical Association*, **188**, 191–192.
53. Jurczynski, K. and Zittlau, E. (2007) Pentobarbital poisoning in Sumatran tigers (Panthera tigris sumatrae). *Journal of Zoo and Wildlife Medicine*, **38**, 583–584.
54. Verster, A., Schroder, H. and Nesbit, J. (1990) Accidental pentobarbital poisoning in a lioness. *Journal of the South African Veterinary Association*, **61**, 37–38.

55. Bischoff, K., Jaeger, R. and Ebel, J. (2011) An unusual case of relay pentobarbital toxicosis in a dog. *Journal of Medical Toxicology*, **7**, 236–239.
56. Otten, D. (2001) Advisory on proper disposal of euthanized animals. *Journal of the American Veterinary Medical Association*, **219**, 1677–1678.
57. O'Connor, J., Stowe, C. and Robinson, R. (1985) Fate of sodium pentobarbital in rendered products. *American Journal of Veterinary Research*, **46**, 1721–1724.
58. Bren, L. (2002) Pentobarbital in dog food. *FDA Veterinarian Newsletter*, **16**, 8.
59. Service UFaW (2003) *Secondary Pentobarbital Poisoning of Wildlife*. US Fish and Wildlife Service, Stafford. http://cpharm.vetmed.vt.edu/USFWS/USFWSFPentobarbFactSheet.pdf (accessed January 22, 2014).

Index

Note: Page numbers in *Italics* refer to figures; those in **bold** to Tables

Farm Animal Anesthesia: Cattle, Small Ruminants, Camelids, and Pigs, First Edition.
Edited by HuiChu Lin and Paul Walz.

TJI66084-9781118474358-23-02-18